Study Guide for

Brunner & Suddarth's Textbook of Medical-Surgical Nursing

15th EDITION

T0364680

 Wolters Kluwer

Philadelphia • Baltimore • New York • London
Buenos Aires • Hong Kong • Sydney • Tokyo

Vice President, Nursing Segment: Julie K. Stegman
Director, Nursing Education and Practice Content: Jamie Blum
Senior Acquisitions Editor: Jonathan Joyce
Senior Development Editor: Meredith L. Brittain
Senior Editorial Coordinator: Julie Kostelnik
Marketing Manager: Brittany Clements
Editorial Assistant: Molly Kennedy
Senior Production Project Manager: David Saltzberg
Manager, Graphic Arts and Design: Steve Druding
Art Director: Jennifer Clements
Manufacturing Coordinator: Margie Orzech
Prepress Vendor: Aptara, Inc.

15th Edition

9 8 7 6 5 4 3 2 1

Printed in Singapore

ISBN: 978-1-9751-6325-9

Contributor

Leigh W. Moore, MSN, RN, CNOR, CNE
Associate Professor of Nursing
ADN Program
Southside Virginia Community College
Alberta, Virginia

Preface

This Study Guide was developed by Leigh W. Moore, MSN, RN, CNOR, CNE, to accompany *Brunner and Suddarth's Textbook of Medical-Surgical Nursing*, 15th Edition, by Janice L. Hinkle, Kerry H. Cheever, and Kristen J. Overbaugh. The Study Guide is designed to help you review and apply important concepts from the textbook to prepare for exams as well as for your nursing career. The following types of exercises are provided in each chapter of the Study Guide.

ASSESSING YOUR UNDERSTANDING

The first section of each Study Guide chapter reviews the basic information of the textbook chapter and helps you to remember key concepts, vocabulary, and principles.

- **Fill in the Blanks:** Fill-in-the-blank exercises test important chapter information, encouraging you to recall key points.
- **Short Answers:** Short-answer questions cover facts, concepts, procedures, and principles of the chapter. These questions ask you to recall information as well as demonstrate your comprehension of the information.
- **Matching:** Matching questions test your knowledge of the definition of key terms.
- **Labeling:** Labeling exercises are used where you need to remember certain visual representations of the concepts presented in the textbook.
- **Sequencing:** Sequencing exercises ask you to remember particular sequences or orders, such as in normal or abnormal physiologic processes.

APPLYING YOUR KNOWLEDGE

The second section of each Study Guide chapter consists of case study–based exercises that ask you to begin to apply the knowledge you gained from the textbook chapter that was reinforced in the first section of the Study Guide chapter. A case study scenario based on the chapter's content is presented, followed by related short-answer questions. The questions could cover topics such as lab values, next steps in nursing care, and anticipated diagnoses.

PRACTICING FOR NCLEX

The third and final section of each Study Guide chapter helps you practice NCLEX-style questions while further applying the knowledge you have gained and reinforced through reading the textbook chapter and completing the first two sections of the Study Guide chapter. Including both multiple-choice and alternate-item formats, the questions are scenario based, asking you to reflect, consider, and apply what you know and to choose the best answer out of those offered.

ANSWERS

The answers for all of the exercises and questions in the Study Guide are provided at the back of the book, so you can assess your own learning as you complete each chapter.

We hope that you will find this Study Guide to be helpful and enjoyable, and we wish you every success in your studies and future profession.

The Publisher

Contents

Principles of Nursing Practice

CHAPTER 1

Professional Nursing Practice

Learning Outcomes

1. Define nursing, patient, health, wellness, health promotion, and health care.
2. Describe salient influences on the delivery of health care.
3. Discuss practices that improve quality and safety and ensure the use of evidence-based practices within the health care system.
4. Discuss behavioral competencies and characteristics of professional nursing practice and the nurse's role as a collaborative member of the interprofessional health care team.
5. Define the characteristics of critical thinking, the critical thinking process, and clinical decision making.
6. Describe the components of the nursing process.
7. Identify strategies that can be implemented in ethical decision making.

SECTION I: ASSESSING YOUR UNDERSTANDING

Activity A *Fill in the blanks.*

1. Quality and Safety Education for Nurses (QSEN) prepares future nurses with the _____, _____, and _____ to continuously improve the quality and safety of the health care system.

2. Chronic diseases that account for 7 out of 10 leading causes of death include _____, _____, _____, and _____.

3. When the nurse is performing an assessment for a patient: _____, _____, and _____ will be used to determine the health status and any actual or potential health problems.

4. Moral integrity is a virtue that is composed of _____, _____, _____, _____, and _____.

Activity B *Briefly answer the following.*

1. Wellness involves proactively working toward physical, psychological, and spiritual well-being. Four components of wellness are

_____

_____

_____

_____

2. List four significant changes that have impacted health care delivery and the practice of nursing.

_____,

_____,

_____,

_____.

3. Choose four health and illness problems and write a human response to each that would require nursing intervention. An example is provided.

Health and Illness Problems	Human Response Requiring Nursing Intervention
Fractured right arm (Example)	Self-care limitations (Example)
1. _____	_____
2. _____	_____
3. _____	_____
4. _____	_____

4. The nursing process is a deliberate problem-solving approach for meeting people's health care and nursing needs. List the common components of the nursing process in order:

1. _____

2. _____

3. _____

4. _____

5. _____

5. List Maslow hierarchy of needs, and give an example for each need. The first need is provided as an example.

Need	Example
Physiologic (Example)	Food and water (Example)
_____	_____
_____	_____
_____	_____
_____	_____
_____	_____
_____	_____

6. Which two virtues are inherent within the moral foundation for professional practice?

_____ and

_____ .

7. What does the principle of autonomy entail?

_____

_____

8. Define the term *evidence-based practice* (EBP).

_____

_____

_____

9. When the nurse is faced with two conflicting alternatives in an ethical dilemma, what is the nurse's moral responsibility?

_____

_____

_____

10. Identify at least three common health care problems veterans are experiencing.

_____

_____

11. Identify at least three recent key advances in health information technologies.

_____

_____

12. Identify at least three of the evidence-based practice tools that are currently used for planning patient care.

_____

_____

13. Clinical reasoning is the core of the nursing process and guides decision making. Name at least three factors that are critical components of clinical reasoning.

_____

_____

SECTION II: APPLYING YOUR KNOWLEDGE

Activity C *Consider the scenario and answer the questions.*

The nurse is caring for an older adult patient recently diagnosed with pancreatic cancer. The family has been informed of the diagnosis and states to the nurse, "We don't want anyone to tell our parent what the diagnosis is. We are just going to say that it is a stomach issue that will get better with time." When the family leaves, the patient asks the nurse, "What is wrong with me?"

1. What is the best response by the nurse to address this ethical dilemma?
   a. "I don't know, so it would be best to ask your family what the health care provider said."
   b. "Your family would rather you not know what the diagnosis is, and I can't say without permission."
   c. "I will talk with your family and health care provider and inform them of your request for a diagnosis."
   d. "Don't worry about your diagnosis right now; let's just help you get better and take care of the pain."

2. What strategies can the nurse use to respect the patient's rights? (Select all that apply.)
   a. Provide all information related to nursing procedures and diagnoses.
   b. Avoid lying to the patient when asked a direct question.
   c. Make a referral to the institution's ethics committee.
   d. Act as an advocate for the patient's rights.
   e. Encourage the family to make decisions for the patient.

3. The nurse talks with family members about the patient's desire to be informed of the diagnosis. The patient's family states, "We just don't know the right words to say." What is the best response by the nurse?
   a. "Maybe it would be better to postpone telling the patient until you can say it correctly."
   b. "Would you like for me to contact your clergy to be present with you?"
   c. "I will wait outside of the room, and you can call me when you are finished."
   d. "Would you like me to give the patient a sedative prior to the discussion?"

SECTION III: PRACTICING FOR NCLEX

Activity D *Answer the following questions.*

1. The registered nurse has a responsibility to practice nursing according to the Social Policy Statement (2015) of the American Nurses Association (ANA). What definition by the ANA best describes the role of registered nurses?
   a. To diagnose and treat medical conditions
   b. To prescribe medications in order to treat a variety of medical conditions
   c. To prevent illness and maintain health
   d. To diagnose and treat the human responses to health and illness

2. What underlying focus in any definition of nursing is the registered nurse's responsibility in practice?
   a. Appraise and enhance a person's health-seeking perspective
   b. Coordinate a patient's total health management with all disciplines
   c. Diagnose acute pathology
   d. Treat acute clinical reactions to chronic illness

3. Using the concept of the wellness–illness continuum, what would the nurse include in the development of a nursing care plan for a chronically ill patient?
   a. Educate the patient about every possible complication associated with the specific illness
   b. Encourage positive health characteristics within the limits of the specific illness
   c. Limit all activities because of the progressive deterioration associated with all chronic illnesses
   d. Recommend activity beyond the scope of tolerance to prevent early deterioration

4. What does the nurse identify as the primary purpose of CQI?
   a. Identify measures to ensure minimal expectations of care
   b. Assess the impact of financial decisions on patient care delivery
   c. Examine processes that affect patient care and the need for improvement
   d. Review medication errors for individual patients

5. The nurse is using a bundle to prevent the occurrence of ventilator-associated pneumonia in intensive care patients who are on ventilators. Which is the priority goal for the use of this bundle in patient care?
   a. To improve patient outcomes
   b. To ensure that all nurses provide the same care
   c. To alleviate the use of ventilators in the ICU
   d. To provide a universal documentation system

6. When an ethical decision is made based on the reasoning of the "greatest good for the greatest number," which theory is the nurse following?
   a. Deontologic theory
   b. Formalist theory
   c. Moral justification theory
   d. Utilitarian theory

7. The nurse prepares to administer medication to the patient. The patient states, "I would prefer not to take that medication until I speak with my health care provider." The nurse honors the patient's desire to make decisions, following which common ethical principle?
   a. Autonomy
   b. Beneficence
   c. Fidelity
   d. Paternalism

8. Which does the nurse determine is a moral problem rather than a moral dilemma?
   a. Family members tell the health care provider that they do not want their father informed of his terminal diagnosis.
   b. A 32-year-old father of three with advanced cancer of the lungs asks that everything be done to prolong his life, even though his chemotherapy treatments are no longer effective.
   c. A confused 80 year old needs restraints for protection from injury, even though the restraints increase agitation.
   d. A young patient with AIDS has asked not to receive tube feedings to prolong life because of intense pain.

9. The nurse is developing a plan of care for a patient. Which is the end result of data analysis during the assessment process?
   a. Actualization of the plan of care
   b. Determination of the patient's responses to care
   c. Collection and analysis of data
   d. Identification of actual or potential health problems

10. Which therapeutic communication technique validates what the nurse believes to be the main idea of an interaction?
    a. Acknowledgment
    b. Focusing
    c. Restating
    d. Summarizing

11. Which statement does the nurse identify as a medical diagnosis rather than a nursing diagnosis?
    a. Fever of unknown origin
    b. Fluid volume excess
    c. Risk for falls
    d. Sleep pattern disturbances

CHAPTER 2

Medical-Surgical Nursing

Learning Outcomes

1. Discuss principles of medical-surgical nursing practice as well as characteristics and settings of select nursing practice specialties in today's health care delivery system.
2. Describe the significance of the nurse as coordinator of care transitions.
3. Specify the components of a comprehensive assessment of functional capacity.
4. Use the nursing process as a framework for care of the patient with self-care deficits or with impaired physical mobility.
5. Describe the role and practice settings of home health nursing and the significance of continuity of care in transition into community or home settings.

SECTION I: ASSESSING YOUR UNDERSTANDING

Activity A *Fill in the blanks.*

1. _____ is a process of ensuring consistency and coordination of care as patients move within and between health care settings.

2. Rehospitalizations raise concerns about _____ and _____.

3. Functional capacity is the ability to perform _____ and _____.

4. Case management is a system of coordinating health care services to ensure

_____, _____, and _____.

5. One of the most frequently used tools to assess the patient's level of independence is the _____.

6. _____ is a deformity in which the foot is plantarflexed.

7. _____ is a primary concern during a transfer of patient.

Activity B *Briefly answer the following.*

1. What are some of the causes for rehospitalization?

_____

_____

_____

_____

_____

2. What is the role of a nurse navigator?

_____

_____

_____

3. Types of assistive technology include

_____ and _____.

4. Identify the focus of rehabilitation nursing.

_____

_____

5. What is the first step in preparation for an initial visit by the home health nurse?

_____

_____

6. Explain the purpose of the initial home visit.

_____

_____

7. Compare and contrast active and passive range-of-motion exercises.

_____

_____

8. If a patient is readmitted to the acute care setting within 30 days of being discharged, what may occur?

_____

_____

9. What is critical-care nursing and how does it differ from medical-surgical nursing?

_____

_____

_____

_____

_____

10. What is a major financial incentive for hospitals and other health care organizations to discharge a patient in the early stages of recovery?

_____

_____

_____

_____

SECTION II: APPLYING YOUR KNOWLEDGE

Activity C _Consider the scenario and assess the patient's need for a home visit._

CASE STUDY: Assessing the Need for a Home Visit

Question 1. Mrs. Flynn is an 85-year-old woman who suffered a stroke on December 28. She was admitted to the emergency department and suffered another stroke on December 30. The left occipital area and the cerebellum were affected, resulting in the loss of 50% of vision (right half of each eye) and loss of balance. After 2 weeks in the hospital and 10 days in a rehabilitation treatment center, Mrs. Flynn will be discharged to her one-floor home, where she lives alone. Her son and daughter both live an hour away. She is capable of walking with a walker. Before the stroke, Mrs. Flynn was independent, an active member of several citizens' groups, and participated in water aerobics at the YMCA three times a week. Her driver's license was revoked. Using Chart 2-3, Assessing the Home Environment, in the textbook, complete the outline to assess Mrs. Flynn's need for a home visit. Create your own answers to several of the questions so that you can complete the assessment.

Current Health Status

1. How well is the patient progressing?
2. How serious are the present signs and symptoms?
3. Has the patient shown signs of progressing as expected, or does it seem that recovery will be delayed?

_____

_____

Home Environment

1. Are worrisome safety factors apparent?
2. Are family or friends available to provide care, or is the patient alone?

_____

_____

Level of Self-Care Ability

1. Is the patient capable of self-care?
2. What is the patient's level of independence?
3. Is the patient ambulatory or bedridden?
4. Does the patient have sufficient energy or is she frail and easily fatigued?

_____

_____

Level of Nursing Care Needed

1. What level of nursing care does the patient require?
2. Does the care require basic skills or more complex interventions?

_____

_____

Prognosis

1. What is the expectation for recovery in this particular instance?
2. What are the chances that complications may develop if nursing care is not provided?

_____

_____

Educational Needs

1. How well has the patient or family grasped the teaching points made?
2. Is there a need for further follow-up and retraining?
3. What level of proficiency does the patient or family show in carrying out the necessary care?

_____

_____

Mental Status

1. How alert is the patient?
2. Are there signs of confusion or thinking difficulties?

_____

_____

Level of Adherence

1. Is the patient following the instructions provided?
2. Does the patient seem capable of following the instructions?
3. Are the family members helpful, or are they unwilling or unable to assist in caring for the patient as expected?

_____

_____

SECTION III: PRACTICING FOR NCLEX

Activity D _Answer the following questions._

1. When would be the best time to begin discharge planning for a patient who will require assistance in the home after leaving the acute care facility?

   a. As the patient is preparing to be picked up from the hospital by family members

   b. At the time of the patient's admission to the hospital

   c. When the patient recovers from the acute phase of the illness

   d. After the patient is discharged from the hospital

2. The nurse is making an initial home visit to assess a patient for home health services. Which patients most frequently require home health services?

   a. Children with chronic, debilitating disorders

   b. Newborns who are sent home with apnea monitors

   c. The older adult patient who needs skilled care

   d. Young adults on prolonged intravenous therapy

3. An older adult patient admitted to the hospital for a total left hip arthroplasty is unable to independently participate in the rehabilitation process after discharge. Which providers to coordinate and transition care will the nurse refer the patient to? (Select all that apply.)

   a. A nurse navigator

   b. A critical-care nurse

   c. A case manager

   d. A clinical nurse leader (CNL)

   e. A nursing home administrator

4. The nurse is caring for a group of patients at the hospital medical-surgical unit. Which patient assessed by the nurse is considered to have a severe disability? (Select all that apply.)

a. A patient that requires glasses to read fine print

b. A patient that is receiving federal benefits due to an inability to work

c. A patient that has to use an assistive device to ambulate

d. A patient that has a family member assist with all personal hygiene needs

e. A patient with a speech impediment

5. The nurse is caring for a patient who had a stroke with left-sided paralysis. Which nursing intervention implemented will assist in the prevention of contractures?

a. Maintain proper body positioning while in bed.

b. Offer fluids every 2 hours while awake.

c. Clean the patient immediately after incontinence.

d. Have the patient sit on the side of the bed before ambulating.

6. A patient is identified to be at risk for the development of external rotation of the hip while on bed rest. Which nursing action would be best to implement to prevent this occurrence?

a. Turn the patient every 2 hours.

b. Provide a trochanter roll.

c. Promote active range-of-motion exercises.

d. Massage the hip areas every 4 hours.

7. The nurse is performing passive range-of-motion exercises for a patient to prevent complications of immobility. When the nurse moves the leg away from the body, which movement is the nurse performing?

a. Flexion

b. Adduction

c. Abduction

d. Rotation

CHAPTER 3

Health Education and Health Promotion

Learning Outcomes

1. Describe the purposes and significance of health education.
2. Distinguish between the concepts of adherence to a therapeutic regimen and health literacy.
3. Explain the variables that affect learning and apply them to the teaching–learning process.
4. Describe the components of health promotion and discuss major health promotion models.
5. Specify the variables that affect health promotion activities across the life cycle, and describe the role of the nurse in health promotion.

SECTION I: ASSESSING YOUR UNDERSTANDING

Activity A *Briefly answer the following.*

1. List three significant factors for a nurse to consider when planning patient education.

   _____

   _____

   _____

2. Explain why health education is so essential for those with a chronic illness.

   _____

   _____

3. List five common examples of specific activities that promote and maintain health.

   _____   _____

   _____   _____

   _____

4. How does *adherence* relate to a person's therapeutic regimen?

   _____

5. Name four classifications of variables (factors) that influence a person's ability to adhere to a program of care.

   _____   _____

   _____   _____

6. There is a positive correlation between patient motivation and adherence to a teaching plan. Name three significant variables affecting motivation and learning.

   _____   _____

   _____

7. List the six stages of personal change that a person experiences as they move toward a healthy behavior.

   _____   _____

   _____   _____

   _____   _____

8. Describe the nature of the teaching–learning process.

   _____

   _____

9. List at least six variables that make adherence to a therapeutic regimen difficult for the older adult.

   _____ _____

   _____ _____

   _____ _____

10. What factors serve as a basis for evaluating the effectiveness of teaching strategies?

    _____

11. Discuss how learner readiness affects a learner and the learning situation.

    _____

    _____

    _____

12. Identify six teaching techniques that nurses frequently use.

    _____ _____

    _____ _____

    _____ _____

13. Identify two select topics from the proposed objectives for *Healthy People 2030*.

    _____

    _____

14. Which are the four active processes for health promotion?

    _____ _____

    _____ _____

15. Explain at least five ways that exercise can promote health.

    _____ _____

    _____ _____

    _____

Activity B *Rewrite each statement correctly. Underline the key concepts.*

1. Health education is a dependent function of nursing practice that requires primary provider approval.

   _____

   _____

2. The largest groups of people in need of health education today are children and those with infectious diseases.

   _____

   _____

3. Patients are encouraged to evidence adherence with their therapeutic regimen.

   _____

   _____

4. Evaluation, the final step in the teaching process, should be summative (done at the end of the teaching process).

   _____

   _____

5. Older adults rarely experience significant improvement from health promotion activities.

   _____

   _____

6. About 50% of older adults have one or more chronic illnesses.

   _____

   _____

SECTION II: APPLYING YOUR KNOWLEDGE

Activity C *Consider the scenario and answer the questions.*

The nurse is admitting a patient into the intensive care unit with acute congestive heart failure. The patient was discharged 8 days ago with the same diagnosis. The patient had been instructed prior to discharge to follow up with the primary provider within 1 week, follow a low sodium/1.5-L fluid restriction diet, and begin taking two new medications. When performing the assessment of the patient, the nurse found that the patient had not followed the discharge instructions and had been eating and drinking without restriction. The medications had not been started, and the patient had not seen the primary provider.

1. What variables can determine the patient's adherence to the therapeutic regimen?

   _____

   _____

   _____

2. How can the nurse increase the success of the patient's adherence to the therapeutic regimen after discharge?

   _____

   _____

SECTION III: PRACTICING FOR NCLEX

Activity D *Answer the following questions.*

1. The nurse is caring for several patients. Which patient is most in need of health education by the nurse?
   a. A 28-year-old female with abdominal pain
   b. A 62-year-old male with chronic kidney injury
   c. A 42-year-old male with acute pericarditis
   d. A 72-year-old female with a respiratory infection

2. Which is the priority responsibility for the nurse providing patient education? (Select all that apply.)
   a. Determining individual needs for education
   b. Motivating each person to learn
   c. Giving a test at the end of an educational session
   d. Waiting until the patient expresses a desire to learn
   e. Presenting information at the level of the learner

3. The nurse is preparing to educate a patient about the home care of an abdominal wound. Which patient behaviors does the nurse assess that demonstrate readiness to learn? (Select all that apply.)
   a. The patient shows the motivation to learn
   b. The patient has accepted the therapeutic regimen
   c. The patient is unable to look at the wound
   d. The patient tells the nurse the family member will take care of it
   e. The patient requests a contact number if there are questions

4. Which action by the nurse can negatively affect the patient's ability to learn?
   a. Feedback in the form of constructive encouragement when a person has been unsuccessful in the learning process
   b. Negative criticism when the patient is unsuccessful so that inappropriate behavior patterns will not be learned
   c. The creation of a positive atmosphere in which the patient is encouraged to express anxiety
   d. The establishment of realistic learning goals based on individual needs

5. Since normal aging results in changes in cognition, how will the nurse teach an older adult patient to administer insulin?

   a. Repeat the information frequently for reinforcement

   b. Present all the information at one time so that the patient is not confused by pieces of information

   c. Speed up the demonstration because the patient will tire easily

   d. The older patient is not capable of learning self-administration and someone else should be instructed

6. The home health nurse reviews a medication administration calendar with an older adult patient. In order to consider sensory changes that occur with aging, how will the nurse proceed?

   a. Print directions in large, bold type, preferably using black ink

   b. Highlight or shade important dates and times with contrasting colors

   c. Use several different colors to emphasize special dates

   d. Type out the information on the computer

7. The nurse has modified a teaching program for a learner that is not experientially prepared. Which nursing action is appropriate?

   a. Changing the wording in a teaching pamphlet so that a patient with a fourth-grade reading level can understand it

   b. Contacting family members to assist in goal development to help stimulate motivation

   c. Postponing a teaching session with a patient until pain has subsided

   d. Notifying the primary provider that the patient will not yet be eligible for discharge

8. The nurse identifies a patient's inability to pour a liquid medication into a measuring spoon. Which part of the nursing process is this?

   a. Assessment

   b. Planning

   c. Implementation

   d. Evaluation

9. The nurse develops a program of increased ambulation for a patient with an orthopedic disorder. Which component of the nursing process is this?

   a. Assessment

   b. Planning

   c. Implementation

   d. Evaluation

10. The nurse develops outcome criteria for a patient with chronic obstructive pulmonary disease. Which outcome criteria are appropriate for this patient?

    a. The patient will have the ability to climb a flight of stairs without experiencing difficulty in breathing

    b. The patient will not experience an alteration in skin integrity

    c. The patient will perform passive range-of-motion exercises once daily

    d. The nurse will obtain a pulse oximetry reading twice a day

11. Which health promotion model does the nurse identify is the reason some people choose actions to foster health and others refuse to participate?

    a. Health Belief Model

    b. Resource Model of Preventive Health

    c. Achieving Health for All Model

    d. Social Learning Theory Model

12. What does the nurse determine is the single most important factor in determining health status and longevity?

    a. Adherence to a plan

    b. Good nutrition

    c. Motivation to change

    d. Stress reduction

CHAPTER 4

Adult Health and Physical, Nutritional, and Cultural Assessment

Learning Outcomes

1. Describe the components of a holistic and comprehensive health history and assessment.
2. Describe the techniques of inspection, palpation, percussion, and auscultation to perform a basic physical assessment.
3. Discuss the techniques of measurement of body mass index, biochemical assessment, clinical examination, and assessment of food intake to assess a person's nutritional status.
4. Describe the techniques of conducting a cultural assessment.

SECTION I: ASSESSING YOUR UNDERSTANDING

Activity A *Fill in the blanks.*

1. The role of the nurse in assessment includes two primary responsibilities: _____ and _____.

2. When questioning a patient about lifestyle and health-related behaviors, the nurse should ask about _____,

   _____, _____,

   _____, and _____.

3. The *three leading causes of death* in the United States that are related in part to poor nutrition

   are _____, _____,

   and _____.

4. Adolescent girls are particularly at risk for nutritional deficits in minerals, such as

   _____, _____, and

   _____.

Activity B *Briefly answer the following.*

1. Describe five basic guidelines that a nurse should use while conducting a health assessment.

   _____   _____

   _____   _____

   _____

2. Explain how mutual trust and confidence between the interviewer and the patient facilitate the communication process.

   _____

   _____

3. What are the four basic characteristics of ethnic culture?

   _____

   _____

15

4. A number of diseases of first- or second-order relatives are significant when a nurse takes a patient's family history. List six diseases that are considered significant.

_____   _____

_____   _____

_____   _____

5. Which cultures require the most personal space?

_____

_____

6. Which type of nutritional assessment tool would be best for an older adult patient who is malnourished or at risk for becoming malnourished?

_____

_____

7. List six questions that a nurse could incorporate into a genetic health assessment.

_____

_____

_____

_____

_____

_____

Activity C
PART I

Identify which type of assessment was most likely used to obtain the data. Write the word on the line provided.

Column I

_____ **a.** Asymmetry of movement is associated with a central nervous system disorder

_____ **b.** Clubbing of the fingers is a diagnostic symptom of chronic pulmonary disorders

_____ **c.** Tenderness is present in the area of the thyroid isthmus

_____ **d.** Tactile fremitus is diagnostic of lung consolidation

_____ **e.** Tympanic or drumlike sounds are produced by pneumothorax

_____ **f.** The first heart sound is created by the simultaneous closure of the mitral and tricuspid valves

_____ **g.** A friction rub is present with pericarditis

_____ **h.** Nodules present with gout lie adjacent to the joint capsule

Column II

a. Inspection

b. Palpation

c. Percussion

d. Auscultation

PART II

Match the body area listed in Column II with the descriptive sign of poor nutrition listed in Column I.

Column I

____ 1. Atrophic papillae

____ 2. Brittle, dull, depigmented

____ 3. Cheilosis

____ 4. Flaccid, underdeveloped

____ 5. Fluorosis

____ 6. Xerophthalmia

Column II

a. Abdomen

b. Eyes

c. Hair

d. Lips

e. Muscles

f. Skeleton

g. Teeth

h. Tongue

SECTION II: APPLYING YOUR KNOWLEDGE

Activity D *Consider the scenario and answer the questions.*

CASE STUDY: Estimate Ideal Body Weight

Mrs. Allred is a 40-year-old Hispanic woman, 5 ft 5 inch tall, with three children younger than 5 years of age. She weighs 79.5 kg (175 lb). She had no known history of any physical illness before experiencing fatigue and irritability that she believed was the result of her parenting responsibilities. Mrs. Allred does not exercise regularly, eats snack foods while watching television with her children, and is too tired to prepare balanced meals for her family. She orders fast food or pizza for dinner at least three times a week.

1. Calculate Mrs. Allred's frame size based on a waist circumference of 16 cm.

   a. Small frame

   b. Medium frame

   c. Large frame

2. Mrs. Allred's ideal body weight (IBW) is _____ lb. Therefore, she needs to _____ (gain/lose) approximately _____ lb.

3. Her body mass index (BMI) is _____, which is considered (ideal, overweight, obese) _____.

CASE STUDY: Cultural and Nutritional Assessment

Activity D *Consider the scenario and answer the questions.*

A 72-year-old Egyptian woman who speaks no English and is a devout Muslim is visiting her son in the United States for 2 months. While she is going down the steps of her son's home, her foot misses the top step, and she falls down nine steps and fractures her left femur. She has an open reduction and internal fixation of her left hip and is admitted to the surgical unit.

1. What activities could the nurse use to overcome language barriers when interacting with this patient?

   _____

   _____

   _____

2. The patient receives a lunch tray that she pushes away. The nurse observes the food on the tray and determines why the patient refuses to eat it. What food item may be offensive to this patient?

   _____

   _____

SECTION III: PRACTICING FOR NCLEX

Activity E *Answer the following questions.*

1. The nurse is obtaining a health history from a patient. Which will be the primary focus of the assessment? (Select all that apply.)

   a. The primary method of payment

   b. A comprehensive body systems review

   c. What the patient ate prior to coming to the clinic

   d. Current and past medical problems

   e. Family history

2. Which does the patient have the right to know about the data collected by the nurse? (Select all that apply.)
   a. How the information will be used
   b. Why the information is being obtained
   c. What type of document is being used
   d. Whether the information will be held in confidence
   e. When the facility will be using electronic order entry

3. The nurse is performing a pain assessment for a patient. Which question asked by the nurse is considered an open-ended question?
   a. "Are you having pain?"
   b. "Is the pain sharp and piercing?"
   c. "Point to where it hurts."
   d. "Describe the pain."

4. Which priority factor regarding the patient may help the health care provider arrive at a diagnosis?
   a. Family history
   b. History of the present illness
   c. Past health history
   d. Results of the systems review

5. Which question by the nurse may be used to obtain educational or occupational information?
   a. "Are you a blue-collar worker?"
   b. "Do you have difficulty meeting your financial commitments?"
   c. "Is your income more than $20,000 per year?"
   d. "What college did you attend?"

6. Which statement made by the nurse would be a nontherapeutic response when the patient states, "I will not take pain medication when I am in pain"?
   a. "Is there another way you have learned to lessen pain when you experience it?"
   b. "Let a nurse know when you are in pain so you can be helped to decrease stimuli that may exaggerate your pain experience."
   c. "Refusing medication can only hurt you by increasing your awareness of the pain experience."
   d. "You have the right to make that decision. How can the nurses help you cope with your pain?"

7. Which question asked by the nurse will provide information about a patient's lifestyle? (Select all that apply.)
   a. "Have you always lived in this geographic area?"
   b. "Do you have any food preferences?"
   c. "How many hours of sleep do you require each day?"
   d. "What type of exercise do you prefer?"
   e. "What are the names of your children?"

8. The nurse is obtaining a health history from an older adult patient. Which nursing actions are appropriate when conducting the history? (Select all that apply.)
   a. Ask questions slowly, directly, and in a voice loud enough to be heard by those who are hearing impaired.
   b. Clarify the frequency, severity, and history of signs and symptoms of the present illness.
   c. Conduct the interview in a calm, unrushed manner using eye-to-eye contact.
   d. Have a family member in the room when asking questions to make sure the patient's answers are accurate.
   e. Frequently touch the patient so that you may bring their attention back to the interview.

9. The nurse assesses the patient's posture, stature, and body movements. Which part of the physical examination process is this?
   a. Auscultation
   b. Inspection
   c. Palpation
   d. Percussion

10. When the nurse is percussing for measurement of the patient's liver span, which type of response should be heard?
   a. Dull sound
   b. Flat sound
   c. Resonant sound
   d. Tympanic sound

11. The nurse notes hyperresonance over inflated lung tissue when performing a physical assessment on a patient with emphysema. Which process does the nurse use for this assessment?
    a. Auscultation
    b. Inspection
    c. Palpation
    d. Percussion

12. The nurse detects a heart murmur when performing a physical assessment on a patient. Which process does the nurse use for this assessment?
    a. Auscultation
    b. Inspection
    c. Palpation
    d. Percussion

13. The nurse is assigned to care for a patient with a cultural background that is different than the nurse's. Prior to delivering care, which is important for the nurse to do?
    a. The nurse should explore their own cultural beliefs
    b. Request to be reassigned to a patient with a culture the nurse is familiar with
    c. Be determined to provide care the same way to every patient, regardless of cultural background
    d. Determine what type of dietary restrictions the patient will have

14. The nurse observes a serum albumin level of 2.50 g/dL in an older adult patient who lives at home alone. What does this level indicate to the nurse?
    a. A severe protein deficiency
    b. Low levels of serum protein
    c. An acceptable amount of protein
    d. An extremely high measurement of protein

15. Which primary nutritional nursing consideration should be included in the physical assessment of an older adult patient?
    a. Altered metabolism and nutrient use secondary to an acute or chronic illness
    b. Decreased appetite related to loneliness
    c. Limited financial resources
    d. The patient's ability to shop for and prepare food

16. When performing a physical assessment, the nurse should be aware that in which culture would it be impolite to touch the patient's head?
    a. Arabian
    b. Hispanic
    c. Jewish
    d. Asian

Stress and Inflammatory Responses

Learning Outcomes

1. Describe the significance of the principles of internal constancy, homeostasis, stress, and adaptation in promoting and maintaining steady state in the body.
2. Describe the General Adaptation Syndrome and the sympathetic–adrenal–medullary and hypothalamic-pituitary responses to stress.
3. Identify ways in which maladaptive responses to stress can increase the risk of illness and cause disease.
4. Compare the adaptive processes of atrophy, hypertrophy, hyperplasia, metaplasia, and dysplasia within the body's inflammatory and reparative processes.
5. Assess the health patterns of individuals and families, identifying strategies that are useful in reducing stress.

SECTION I: ASSESSING YOUR UNDERSTANDING

Activity A *Fill in the blanks.*

1. Stress is a change in the environment that is perceived as _____, _____, or _____.

2. Maladaptive compensatory mechanisms result in disease processes in which cells may be _____, _____, or _____.

3. The neural and hormonal activities that respond to stress and maintain homeostasis are located in the _____.

4. Cell injury results when stressors interfere with the body's optimal balance by altering cellular ability to _____, _____, and _____.

5. Research has shown that the single most important factor influencing a person's health is _____.

6. Four concepts that are key to understanding a steady state of dynamic balance are _____, _____, _____, and _____.

7. Five bodily functions that are regulated by negative feedback mechanisms include the following: _____, _____, _____, _____, and _____.

8. The five cardinal signs of inflammation are _____, _____, _____, _____, and _____.

Activity B *Briefly answer the following.*

1. Define a *maladaptive* response to a stressor.

_____

_____

2. Explain why *hyperpnea,* after intense exercise, is considered an adaptive response to a physiologic stressor.

_____

_____

3. Give several examples of acute, *time-limited* stressors and chronic, *enduring* stressors.

_____

_____

4. Psychosocial stressors are classified as day-to-day occurrences (daily hassles), major events that affect large groups, and those infrequently occurring situations that directly affect a person. List two examples from your personal experiences that could be included under each classification.

   a. Day-to-day occurrences.

   _____

   _____

   b. Major events that affect large groups of people.

   _____

   _____

   c. Infrequently occurring major stressors.

   _____

   _____

5. Discuss the correlation between stress, illness, and critical life events.

_____

_____

6. Discuss how internal cognitive processes and external resources are used by a person to manage stress.

_____

_____

7. Define stress according to Hans Selye's Theory of Adaptation (1976).

_____

_____

8. According to Hans Selye's Theory of Adaptation (1976), there are about 12 diseases of maladaptation. List six.

   _____   _____

   _____   _____

   _____   _____

9. List four possible nursing diagnoses for individuals suffering from stress.

   _____   _____

   _____   _____

10. How does a person with positive self-esteem, energy, and health typically respond to stressors in a positive way?

_____

_____

11. What is the difference between physical, physiologic, and psychosocial stressors?

_____

_____

Activity C *Match the primary category of stressors listed in Column II with its associated stressors listed in Column I.*

Column I	Column II
____ **1.** Anxieties	**a.** Physiologic
____ **2.** Genetic disorders	**b.** Psychosocial
____ **3.** Hypoxia	
____ **4.** Infectious agents	
____ **5.** Life changes	
____ **6.** Nutritional imbalance	
____ **7.** Social relationships	
____ **8.** Trauma	

SECTION II: APPLYING YOUR KNOWLEDGE

Activity D *Consider the scenario and answer the questions.*

Mr. David, a 52-year-old corporate attorney, comes to the clinic and informs the nurse that he has been suffering from chest pain, an inability to sleep at night, and anxiety. He states, "I am working 70 or more hours a week and there is no time to enjoy life." Mr. David has a physical examination with an electrocardiogram and laboratory studies that rule out any physical cause for the symptoms.

1. The nurse attempts to educate Mr. David about relaxation techniques. What is the goal of relaxation techniques?

   _____

   _____

2. What type of commonly used relaxation techniques can the nurse educate Mr. David about?

   _____

   _____

3. What four similar factors in all relaxation techniques does the nurse identify?

   _____

   _____

SECTION III: PRACTICING FOR NCLEX

Activity E *Answer the following questions.*

1. A patient has been paralyzed from the chest down for 7 years and is now diagnosed with pneumonia. For which reason would the patient need additional support to cope with the infection?
   a. Coping measures become less effective with advancing age
   b. The patient's available coping resources are already being used to manage the problems of immobility
   c. An acute infectious process requires more adaptive mechanisms than a chronic stressor does
   d. This additional physical stressor places unmanageable demands on the patient's internal and external resources

2. A patient is admitted to the medical unit with periodic episodes of shortness of breath, choking sensation, and is crying. Which will the nurse do to evaluate the impact of physiologic and psychological components on the patient's illness?
   a. Perform a thorough physical examination and include subjective patient statements as well as objective laboratory data
   b. Focus primary attention on the respiratory system, because this is the patient's chief complaint
   c. Determine that the patient is not in acute distress, then perform a complete physical examination, including data about the patient's lifestyle and social relationships
   d. Attempt to discover the reasons behind the patient's anxieties, because stress can cause breathing difficulties

3. The nurse is interviewing a patient with shortness of breath who reveals they are in the process of obtaining a divorce. Which is the priority action by the nurse?
   a. Try to determine whether there is a psychological basis for the patient's physical symptoms
   b. Restrict family members from visiting, because their presence may aggravate the patient's symptoms
   c. Teach the patient specific breathing exercises that can be used to manage symptoms
   d. Request that the health care provider recommend counseling services

4. A patient is admitted to the emergency department (ED) for observation after a minor automobile crash. In reaction to the sympathetic nervous system's response to stress, which expected finding will be assessed? (Select all that apply.)
   a. Cold, clammy skin
   b. Decreased heart rate
   c. Rapid respirations
   d. Skeletal muscle tension
   e. Seizure activity

5. A patient is experiencing lower leg pain associated with lactic acid accumulation. When does the nurse expect the pain to decrease?
   a. When aerobic metabolism is reinstated
   b. When anaerobic metabolism becomes the major pathway for energy release
   c. When muscle use and subsequent glucose catabolism increase
   d. When vasoconstriction diminishes blood flow, thereby slowing the removal of waste products

6. A patient has a diagnosis of hypertrophy of the heart muscle, which correlates with cellular adaptation to injury. Which findings does the nurse expect to occur? (Select all that apply.)
   a. Compromised cardiac output
   b. Muscle mass changes evident on radiologic examination
   c. Cellular alteration compensatory to some stimulus
   d. Decreased cell size, leading to more effective ventricular contractions
   e. Increased cardiac output

7. A patient who is pregnant is having changes in her breast and asks the nurse if this should be cause for concern. Which does the nurse explain to the patient is the cellular adaptation to stress?
   a. Dysplasia
   b. Hyperplasia
   c. Hypertrophy
   d. Metaplasia

8. A patient has a hemoglobin level of 7 g/dL. Which is the priority assessment finding by the nurse that should be immediately reported to the health care provider?
   a. Hyperemia
   b. Hypertension
   c. Hypoglycemia
   d. Hypoxia

9. A patient with diabetes is admitted to the hospital with a blood sugar level of 320 mg/dL. Why will the nurse monitor fluid intake and output for this patient?
   a. Decreased blood osmolarity causes fluid to shift into the interstitial spaces, resulting in polydipsia
   b. Polydipsia occurs when glucose catabolism is accelerated, thereby increasing the body's need for fluids
   c. Polyuria results from osmotic diuresis, which is compensatory to hyperglycemia
   d. The blood's hypotonicity will result in tissue fluid retention and weight gain

10. The nurse is caring for a patient with a fever. Care for this patient will be based on what body responses? (Select all that apply.)
    a. Diaphoresis, which is a compensatory mechanism that cools the body
    b. Vasodilation of surface blood vessels, which prevents excessive heat loss
    c. Increased heart rate, which helps to meet increased metabolic demands
    d. Increased nutrient catabolism, which influences the body's caloric needs
    e. Decrease in cellular metabolism, which decreases metabolic demand

11. The patient wants to be prescribed an anti-infective drug for the flu. The nurse explains to the patient that anti-infective medications would not be useful against which biologic agents?
    a. Bacteria
    b. Fungi
    c. Mycoplasmas
    d. Viruses

12. The nurse is talking with a patient who is considering becoming pregnant and is concerned about genetic disorders. Which genetic disorders does the nurse inform the patient arise from inherited traits? (Select all that apply.)
    a. Hemophilia
    b. Meningitis
    c. Phenylketonuria
    d. Sickle cell disease
    e. Encephalitis

13. A nurse is caring for a patient with a localized response to bee stings. Which symptoms will the nurse assess for? (Select all that apply.)
    a. Hyperemia due to increased blood flow
    b. Cool skin around the site of the sting
    c. Blanching due to compensatory vasoconstriction
    d. Pain due to pressure on the nerve endings
    e. Swelling due to increased vascular permeability

14. The nurse is caring for a patient with an infected surgical incision. Which signs demonstrating systemic response does the nurse observe? (Select all that apply.)
    a. A febrile state caused by the release of pyrogens
    b. Anorexia, malaise, and weakness
    c. Leukopenia owing to increased white blood cell production
    d. Loss of appetite and complaints of aching
    e. Subnormal body temperature caused by vasoconstriction

15. The nurse is performing an assessment to determine the patient's social support systems. Which question is important for the nurse to ask?
    a. Does the patient believe that they belong to a group that is mutually dependent and communicative?
    b. Does the patient have adequate insurance coverage to take care of health costs?
    c. What does the patient do for a living?
    d. Does the patient have any significant past medical problems?

16. A patient with a strong history of breast malignancy in her family is scheduled for a breast biopsy in the morning. Which is the nursing priority action when caring for this patient the evening before surgery?
    a. Give a soothing back massage to promote relaxation and decrease stress
    b. Make sure she eats all of her evening meal, because she will be NPO after midnight
    c. Minimize the emotional impact of surgery by encouraging her to socialize with other patients
    d. Sit with her and provide an opportunity for her to talk about her concerns

CHAPTER 6

Genetics and Genomics in Nursing

Learning Outcomes

1. Describe the role of the nurse in integrating genetics and genomics in nursing care.
2. Identify the common patterns of inheritance of genetic disorders.
3. Conduct a comprehensive genetic- and genomic-based assessment.
4. Apply the principles, concepts, and theories of genetics and genomics to individuals, families, groups, and communities.
5. Identify ethical, legal, and social issues in nursing related to genetics and genomics.

SECTION I: ASSESSING YOUR UNDERSTANDING

Activity A *Fill in the blanks.*

1. A person's individual genetic makeup (composed of approximately 25,000 genes) is called a _____; the person's set of characteristics of physical appearance and other traits is called a _____.

2. Genes are working subunits of DNA. Genes are arranged in linear order within _____. Twenty-two pairs of chromosomes, also called _____, are the same in males and females. The 23rd pair, the _____, is composed of two _____ for the female and _____ for the male. At conception, the gender of a child is determined because each parent gives _____.

3. With autosomal dominant inheritance, a woman with the *BRCA1* hereditary breast cancer gene has a lifetime risk of _____% of acquiring breast cancer and a _____% chance of passing the gene to each child.

4. _____ is a common chromosomal condition that occurs with greater frequency in pregnancies of women who are 35 years of age or older.

5. The frequency of chromosomal abnormalities in newborns is _____; this accounts for _____% of all spontaneous first-trimester pregnancy losses.

6. _____, which can be identified with parasympathetic testing, is the most common adult-onset condition in the Caucasian population.

7. _____ is the study of all the genes in the human genome and their interactions.

8. Chromosomes are located within the nucleus of a cell. The human body has _____ chromosomes.

9. Gene mutations have significant implications for health and illness. _____ is a mutation in protein structure that alters the configuration of hemoglobin.

10. _____ is a multifactorial genetic condition that tends to cluster in families.

11. Three examples of adult-onset conditions believed to be the result of multifactorial genetic mutations include _____, _____, and _____.

Activity B *Briefly answer the following.*

1. Define the term *genomic medicine.*

   _____

   _____

   _____

2. What are the essential nursing competencies for genetics and genomics?

   _____

   _____

3. Cite five examples of multifactorial inherited conditions.

   _____   _____

   _____   _____

   _____

4. Define the term *pharmacogenetics.*

   _____

   _____

5. List five nursing activities in genetics-related nursing practice.

   _____   _____

   _____   _____

   _____

Activity C

PART I: Terminology

Match the genetic term listed in Column II with its specific definition listed in Column I.

Column I

____ 1. The number of chromosomes normally present in humans ($N = 46$)

____ 2. The presence of one extra chromosome (e.g., Down syndrome)

____ 3. The genes and variations that a person inherits from his or her parents

____ 4. A single chromosome from any of the 22 pairs not involved in gender determination (XX or XY)

____ 5. A person's entire physiologic and biologic makeup as determined by genotype and environment

____ 6. Primary genetic material (DNA)

____ 7. A heterozygous person who carries two different alleles of a gene pair

____ 8. The microscopic cell nucleus that contains genetic information

Column II

a. Autosome

b. Carrier

c. Chromosome

d. Deoxyribonucleic acid

e. Diploid

f. Genotype

g. Phenotype

h. Trisomy

PART II: Adult-Onset Disorders

Match the age of adult onset in Column II with the specific disorder listed in Column I.

Column I	Column II
_____ 1. Spinocerebellar ataxia, type 2	a. Mean age of 30 years
_____ 2. Huntington disease	b. 30 to 40 years
_____ 3. Early-onset familial Alzheimer's disease	c. 35 to 44 years
	d. 40 to 60 years
_____ 4. Hereditary hemochromatosis	e. 60 to 65 years
	f. 50 to 70 years
_____ 5. Spinocerebellar ataxia, type 3	
_____ 6. Polycystic kidney disease	
_____ 7. Familial hypercholesterolemia	
_____ 8. Amyotrophic lateral sclerosis (ALS)	

SECTION II: APPLYING YOUR KNOWLEDGE

Activity D *Consider the scenario and answer the questions.*

Maggie and Josh are planning to have another child. Maggie has had four spontaneous abortions prior to week 16, and they have a 3-year-old son with Down syndrome.

1. Maggie has a "balanced" chromosomal rearrangement. What can this mean for future pregnancies?

   _____

   _____

2. Prior to Maggie becoming pregnant, what should the nurse suggest to the couple?

   _____

3. Why would fluorescent in situ hybridization (FISH) be performed?

   _____

SECTION III: PRACTICING FOR NCLEX

Activity E *Answer the following questions.*

1. A patient at 22 weeks' gestation had an amniocentesis and was told that the fetus has a condition in which cellular division results in an extra chromosome. Which condition may affect the fetus?

   a. Down syndrome
   b. Sickle cell disease
   c. Tay-Sachs disease
   d. Turner syndrome

2. A patient understands that her diagnosis of ovarian cancer syndrome is an autosomal dominant inherited condition. What is the chance that her daughter will inherit the gene mutation for this disease?

   a. 10%
   b. 25%
   c. 50%
   d. 80%

3. A patient has an autosomal recessive inherited condition. For which type of disorder does the nurse anticipate the patient will be treated?

   a. Cystic fibrosis
   b. Hereditary breast cancer
   c. Huntington disease
   d. Familial hypercholesterolemia

4. A 32-year-old patient has just been told that she has the *BRCA1* hereditary breast cancer gene mutation. What is her risk of developing cancer by the age of 65 years?

   a. 25%
   b. 50%
   c. 80%
   d. 100%

5. A couple considering starting a family is told that they are both carriers for thalassemia. What does the nurse tell them is the risk that their child will inherit the gene?

   a. 25%
   b. 50%
   c. 75%
   d. 100%

6. A couple is preparing for pregnancy and concerned about the risk of Tay-Sachs disease. Which cultural group does the nurse identify is at most risk for the disease?

   a. Ashkenazi Jewish

   b. Italian Americans

   c. Native Americans

   d. African Americans

7. Which target cultural population is a priority for the nurse to educate about prevention of hypertension?

   a. Italian Americans

   b. Native Americans

   c. African Americans

   d. Hispanics

8. Parents request that a test be done to determine if the fetus has Down syndrome. Which type of test does the nurse anticipate the primary provider will prescribe?

   a. Presymptomatic testing

   b. Prenatal screening

   c. Predisposition testing

   d. A family pedigree

9. The daughter of a patient with Huntington disease has requested testing for the disease even though she has no symptoms at this time. Which type of test does the nurse anticipate the health care provider will prescribe?

   a. Presymptomatic testing

   b. Prenatal testing

   c. Predisposition testing

   d. A family pedigree

10. In order to develop an awareness of genetics and genomic concepts, which is essential that the nurse do first?

    a. Examine their own beliefs and values.

    b. Make judgments based on the type of patients being treated.

    c. Do an Internet search on genetics.

    d. Ask the primary provider what they think.

CHAPTER 7

Disability and Chronic Illness

Learning Outcomes

1. Compare and contrast the concepts of disability, chronic illness, and chronic disease.
2. Differentiate between models of disability.
3. Critically analyze the influence of disability on nursing care decisions and actions for patients.
4. Identify factors related to the increasing incidence of chronic conditions.
5. Describe characteristics of chronic conditions and nursing implications for people with chronic conditions and for their families.

SECTION I: ASSESSING YOUR UNDERSTANDING

Activity A *Fill in the blanks.*

1. The four causes of major chronic illnesses that are preventable by lifestyle changes are
_____, _____, _____, and _____.

2. Disparities in health and health outcomes are associated with _____, _____, and _____ factors.

3. The three most frequently occurring chronic diseases that result from four preventable causes are _____, _____, and _____.

4. The three categories used to classify disabilities are _____, _____, and _____.

Activity B *Briefly answer the following.*

1. List three characteristics common to all forms of chronic illness.

_____

_____

_____

2. Identify six challenges commonly associated with chronic conditions.

_____ _____

_____ _____

_____ _____

3. List six common medical and nursing management problems related to chronic conditions.

_____ _____

_____ _____

_____ _____

4. What two interventions can be provided to address health promotion for the risk factor of cancer?

_____

_____

5. What is the difference between the terms *disability* and *impairment* according to the definitions approved by the World Health Organization's (2018) classification system?

_____

_____

6. What psychological and emotional reactions to chronic illness and its consequences (e.g., lifestyle changes, financial resources) affect adjustment?

_____

_____

7. What is the difference between the Rehabilitation Act of 1973 and the Disabilities Act of 1990, and how they have helped protect disabled people from discrimination?

_____

_____

Activity C *The following statements list some characteristics of chronic illness. For each statement, write an explanation of how nursing care can improve the patient's and family's response to management and adaptation.*

1. Managing chronic illness involves more than managing medical problems.

_____

_____

2. Chronic conditions are associated with different phases over a course of time.

_____

_____

3. Managing chronic conditions requires persistent adherence to a therapeutic regimen.

_____

_____

4. Chronic illness affects the whole family.

_____

_____

SECTION II: APPLYING YOUR KNOWLEDGE

Activity D *Consider the scenario and answer the questions.*

Mrs. Mercer, a 32-year-old mother of two, works part time as a teacher assistant and has just been diagnosed with end-stage kidney disease. The nephrologist has informed her that it is most likely that she will have to have hemodialysis 3 days a week.

1. What barriers related to this disability will Mrs. Mercer likely encounter?

_____

_____

2. What federal assistance programs should the case worker discuss with Mrs. Mercer to assist with the cost of health care?

_____

_____

SECTION III: PRACTICING FOR NCLEX

Activity E *Answer the following questions.*

1. The nurse is caring for a patient who had a stroke and has right-sided hemiparesis. The patient is receiving physical therapy that will continue when discharged through home health care services. After what minimum period of time will this patient's medical condition be termed *chronic*?

   a. 8 weeks
   b. 3 months
   c. 16 weeks
   d. 6 months

2. The nurse is developing a program to address a chronic illness on the rise that is directly related to an unhealthy lifestyle. Which will the nurse prepare to educate the community about?

   a. Diabetes mellitus
   b. Breast cancer
   c. Emphysema
   d. Colorectal cancer

3. Which aspect of a healthy lifestyle can the nurse encourage a patient to improve that can significantly enhance quality of life with a chronic condition?
   a. Diet
   b. Exercise
   c. Hydration
   d. Rest

4. Which model of disability is viewed as promoting dependency and passivity?
   a. Medical model
   b. Rehabilitation model
   c. Social model
   d. Functional model

5. The nurse is caring for a patient admitted to the hospital that is visually impaired and requires safety measures to be immediately implemented. Which type of disability will be addressed?
   a. Cognitive
   b. Sensory
   c. Developmental
   d. Psychiatric

6. When documenting a patient admitted for diabetes, which is the appropriate "people-first" language?
   a. The diabetic patient has a blood glucose of 324 mg/dL.
   b. The diabetic in room 240 is going down for a chest x-ray.
   c. The patient with diabetes has been admitted to room 222.
   d. Has the diabetic patient had dinner so I can give medication?

7. The nurse recognizes which disorder as a developmental disability in a patient?
   a. Cerebral palsy
   b. Spinal cord injury
   c. Stroke
   d. Osteoarthritis

8. Which disability model is most appropriate for the nurse to use as a guide for planning care?
   a. Biopsychosocial Model
   b. Interface Model
   c. Medical and Rehabilitation Model
   d. Social Model

9. When providing education to the patient with a chronic illness, which is a priority intervention for the nurse to perform?
   a. Educate all patients the same.
   b. Provide written information only so that patients will have a reference.
   c. Adapt teaching strategies and materials to the individual patient.
   d. If the patient is hearing impaired, teach a family member instead.

10. A patient has had a traumatic amputation of the left leg above the knee following an industrial accident. Which type of disability does this patient have?
    a. Chronic disability
    b. Impaired disability
    c. Developmental disability
    d. Acquired disability

Management of the Older Adult Patient

1. Specify the demographic trends and the physiologic aspects of aging in the United States.
2. Describe the significance of preventive health care and health promotion for the older adult.
3. Compare and contrast the common physical and mental health problems of aging and their effects on the functioning of older adults and their families.
4. Identify the role of the nurse in meeting the health care needs of the older patient.
5. Examine common health issues of older adults and their families in the home and the community, in the acute care setting, and in the long-term care facility.

SECTION I: ASSESSING YOUR UNDERSTANDING

Activity A Fill in the blanks.

1. Bone changes associated with aging frequently result from a loss of _____.

2. The primary cause of age-related vision loss in the older adult is _____.

3. With aging, there is a gradual decline in _____ and _____; _____ skills tend to remain intact.

4. _____ is the most common affective or mood disorder of the older adult patient.

5. _____ are the leading cause of injury in the older adult.

6. _____, the primary source of federal funding, provides nursing home care for the older adult poor.

Activity B Briefly answer the following.

1. Define the term geriatric syndromes.

   _____

   _____

2. Age-related changes reduce the efficiency of the cardiovascular system. These changes include _____, _____, _____, and _____, which result in _____.

3. Name two age-related alterations in metabolism.

   _____

   _____

4. List the five most common infections in the older adult: _____, _____, _____, _____, and _____.

5. Describe the concept of continuing care retirement communities.

_____

_____

_____

6. What nursing interventions can be used to help older adults with learning and memory?

_____

_____

7. Determine what nursing interventions can be used to help patients manage their medications and adhere to the prescribed medication regimen.

_____

_____

_____

8. What is the most common form of dementia?

_____

_____

9. What is the purpose of the Older Americans Act, and what services does it provide to the older adult?

_____

_____

10. What is the difference between Medicare and Medicaid?

_____

_____

11. What is the purpose of a living will and a durable power of attorney, and what are their limitations?

_____

_____

12. Describe the Patient Self-Determination Act (PSDA).

_____

_____

_____

SECTION II: APPLYING YOUR KNOWLEDGE

Activity C *Consider the scenarios and answer the questions.*

CASE STUDY: Loneliness

Mrs. Shelly is an 80-year-old retired schoolteacher. She was recently widowed and lives alone. She is financially secure but socially isolated, because she has outlived most of her friends. Her children are self-sufficient and are very busy with their own lives.

1. What psychological threats may Mrs. Shelly experience?

_____

_____

2. Mrs. Shelly is concerned about the dryness of her skin. What suggestions can the nurse make for care of her skin?

_____

_____

3. Mrs. Shelly notices that food does not taste the same as before. What does she need to be aware that this sensory change is probably related to?

_____

_____

4. An analysis of Mrs. Shelly's diet shows that it does not contain adequate protein. For a body weight of 60 kg (134 lb), what should her daily protein intake be?

_____

_____

5. Most accidents among older adults involve falls within the home. What preventive measures can the nurse advise Mrs. Shelly to take?

_____

_____

CASE STUDY: Alzheimer's Disease

Mr. Thomas, a 75-year-old retired bricklayer, lives at home with his 65-year-old wife, who is healthy and active. Lately she has noticed that Mr. Thomas is negative, hostile, and suspicious of her. He gets lost in his own home, and his conversations have been accompanied by forgetfulness. Recently, Mr. Thomas's health care provider has indicated a probable diagnosis of Alzheimer's disease.

1. What can the nurse suggest to help Mrs. Thomas deal with Mr. Thomas's behavior?

   _____

   _____

2. What is an important point for the nurse to communicate to Mrs. Thomas?

   _____

   _____

3. What can the nurse make patient caregivers aware of regarding psychosocial support?

   _____

   _____

4. The health care provider explains that there is no cure for the disease and no way to slow its progression, which intensifies symptoms. What complications should the family be aware of that are the cause of death in patients with Alzheimer's?

   _____

   _____

CASE STUDY: Dehydration

Mrs. Vega, an 89-year-old widow, was transferred from a nursing home to the local hospital with a diagnosis of dehydration. She needs to be on bed rest because of her generalized weakness. She is occasionally confused and disoriented.

1. What interventions should the nurse provide to ensure adequate temperature regulation?

   _____

   _____

2. Mrs. Vega has been incontinent of urine since admission. What nursing intervention would be important for the nurse to implement?

   _____

   _____

3. The nurse suggests that Vega sit in a rocking chair for 20 minutes, four times a day. Why does the nurse suggest this for her?

   _____

   _____

SECTION III: PRACTICING FOR NCLEX

Activity D *Answer the following questions.*

1. The nurse is working in a long-term care facility. When assessing the patients, which body system dysfunction should the nurse look for as the leading cause of morbidity and mortality in the older adult population?

   a. Cardiovascular

   b. Genitourinary

   c. Gastrointestinal

   d. Respiratory

2. The nurse is performing a respiratory assessment for an older adult patient. Which age-related findings could be identified with this patient? (Select all that apply.)

   a. Increased residual volume

   b. Decreased residual volume

   c. Loss of elastic tissue surrounding the alveoli

   d. Reduced vital capacity

   e. Decreased pulmonary resistance

3. The nurse is assessing the genitourinary status of an older adult female patient who is experiencing stress incontinence. Which finding is a common age-related finding for this population?

   a. Bladder capacity decreases with advanced age.

   b. All patients develop urinary tract infections.

   c. Renal filtration rate increases.

   d. Urine is more dilute in the older population.

4. The nurse is assisting an older adult patient with dietary planning. Which will the patient's daily carbohydrate intake be?
   a. 20% to 25%
   b. 40% to 45%
   c. 55% to 60%
   d. 70% to 75%

5. A patient asks the nurse why she seems to have bone changes since getting older. Which is the best response by the nurse?
   a. "Bone changes from aging result from a loss of calcium."
   b. "Bone changes from aging result from a loss of magnesium."
   c. "Bone changes from aging result from a loss of vitamin A."
   d. "Bone changes from aging result from a loss of vitamin C."

6. When administering medications to an older adult patient, which medication does the nurse understand may remain in the body longer due to increased body fat?
   a. Anticoagulants
   b. Barbiturates
   c. Digitalis glycosides
   d. Diuretics

7. An older adult female patient informs the nurse that she is sexually active but has a problem with vaginal dryness. What can the nurse suggest to the patient that may help relieve this problem?
   a. Use vaginal douche daily.
   b. Use Monistat vaginal cream to treat the fungal infection she probably has.
   c. Use a water-based lubricant when having sexual intercourse.
   d. Find other methods of sexual expression.

8. An older adult female patient tells the nurse, "I have lost an inch of height and have a hump on my back. What can I do about this?" Which is the best response by the nurse?
   a. "In order to prevent further bone loss, eat a diet high in calcium and low in phosphorus."
   b. "In order to prevent further bone loss, eat a diet high in magnesium and high in phosphorus."
   c. "You can reverse the bone loss with surgical intervention."
   d. "Supplement your diet with a multivitamin."

9. An older adult male patient tells the nurse that he wakes several times a night to pass his urine but never feels as though he fully empties his bladder. Which suggestion can the nurse make to help control this in the evening?
   a. Drink several glasses of fluid prior to going to bed in the evening to dilute the urine.
   b. He probably has developed a urinary tract infection and requires an antibiotic.
   c. Limit drinking a lot of fluid in the evening, especially caffeinated beverages.
   d. Wear a condom catheter at night so that he will not have to get up so much.

10. The nurse brings the older adult patient a dinner tray and observes the patient placing excess amounts of salt on the food. Which suggestions for flavoring can the nurse provide to decrease the amount of salt the patient is placing on the food? (Select all that apply.)
   a. Drink water before the meal.
   b. Use low-sodium herbs and spices.
   c. Use an alcohol-based mouthwash prior to eating.
   d. Use pepper instead of salt.
   e. Use lemon instead of salt to flavor food.

Concepts and Principles of Patient Management

Pain Management

Learning Outcomes

1. Describe the fundamental concepts of pain including the types of pain, the four processes of nociception, and neuropathic pain.
2. Explain and demonstrate methods to perform a pain assessment.
3. List the first-line agents from the three groups of analgesic agents.
4. Identify the unique effects of select analgesic agents on older adults.
5. Describe practical nonpharmacologic methods that can be used in the clinical setting in patients with pain.
6. Use the nursing process as a framework for care of the patient with pain.

SECTION I: ASSESSING YOUR UNDERSTANDING

Activity A *Fill in the blanks.*

1. Pain can be defined according to its
   _____, _____, and
   _____.

2. _____, _____, and _____
   are the three basic categories of pain.

3. A person's reported intensity of pain is determined by a person's _____
   (the smallest stimulus where pain is felt) and
   _____ (the maximum amount of pain a person can tolerate).

4. Although the criterion is arbitrary, acute pain can be classified as chronic when it has persisted for _____.

5. After administration of an epidural opioid, the nurse needs to assess for _____,
   which may occur up to _____ hours but usually peaks between _____
   hours.

6. A chemical substance thought to inhibit the transmission of pain is _____.

Activity B *Briefly answer the following.*

1. Pain can be categorized by its etiology. List four of eight pain syndromes.

   _____   _____

   _____   _____

2. Name one pathophysiologic response to chronic pain.

   _____

3. List five algogenic substances that are released into the tissues and affect the sensitivity of nociceptors: _____, _____,

   _____, _____, and _____.

4. List seven factors that directly influence a person's response to pain: _____,

   _____, _____, _____,

   _____, _____, and _____.

5. Identify seven factors that a nurse needs to consider for complete pain assessment:

   _____, _____,

   _____, _____,

   _____, _____,

   and _____.

6. List eight common physiologic responses to pain: _____, _____,

   _____, _____,

   _____, _____,

   _____, and _____.

7. Define the term *balanced analgesia*.

   _____

   _____

8. Define the term *placebo effect*.

   _____

   _____

9. List four nonpharmacologic interventions for pain management: _____,

   _____, _____, and

   _____.

10. Distinguish among acute, chronic (persistent, nonmalignant), and cancer-related pain and cite an example of each.

    _____

    _____

11. What pain management strategies may be used for those at the end of their life?

    _____

    _____

12. Compare and contrast the precautions and contraindications for the following opioids.

	Precautions	Contraindications
Morphine		
Codeine		
Oxycodone		
Demerol		
Darvon		
Vicodin		

13. What are the nursing responsibilities for management of patient-controlled analgesia?

    _____

    _____

14. How does the technique of *distraction* work to relieve acute and chronic pain?

    _____

    _____

Activity C *Match the term listed in Column II with its definition in Column I.*

Column I

____ 1. Pain receptors sensitive to noxious stimuli

____ 2. Nonsteroidal agents that decrease inflammation

____ 3. The only commercially available transdermal opioid medication

____ 4. Significantly increases a person's response to pain

____ 5. Chemicals known to inhibit the transmission or perception of pain

____ 6. This substance, released in response to painful stimuli, causes vasodilation

____ 7. An inactive substance given in place of pain medication

____ 8. Medication administered directly into the subarachnoid space and cerebrospinal fluid

____ 9. Transcutaneous stimulation of non-pain receptors in the same area of an injury

____ 10. Term used to describe a pain's rhythm

Column II

a. Fentanyl

b. Endorphins

c. Placebo

d. Waning

e. TENS

f. Nociceptors

g. Histamine

h. Anxiety

i. Epidural

j. NSAIDs

SECTION II: APPLYING YOUR KNOWLEDGE

Activity D *Consider the scenario and answer the questions.*

CASE STUDY: Pain Experience

Courtney is a young, healthy adult who slipped off the stairs going down to the basement and struck her forehead on the cement flooring. Courtney did not lose consciousness but did sustain a mild concussion and a hematoma that was 5 cm in width and protruded outward approximately 6 cm. She experienced immediate acute pain at the site of injury plus a pounding headache.

1. After an immediate assessment of the localized pain, based on the patient's description, what does the nurse expect the patient to report during the pain assessment?

2. During the assessment process, the nurse attempts to determine Courtney's physiologic and behavioral responses to her pain experience. The nurse is aware that a patient can be in pain yet appear to be "pain free." Which behavioral response by Courtney indicates she is experiencing acute pain?

3. The nurse uses distraction techniques to help Courtney cope with her pain experience. What suggested activities would be best to help her cope?

4. After treatment, Courtney is discharged to home while still in pain. What education will the nurse provide upon discharge?

SECTION III: PRACTICING FOR NCLEX

Activity E *Answer the following questions.*

1. A patient slipped and fell on the floor in the hospital room, causing a back injury, and the patient now reports pain. How will the nurse determine that the pain is characteristic of acute pain?
   a. It does not respond well to treatment.
   b. It is associated with a specific injury.
   c. It serves no useful purpose.
   d. It responds well to placebos.

2. The nurse is caring for a patient who has been hospitalized on several occasions for lower abdominal pain related to Crohn's disease. How may this chronic pain be identified?
   a. It is attributable to a specific cause.
   b. It is prolonged in duration.
   c. It occurs rapidly and subsides with treatment.
   d. It is separate from any central or peripheral pathology.

3. A patient comes into the clinic frequently with reports of pain. Which will the nurse recognize as chronic benign pain in this patient?
   a. A migraine headache
   b. An exacerbation of rheumatoid arthritis
   c. Low back pain
   d. Sickle cell crisis

4. The nurse is performing an assessment for a patient reporting pain but finds no physical cause. Which nursing action is appropriate with the patient's continued report of pain?
   a. Believe a patient when they state that pain is present.
   b. Doubt that pain exists when no physical origin can be identified.
   c. Realize that patients frequently imagine and state that they have pain without actually feeling painful sensations.
   d. Assume that the patient may be a drug seeker and should be given other methods for pain control.

5. When a nurse asks a patient to describe the quality of the pain, which type of descriptive term does the nurse expect the patient to use?
   a. Burning
   b. Chronic
   c. Intermittent
   d. Severe

6. The nurse is assessing a patient reporting severe pain. Which physiologic indicator does the nurse recognize as significant of acute pain?
   a. Diaphoresis
   b. Bradycardia
   c. Hypotension
   d. Decreased respiratory rate

7. The nurse is assessing an older adult patient just admitted to the hospital. Why is it important that the nurse carefully assess pain in the older adult patient?
   a. Older adults are expected to experience chronic pain.
   b. Older adults have a decreased pain threshold.
   c. Older adults experience reduced sensory perception.
   d. Older adults have increased sensory perception.

8. The nurse is administering an analgesic to an older adult patient. Why is it important for the nurse to assess the patient carefully prior to administering the medication?
   a. Older adults metabolize drugs more rapidly.
   b. Older adults have increased hepatic, renal, and gastrointestinal function.
   c. Older adults are more sensitive to drugs.
   d. Older adults have lower ratios of body fat and muscle mass.

9. The nurse administers an opioid analgesic to a patient. Which serious side effect should the nurse carefully monitor for?
   a. Renal toxicity
   b. Respiratory depression
   c. Seizure activity
   d. Hypertension

10. The nurse informs the patient that a preventive approach for pain relief will be used, involving nonsteroidal anti-inflammatory drugs. Which will the nurse educate the patient about regarding this method?
    a. The pain medication will be administered before the pain becomes severe.
    b. The pain medication will be administered before the pain is experienced.
    c. The pain medication will be administered when the pain is at its peak.
    d. The pain medication will be administered when the level of pain tolerance has been exceeded.

11. The nurse's major area of assessment for a patient receiving patient-controlled analgesia is assessment of which system?
    a. Cardiovascular
    b. Integumentary
    c. Neurologic
    d. Respiratory

12. What does the nurse understand is the advantage of using intraspinal infusion to deliver analgesics? (Select all that apply.)
    a. It is easily accessible by the nurse.
    b. Higher doses may be administered.
    c. Side effects of systemic analgesia are reduced.
    d. Effects on pulse, respirations, and blood pressure are reduced.
    e. The need for injections decreases in frequency.

13. The nurse observes the anesthesiologist administer a single-dose extended-release drug in an epidural catheter for a patient undergoing a major surgical procedure. Which drug does the nurse determine is being administered?
    a. Codeine
    b. Demerol
    c. Dilaudid
    d. Depodur

14. The nurse is assisting the anesthesiologist with the insertion of an epidural catheter and the administration of an epidural opioid for pain control. Which adverse effect of epidural opioids should the nurse monitor for?

    a. Asystole
    b. Hypertension
    c. Bradypnea
    d. Tachycardia

15. Prior to starting a peripheral intravenous line on a patient, which intervention can the nurse provide to decrease the pain from the needle puncture?

    a. Give an oral opioid analgesic 30 minutes before the procedure.
    b. Apply diclofenac gel over the site 1 hour before the procedure.
    c. Apply eutectic mixture of local anesthetic cream 30 minutes prior to the procedure.
    d. Inject lidocaine 2% with epinephrine locally around the potential procedure site.

16. Which medication can the nurse administer to the patient intravenously for the control of pain and fever?

    a. Hydrocodone
    b. Acetaminophen/oxycodone
    c. Hydromorphone
    d. Acetaminophen

17. The primary provider has prescribed a μ-opioid analgesic for a patient with pain. What drug does the nurse anticipate administering?

    a. Nalbuphine hydrochloride
    b. Butorphanol
    c. Buprenorphine
    d. Fentanyl

18. The patient develops respiratory depression after the nurse administers fentanyl for pain. Which medication can the nurse anticipate administering to counteract the effects of the fentanyl?

    a. Nalbuphine hydrochloride
    b. Morphine
    c. Naloxone
    d. Lidocaine

19. The nurse applies a transdermal patch of fentanyl for a patient with pain due to cancer of the pancreas. The patient puts the call light on 1 hour later and tells the nurse that it has not helped. Which is the best response by the nurse?

    a. "It will take approximately 12 to 18 hours for the medication to begin to work, so I will give you something else now to relieve the pain."
    b. "It should have begun working 30 minutes ago. I will ask the primary provider to prescribe something stronger."
    c. "You have probably developed a tolerance to the medication."
    d. "It will take about 24 hours for the medication to work. I can't give you anything else or you will overdose."

CHAPTER 10

Fluid and Electrolytes

Learning Outcomes

1. Differentiate between osmosis, diffusion, filtration, and active transport.
2. Describe the role of the kidneys, lungs, and endocrine glands in regulating the body's fluid composition and volume.
3. Plan effective care of patients with the following imbalances: fluid volume deficit and fluid volume excess, sodium deficit (hyponatremia) and sodium excess (hypernatremia), and potassium deficit (hypokalemia) and potassium excess (hyperkalemia).
4. Describe the cause, clinical manifestations, management, and nursing interventions for the following imbalances: calcium deficit (hypocalcemia) and calcium excess (hypercalcemia), magnesium deficit (hypomagnesemia) and magnesium excess (hypermagnesemia), phosphorus deficit (hypophosphatemia) and phosphorus excess (hyperphosphatemia), and chloride deficit (hypochloremia) and chloride excess (hyperchloremia).
5. Explain the roles of the lungs, kidneys, and chemical buffers in maintaining acid–base balance; and compare metabolic as well as respiratory acidosis and alkalosis with regard to causes, clinical manifestations, diagnosis, and management.
6. Interpret arterial blood gas measurements.

SECTION I: ASSESSING YOUR UNDERSTANDING

Activity A *Fill in the blanks.*

1. About _____% of total body fluid is in the intracellular space; the major positively charged ion in intracellular fluid is _____. The extracellular space is divided into three compartments: _____, _____, and _____; the major positively charged ion in extracellular fluid is _____. About _____% of the _____ L of total blood volume is _____.

2. The primary concentration of phosphorus (85%) is located in the _____, with about 15% located in _____.

3. The normal blood pH is _____.

4. The upper and lower blood pH levels that are incompatible with life are _____ and _____.

5. The average daily urinary output in an adult is _____ L.

6. Cardiac effects of hyperkalemia are usually present when the serum potassium level reaches _____ mEq/L.

7. A normal oxygen saturation value for arterial blood is _____.

8. Sodium, the most abundant electrolyte in extracellular fluid, is primarily responsible for maintaining fluid _____, which

9. Sodium is regulated by _____,
   _____, and the _____
   system.

10. Sodium establishes the electrochemical state
    necessary for _____ and
    the _____.

11. The most common buffer system in the body
    is the _____.

12. The most characteristic manifestation of
    hypocalcemia and hypomagnesemia is
    _____.

Activity B *Briefly answer the following.*

PART I

1. Define the term *osmotic pressure*.

   _____

   _____

2. Distinguish between the terms *urine specific
   gravity, blood urea nitrogen,* and *creatinine*.

   _____

   _____

3. Distinguish between the terms *baroreceptors*
   and *osmoreceptors*.

   _____

   _____

4. How are calcium levels regulated?

   _____

   _____

5. Name the primary complication of hyperphosphatemia which occurs when the calcium–
   magnesium product exceeds 70 mg/dL.

   _____

   _____

6. Write the mathematical formula that a nurse
   would use to approximate the value of serum
   osmolality.

   _____

7. Explain why the administration of a 3% to
   5% sodium chloride solution requires intense
   monitoring.

   _____

   _____

8. List four of six symptoms associated with
   air embolism, a complication of intravenous
   therapy.

   _____

   _____

PART II

1. Indicate which of the following factors contribute to *hyponatremia* by writing "Low"
   in the space provided, and indicate which
   contribute to *hypernatremia* by writing "High"
   in the space provided.
   a. _____ vomiting
   b. _____ diarrhea
   c. _____ watery diarrhea
   d. _____ inability to quench thirst
   e. _____ burns over a large surface area
   f. _____ diuretics
   g. _____ heatstroke
   h. _____ adrenal insufficiency
   i. _____ syndrome of inappropriate antidi-
      uretic hormone
   j. _____ status post therapeutic abortion
   k. _____ diabetes insipidus with water
      restriction
   l. _____ excessive parenteral administration
      of dextrose and water solution

2. Indicate which of the following factors contribute to *hypokalemia* by writing "Low" in
   the space provided, and indicate which contribute to *hyperkalemia* by writing "High" in the
   space provided.
   a. _____ alkalosis
   b. _____ tourniquet too tight when col-
      lecting a blood sample
   c. _____ vomiting
   d. _____ gastric suction
   e. _____ leukocytosis
   f. _____ anorexia nervosa
   g. _____ hyperaldosteronism
   h. _____ furosemide administration
   i. _____ steroid administration
   j. _____ kidney failure
   k. _____ penicillin administration
   l. _____ adrenal steroid deficiency

3. Indicate which of the following factors contribute to *hypocalcemia* by writing "Low" in the space provided, and indicate which contribute to *hypercalcemia* by writing "High" in the space provided.

   a. _____ hyperparathyroidism

   b. _____ massive administration of citrated blood

   c. _____ malignant tumors

   d. _____ immobilization because of multiple fractures

   e. _____ pancreatitis

   f. _____ thiazide diuretics

   g. _____ kidney failure

   h. _____ aminoglycoside administration

4. Indicate which of the following factors contribute to *hypomagnesemia* by writing "Low" in the space provided, and indicate which contribute to *hypermagnesemia* by writing "High" in the space provided.

   a. _____ alcohol abuse

   b. _____ kidney failure

   c. _____ diarrhea

   d. _____ gentamicin administration

   e. _____ untreated ketoacidosis

5. Indicate which of the following factors contribute to *hypophosphatemia* by writing "Low" in the space provided, and indicate which contribute to *hyperphosphatemia* by writing "High" in the space provided.

   a. _____ hyperparathyroidism

   b. _____ kidney failure

   c. _____ major thermal burns

   d. _____ alcohol withdrawal

   e. _____ neoplastic disease chemotherapy

6. For each of the following factors, indicate the probable cause by writing "M-ACID" for metabolic acidosis, "M-ALKA" for metabolic alkalosis, "R-ACID" for respiratory acidosis, or "R-ALKA" for respiratory alkalosis.

   a. _____ sedative overdose

   b. _____ lactic acidosis

   c. _____ ketoacidosis

   d. _____ severe pneumonia

   e. _____ hypoxemia

   f. _____ acute pulmonary edema

   g. _____ diarrhea

   h. _____ vomiting

   i. _____ hypokalemia

   j. _____ gram-negative bacterial infection

Activity C *Correlate the associations between body fluid compartments. Match the fluid space in Column II with an associated factor in Column I.*

Column I	Column II
____ 1. Third-space fluid shift	a. Intracellular space
____ 2. The smallest compartment of the extracellular fluid space	b. Extracellular fluid compartment
____ 3. Space where plasma is contained	c. Intravascular space
____ 4. Comprises the intravascular, interstitial, and transcellular fluid	d. Transcellular space
____ 5. Comprises about 60% of body fluid	e. Interstitial space
____ 6. Comprises fluid surrounding cell	f. Intravascular fluid volume deficit

SECTION II: APPLYING YOUR KNOWLEDGE

Activity D *Consider the scenarios and answer the questions.*

CASE STUDY: Extracellular Fluid Volume Deficit

Ms. Crutchfield, 30 years old, has been admitted to the burn treatment center with full-thickness burns over 30% of her upper body. Her diagnosis is consistent with extracellular fluid volume deficit (FVD).

1. What symptom would indicate to the nurse that the patient may be experiencing an FVD?

   _____

2. What should the nursing plan of care for Harriet include that would indicate to the nurse that there may be an FVD?

   _____

   _____

3. What interventions provided by the nurse would be appropriate for this patient?

   _____

   _____

CASE STUDY: Congestive Heart Failure

Mr. George, 88 years old, has a history of heart failure. He was admitted to the hospital with a diagnosis of extracellular fluid volume excess. He was frightened, slightly confused, and dyspneic on exertion.

1. What symptoms does the nurse find when performing the assessment on this patient?

   _____

2. What manifestation of extracellular fluid volume excess does the nurse assess?

   _____

3. When developing a plan of care for the patient, what interventions will be a priority to include?

   _____

   _____

CASE STUDY: Diabetes

Mr. Isaac, 63 years old, was admitted to the hospital with a diagnosis of uncontrolled diabetes. On admission, the nurse assesses a respiratory rate of 32, confusion, and signs of dehydration.

1. Isaac's arterial blood gas values are pH, 7.27; HCO_3, 20 mEq/L; PaO_2, 33 mm Hg. What do the blood gas results indicate for this patient?

   _____

2. What manifestations will the nurse associate with an alteration in acid–base balance?

   _____

3. In terms of cellular buffering response, what should the nurse determine the major electrolyte disturbance to be?

   _____

4. What prescribed intravenous medication does the nurse anticipate administering to correct the acid–base imbalance?

   _____

CASE STUDY: Intravenous Therapy

Ms. Giles, an 84-year-old patient, was admitted to the hospital for treatment for dehydration. The health care provider immediately prescribes intravenous therapy, 1000 mL of D_5W, q8h.

1. What systemic complications should the nurse monitor for in the patient?

   _____

2. After several attempts to obtain a peripheral IV site, the nurse requests that a central vein be accessed by the health care provider. Which vein will be cannulated when inserting the central line?

   _____

3. The nurse is determining the flow rate of the IV fluids. What would be the correct way to calculate the flow rate?

   _____

SECTION III: PRACTICING FOR NCLEX

Activity E *Answer the following questions.*

1. The nurse will assess the patient for signs of lethargy, increasing intracranial pressure, and seizures when the serum sodium reaches which level?
   a. 115 mEq/L
   b. 130 mEq/L
   c. 145 mEq/L
   d. 160 mEq/L

2. In a patient with excess fluid volume, hyponatremia is treated by restricting fluids to how many milliliters in 24 hours?
   a. 400
   b. 600
   c. 800
   d. 1200

3. A patient who is semiconscious presents with restlessness and weakness. The nurse assesses a dry, swollen tongue and a body temperature of 99.3°F. The urine specific gravity is 1.020. Which is the most likely serum sodium value for this patient?
   a. 110 mEq/L
   b. 140 mEq/L
   c. 155 mEq/L
   d. 165 mEq/L

4. A patient's serum sodium concentration is within the normal range. Which will the nurse estimate the serum osmolality to be?
   a. <136 mOsm/kg
   b. 275 to 300 mOsm/kg
   c. >408 mOsm/kg
   d. 350 to 544 mOsm/kg

5. The nurse is reviewing the laboratory studies for a group of patients. Which patient is most likely to experience a decrease in serum osmolality?
   a. A patient with diabetes insipidus
   b. A patient with a glucose level of 360 mg/dL
   c. A patient with kidney failure
   d. A patient with uremia

6. The nurse notes that a patient's urine osmolality is 980 mOsm/kg. Which will the nurse assess as a possible cause of this finding?
   a. Acidosis
   b. Fluid volume excess
   c. Diabetes insipidus
   d. Hyponatremia

7. The nurse is reviewing the laboratory studies for a patient suspected of acute kidney injury. Which test would be the best indicator of the patient's renal function?
   a. Blood urea nitrogen
   b. Serum creatinine
   c. Specific gravity
   d. Urine osmolality

8. A patient has been involved in a traumatic accident and is hemorrhaging from multiple sites. The nurse expects that the compensatory mechanisms associated with hypovolemia would cause which clinical manifestations? (Select all that apply.)
   a. Hypertension
   b. Oliguria
   c. Tachycardia
   d. Bradycardia
   e. Tachypnea

9. Which laboratory findings does the nurse determine are consistent with hypovolemia in a female patient? (Select all that apply.)
   a. Hematocrit level of >47%
   b. BUN: serum creatinine ratio of >12.1
   c. Urine specific gravity of 1.027
   d. Urine osmolality of >450 mOsm/kg
   e. Urine positive for blood

10. A patient with mild fluid volume excess is prescribed a diuretic that blocks sodium reabsorption in the distal tubule. Which diuretic does the nurse anticipate administering to this patient?
    a. Bumetanide
    b. Torasemide
    c. Hydrochlorothiazide
    d. Furosemide

11. The nurse is caring for a patient with a diagnosis of hyponatremia. Which nursing intervention(s) is/are appropriate to include in the plan of care for this patient? (Select all that apply.)

    a. Assess for symptoms of nausea and malaise.

    b. Encourage the intake of low sodium liquids.

    c. Monitor neurologic status.

    d. Restrict tap water intake.

    e. Encourage the use of salt substitute instead of salt.

12. A patient with abnormal sodium losses is receiving a regular diet. How will the nurse supplement the patient's diet to provide 1600 mg of sodium daily?

    a. One beef cube and 8 oz of tomato juice

    b. Four beef cubes and 8 oz of tomato juice

    c. One beef cube and 16 oz of tomato juice

    d. One beef cube and 12 oz of tomato juice

13. The nurse is caring for a patient with hypernatremia. Which complication of hypernatremia should the nurse continuously monitor for?

    a. Red blood cell crenation

    b. Red blood cell hydrolysis

    c. Cerebral edema

    d. Kidney injury

14. The health care provider has prescribed a hypotonic IV solution for a patient. Which IV solution should the nurse administer?

    a. 0.45% sodium chloride

    b. 0.90% sodium chloride

    c. 5% dextrose in water

    d. 5% dextrose in normal saline solution

15. A patient is admitted with severe vomiting for 24 hours as well as weakness and "feeling exhausted." The nurse observes flat T waves and ST-segment depression on the electrocardiogram. Which potassium level does the nurse observe when the laboratory studies are complete?

    a. 4.0 mEq/L

    b. 8.0 mEq/L

    c. 2.0 mEq/L

    d. 2.6 mEq/L

16. What foods can the nurse recommend for the patient with hypokalemia?

    a. Fruits such as bananas and apricots

    b. Green, leafy vegetables

    c. Milk and yogurt

    d. Nuts and legumes

17. Which medication does the nurse administer as prescribed to antagonize the effects of potassium on the heart for a patient in severe metabolic acidosis?

    a. Sodium bicarbonate

    b. Magnesium sulfate

    c. Furosemide

    d. Calcium gluconate

18. A patient reports tingling in the fingers as well as feeling depressed. The nurse assesses positive Trousseau and Chvostek signs. Which decreased laboratory results does the nurse observe when the patient's laboratory work has returned?

    a. Potassium

    b. Phosphorus

    c. Calcium

    d. Magnesium

19. A patient is admitted with a diagnosis of kidney injury. The patient reports "stomach distress" and describes ingesting several antacid tablets over the past 2 days. Blood pressure is 110/70 mm Hg, face is flushed, and the patient is experiencing generalized weakness. Which is the most likely magnesium level associated with the symptoms the patient is having?

    a. 11 mEq/L

    b. 5 mEq/L

    c. 2 mEq/L

    d. 1 mEq/L

20. Which clinical indication of hypophosphatemia does the nurse assess in a patient?

    a. Bone pain

    b. Paresthesia

    c. Seizures

    d. Tetany

21. The nurse is caring for a patient with diabetes type I who is having severe vomiting and diarrhea. Which condition that exhibits blood values with a low pH and a low plasma bicarbonate concentration should the nurse assess for?

    a. Respiratory acidosis

    b. Respiratory alkalosis

    c. Metabolic acidosis

    d. Metabolic alkalosis

CHAPTER 11

Shock, Sepsis, and Multiple Organ Dysfunction Syndrome

Learning Outcomes

1. Describe the pathophysiology, clinical manifestations, and collaborative management of progressive stages of various types of shock, of sepsis, and of multiple organ dysfunction syndrome.
2. Compare and contrast the pathophysiology, clinical manifestations, and collaborative management of shock states in hypovolemic, cardiogenic, and distributive shock.
3. Identify medical and nursing management priorities in treating patients across the continuum of shock.
4. Describe medical and nursing management priorities in the treatment and prevention of sepsis and septic shock.
5. Discuss the role of nurses in providing psychosocial support to patients experiencing shock, sepsis, and multiple organ dysfunction syndrome, and their families.
6. Discuss the role of nurses in providing transitional care to patients and their families after having been managed in a critical-care unit for shock, sepsis, or multiple organ dysfunction syndrome.

SECTION I: ASSESSING YOUR UNDERSTANDING

Activity A *Fill in the blanks.*

1. The basic, underlying characteristic of shock is _____, which results in _____, _____, _____, _____, and _____.

2. Energy metabolism occurs in the cells, where _____ is primarily responsible for cellular energy in the form of _____.

3. To maintain an adequate blood pressure, three components of the circulatory system must respond effectively: the _____, _____, and _____.

4. The formula for calculating cardiac output is: cardiac output is the product of _____ times _____. Peripheral resistance is determined by the _____.

5. Baroreceptors are located in the _____ and _____, whereas chemoreceptors are located in the _____ and _____.

6. With the progression of shock, damage at the _____ and _____ levels occurs when the blood pressure drops.

7. Two crystalloids commonly used for fluid replacement in hypovolemic shock are _____ and _____.

8. A cardiac marker for ventricular dysfunction, _____, increases when the ventricle is overdistended. It is used to assess the cardiovascular effects of shock.

Activity B *Briefly answer the following.*

1. Define the term *mean arterial pressure* (MAP).

_____

_____

2. Name three medical management goals for cardiogenic shock.

_____

_____

3. Name the causes of circulatory shock.

_____

_____

4. Name the causes of neurogenic shock.

_____

_____

Activity C *Match the type of shock listed in Column II with its associated cause listed in Column I. Some answers may be used more than once.*

Column I

____ 1. Valvular damage

____ 2. Peritonitis

____ 3. Burns

____ 4. Bee sting allergy

____ 5. Immunosuppression

____ 6. Spinal cord injury

____ 7. Arrhythmias

____ 8. Vomiting

____ 9. Pulmonary embolism

____ 10. Penicillin sensitivity

Column II

a. Hypovolemic, owing to an internal fluid shift

b. Hypovolemic, owing to an external fluid loss

c. Cardiogenic

d. Circulatory of a neurogenic nature

e. Circulatory of an anaphylactic nature

f. Circulatory of a septic nature

g. Noncoronary cardiogenic shock

SECTION II: APPLYING YOUR KNOWLEDGE

Activity D *Consider the scenarios and answer the questions.*

CASE STUDY: Hypovolemic Shock

Mr. Mazda is a 57-year-old, 70-kg (154-lb) patient who was received on the nursing unit from the postanesthesia care unit (PACU) after having a hemicolectomy for colon cancer. On initial assessment, Mr. Mazda was alert, yet anxious; his skin was cool, pale, and moist; and his abdominal dressings were saturated with bright red blood. Urinary output was 100 mL over 4 hours. The patient was receiving 1000 mL of lactated Ringer solution at 150 mL/h. Vital signs were blood pressure (BP), 80/60 mm Hg; heart rate, 126 beats per minute (bpm); and respirations 40 breaths/min (baseline vital signs were 130/70, 84, and 22, respectively). The nurse assessed that the patient was experiencing hypovolemic shock.

1. How much intravascular volume does the nurse determine that Mr. Mazda has lost?

_____

2. The nurse is assessing the patient for the signs of the compensatory stage of shock. What assessment data does the nurse determine is significant for the presence of compensatory shock?

_____

_____

3. The nurse is assessing Mr. Mazda's urinary output hourly. What level of output does the nurse identify as indicative of decreased glomerular filtration?

_____

4. What type of fluids will the nurse administer to this patient?

_____

CASE STUDY: Septic Shock

Mr. Dressler, a 43-year-old patient, was admitted to the medical-surgical unit on the third postoperative day after a vertical-banded gastroplasty for the treatment of morbid obesity. He had initially transferred to the intensive care unit from the postanesthesia care unit (PACU). Mr. Dressler had a normal postoperative recovery period until his first afternoon on the unit. The nurse went into his room to assess vital signs and noted that his temperature was 102°F, his HR was >90 bpm, his respirations were >20 breaths/min, and his systolic BP was <90 mm Hg. He was shaking with chills, skin was warm and dry, yet his extremities were cool to the touch. A recent white blood cell count is 32,000 cells/mm^3. The nurse immediately notified the health care provider.

1. Which clinical criteria in the history and physical indicate the patient is experiencing systemic inflammatory response syndrome?

_____

_____

2. Mr. Dressler's condition may advance to severe sepsis. What additional signs and symptoms should the nurse assess for?

_____

_____

3. The nurse expects that the health care provider will request body fluid specimens for culture and sensitivity tests. What specimens should the nurse prepare to collect?

_____

_____

4. What common and serious side effects of fluid replacement should the nurse monitor for?

_____

_____

SECTION III: PRACTICING FOR NCLEX

Activity E *Answer the following questions.*

1. The nurse caring for the patient in shock identifies which physiologic responses that are common to all shock states? (Select all that apply.)
   a. Increased intravascular volume
   b. Activation of the inflammatory response
   c. Hypoperfusion of tissues
   d. Must produce energy through aerobic metabolism
   e. Increase in cellular activity

2. The nurse is calculating a patient's mean arterial pressure (MAP). Which is the patient's MAP, if the blood pressure is 110/70 mm Hg?
   a. 65
   b. 73
   c. 83
   d. 91

3. The nurse is monitoring a patient in the compensatory stage of shock. Which lab values does the nurse observe that will elevate in response to the release of aldosterone and catecholamines?
   a. T$_3$ and T$_4$
   b. Myoglobin and CK-MB
   c. BUN and creatinine
   d. Sodium and glucose levels

4. The nurse obtains a blood pressure of 120/78 mm Hg from a patient in hypovolemic shock. Since the blood pressure is within normal range for this patient, which stage of shock does the nurse identify this patient is experiencing?
   a. Initial stage
   b. Compensatory stage
   c. Progressive stage
   d. Irreversible stage

5. What can the nurse include in the plan of care to ensure early intervention along the continuum of shock to improve the patient's prognosis? (Select all that apply.)

   a. Assess the patient who is at risk for shock.

   b. Administer vasoconstrictive medications to patients at risk for shock.

   c. Administer prophylactic packed red blood cells to patients at risk for shock.

   d. Administer intravenous fluids.

   e. Monitor for changes in vital signs.

6. The nurse assesses a patient in compensatory shock whose lungs have decompensated. Which clinical manifestation will the nurse assess? (Select all that apply.)

   a. A heart rate >100 bpm

   b. Crackles

   c. Lethargy and mental confusion

   d. Respirations <15 breaths/min

   e. Compensatory respiratory acidosis

7. The nurse assesses a BP reading of 80/50 mm Hg from a patient in shock. Which stage of shock does the nurse identify the patient is experiencing?

   a. Initial

   b. Compensatory

   c. Progressive

   d. Irreversible

8. The nurse is caring for a patient in shock that is experiencing a decrease in stroke volume. Which clinical manifestation is identified by the nurse to correlate with this decrease?

   a. Increase in diastolic pressure

   b. Decrease in respiratory rate

   c. Increase in systolic blood pressure

   d. Narrowed pulse pressure

9. The nurse is using continuous central venous oximetry ($Sc\bar{v}O_2$) to monitor the blood oxygen saturation of a patient in shock. Which value would the nurse document as normal for the patient?

   a. 40%

   b. 50%

   c. 60%

   d. 70%

10. A patient is in the progressive stage of shock with lung decompensation. Which treatment does the nurse prepare the patient for?

    a. Pericardiocentesis

    b. Thoracotomy with chest tube insertion

    c. Administration of oxygen via Venturi mask

    d. Intubation and mechanical ventilation

11. The nurse observes a patient in the progressive stage of shock with blood in the nasogastric tube and when connected to suction. Which is occurring with this patient related to the shock state?

    a. The patient has developed a stress ulcer that is bleeding.

    b. The patient is having a reaction to the vasoconstricting medications.

    c. The patient has a tumor in the esophagus.

    d. The patient has bleeding esophageal varices.

12. When a patient in shock is receiving fluid replacement, which will the nurse monitor for frequently? (Select all that apply.)

    a. Urinary output

    b. Mental status

    c. Vital signs

    d. Ability to perform range-of-motion exercises

    e. Visual acuity

13. The nurse is monitoring the patient in shock when bleeding is observed from previous venipuncture sites, in the indwelling catheter, and rectum. There are multiple areas of ecchymosis. Which does the nurse suspect has developed in this patient?

    a. Stress ulcer

    b. Disseminated intravascular coagulation (DIC)

    c. Septicemia

    d. Stevens–Johnson syndrome

14. The nurse receives an order to administer a colloidal solution for a patient experiencing hypovolemic shock. Which common colloidal solution will the nurse administer that will have the best outcome for the patient?

    a. Blood products

    b. 5% albumin

    c. 6% dextran

    d. 6% hetastarch

15. The nurse is performing glucose checks for sliding scale four times per day for a patient in the progressive stage of shock. For optimal glycemic control, which glucose level would the nurse expect to see for the best outcomes in this patient?

    a. 100 mg/dL

    b. 140 mg/dL

    c. 180 mg/dL

    d. 210 mg/dL

16. A patient is in the irreversible state of shock and is unresponsive. The family requests to stay with the patient during this time. Which is the best response by the nurse?

    a. "You don't want to remember your family member this way."

    b. "We have specific visiting hours that must be adhered to."

    c. "I will make arrangements for your family to be able to stay with the patient."

    d. "The health care team needs room to do procedures to help your family member, so it would be best if you stayed in the waiting area."

17. When planning the care of the patient in cardiogenic shock, which does the nurse identify as the primary treatment goal?

    a. Improve the heart's pumping mechanism.

    b. Limit further myocardial damage.

    c. Preserve the healthy myocardium.

    d. Treat the oxygenation needs of the heart muscle.

18. Which priority intervention can the nurse provide to decrease the incidence of septic shock for patients who are at risk?

    a. Insert indwelling catheters for incontinent patients.

    b. Use strict hand hygiene techniques.

    c. Administer prophylactic antibiotics for all patients at risk.

    d. Have patients wear masks in the health care facility.

19. A patient arrives in the emergency department with reports of chest pain radiating to the jaw. Which medication does the nurse administer as prescribed to reduce pain and anxiety as well as reducing oxygen consumption?

    a. Codeine

    b. Meperidine

    c. Hydromorphone

    d. Morphine sulfate

20. A patient presents to the emergency department after being stung by a bee, reporting difficulty breathing. Which vasoconstrictive medication will be administered by the nurse?

    a. Dexamethasone

    b. Betamethasone

    c. Diphenhydramine

    d. Epinephrine

CHAPTER 12

Management of Patients with Oncologic Disorders

Learning Outcomes

1. Differentiate between characteristics of benign and malignant tumors.
2. Discuss the role of the nurse in the prevention and management of cancer.
3. Compare and contrast the goals of cancer care in prevention, diagnosis, cure, control, and palliation.
4. Describe the role of surgery, radiation therapy, chemotherapy, hematopoietic stem cell transplantation, immunotherapy, and targeted therapy in the treatment of cancer.
5. Use the nursing process as a framework for the care of the patient with cancer throughout the disease trajectory, from the time of diagnosis, to survivorship, and at the end of life.

SECTION I: ASSESSING YOUR UNDERSTANDING

Activity A *Fill in the blanks.*

1. In the United States, the three leading causes of cancer deaths are _____, _____, and _____ in men, and _____, _____, and _____ in women.

2. _____ and _____ are two examples of tumor-specific antigens in the altered cell membranes of malignant cells.

3. The two key ways by which cancer is spread are the _____ and the _____.

4. About _____% of all cancers are thought to be related to the environment.

5. The single most lethal chemical carcinogen, accounting for 30% of all cancer deaths, is _____.

6. _____, _____, and _____ are three dietary substances (cruciferous vegetables) that appear to reduce cancer risk. _____, _____, _____, and _____ tend to increase the risk of cancer.

7. The two *most common* side effects of chemotherapy are _____ and _____.

8. Myelosuppression, caused by chemotherapeutic agents, results in _____, _____, _____, and an increased risk of _____ and _____.

9. Three chemotherapeutic agents that are particularly toxic to the renal system are _____, _____, and _____.

Activity B *Briefly answer the following.*

1. Summarize the cause of cancer.

   _____

   _____

2. Name two examples of an inherited cancer susceptibility syndrome.

   _____

3. List four of seven cancers that are associated with an increased intake of alcohol.

   _____   _____

   _____   _____

4. Identify five substances produced by the immune system in response to cancer cells.

   _____   _____

   _____   _____

   _____

5. Toxicity occurs with radiation therapy. For each of the following, list three common side effects.

   a. Skin: _____, _____, and

      _____.

   b. Oral mucosal membrane: _____,

      _____, and _____.

   c. Stomach or colon: _____,

      _____, and _____.

   d. Bone marrow–producing sites: _____,

      _____, and _____.

6. List five of nine signs that indicate that an extravasation of an infusion of a cancer chemotherapeutic agent has occurred.

   _____   _____

   _____   _____

   _____

Activity C

PART I

Match the term listed in Column II with its associated definition listed in Column I.

Column I

____ 1. Growth of new capillaries from the host tissue

____ 2. Innate process of programmed cell death

____ 3. The use of thermal energy to destroy cancer cells

____ 4. Point at which blood counts are their lowest

____ 5. Target antibodies to destroy specific malignant cells

____ 6. A substance that can cause tissue necrosis

____ 7. A dry oral cavity caused by salivary gland dysfunction

____ 8. Substances produced by the immune system cells to enhance the function of the immune system

Column II

a. Angiogenesis

b. Apoptosis

c. Cytokines

d. Monoclonal antibodies

e. Nadir

f. Radiofrequency ablation

g. Vesicant

h. Xerostomia

PART II

Match the term listed in Column II with its associated definition listed in Column I.

Match the type of neoplasm in Column II with its associated description listed in Column I.

Column I

_____ 1. Cells bear little resemblance to the normal cells of the tissue from which they arose

_____ 2. Rate of growth is usually slow

_____ 3. Tumor tissue is encapsulated

_____ 4. Tumor spreads by way of blood and lymph channels to other areas of the body

_____ 5. Growth tends to recur when removed

Column II

a. Benign

b. Malignant

PART III

Match the drug category listed in Column II with an associated antineoplastic agent listed in Column I. For each drug, list a common side effect in Column I. Some answers may be used more than once.

Column I

_____ 1. Cisplatin _____

_____ 2. 5-fluorouracil (5-FU) _____

_____ 3. Estrogens _____

_____ 4. Thiotepa _____

_____ 5. Lomustine (CCNU) _____

_____ 6. Doxorubicin _____

_____ 7. Ifosfamide _____

_____ 8. Methotrexate _____

_____ 9. Vincristine (VCR) _____

_____ 10. Irinotecan _____

_____ 11. Asparaginase _____

Column II

a. Alkylating agent

b. Nitrosourea

c. Antimetabolite

d. Antitumor antibiotic

e. Plant alkaloid/ mitotic spindle

f. Hormonal agent

g. Miscellaneous agent

h. Topoisomerase 1 inhibitors

SECTION II: APPLYING YOUR KNOWLEDGE

Activity D *Consider the scenarios and answer the questions.*

CASE STUDY: Cancer of the Breast

Mrs. Kim is a 45-year-old mother of four who, after a needle aspiration biopsy, is diagnosed as having a malignant breast tumor, stage III. She was scheduled for a modified radical mastectomy. On assessment, her breast tissue had a dimpling or "orange-peel" appearance.

1. The nurse determines by the patient's history that her mother died of breast cancer. What is the correlation with the diagnosis of breast cancer in this patient?

   _____

2. What will the nurse assess in order to assist Kim in adapting to the loss of her breast?

   _____

3. Kim's husband refuses to participate in any discussion about his wife's diagnosis. What defense mechanism does the nurse identify the husband is using?

   _____

4. The nurse assesses Kim's pain postoperatively, with Kim stating the pain is an 8 on a scale of 0 to 10. What other factors can alter Kim's perception of pain?

   _____

   _____

5. Kim is scheduled to begin radiation therapy, followed by chemotherapy with 5-FU. What can the nurse tell Kim about the effects of the radiation therapy so that she will be prepared?

   _____

   _____

6. What measures can the nurse educate Kim to take to assist in protecting her skin between radiation treatments?

   _____

7. After radiation therapy, Kim begins a regimen of chemotherapy with 5-FU. Three weeks after treatment begins, Kim develops a fever, sore throat, and cold symptoms. What does the nurse determine that these symptoms could be related to?

_____

CASE STUDY: Cancer of the Lung

Mr. Donato is a 48-year-old accountant who has been a one-pack-a-day smoker for 23 years. He has had a persistent cough for 1 year that is hacking and nonproductive, and has had repeated unresolved upper respiratory tract infections. He went to see his health care provider with reports of fatigue, loss of appetite, and a weight loss of 5.45 kg (12 lb) over the last 3 months. Diagnostic evaluation led to the diagnosis of a localized tumor with no evidence of metastatic spread. Mr. Donato is scheduled for a lobectomy in 3 days.

1. After Mr. Donato receives a diagnosis of cancer, what will likely be the first reaction in the grieving process?

_____

2. What interventions can the nurse provide to support the patient and family during the grieving process?

_____

_____

3. What assessment data would the nurse identify that indicates a compromised nutritional status?

_____

4. What should the nurse assess for in the postoperative period that may indicate the presence of infection?

_____

SECTION III: PREPARING FOR NCLEX

Activity E *Answer the following questions.*

1. The nurse is caring for patients on the oncology unit. Which priority action would most benefit the patient with cancer?

   a. Identify own perception of cancer and set realistic goals.

   b. Set the same goals for all patients with cancer.

   c. Tell the patient about the things the patient has done to cause cancer.

   d. Ensure that the patient has the financial means to afford their care.

2. A patient, age 67 years, is admitted for diagnostic studies to rule out cancer. The patient is Caucasian, has been employed as a landscaper for 40 years, and has a 36-year history of smoking a pack of cigarettes daily. Which significant risk factors does the nurse recognize this patient has? (Select all that apply.)

   a. Age

   b. Cigarette smoking

   c. Occupation

   d. Race

   e. Marital status

3. Which foods will the nurse suggest that the patient consume less of in order to reduce nitrate intake because of the possibility of carcinogenic action?

   a. Eggs and milk

   b. Fish and poultry

   c. Ham and bacon

   d. Green, leafy vegetables

4. A patient will be having an endoscopic procedure with a diagnostic biopsy. Which type of biopsy does the nurse explain will remove an entire piece of suspicious tissue?

   a. Excisional biopsy

   b. Incisional biopsy

   c. Needle biopsy

   d. Punch biopsy

5. A patient is admitted for an excisional biopsy of a breast lesion. Which intervention should the nurse provide for the care of this patient?
   a. Clarify information provided by the health care provider.
   b. Provide aseptic care to the incision postoperatively.
   c. Provide time for the patient to discuss her concerns.
   d. Counsel the patient about the possibility of losing her breast.

6. A patient is scheduled for cryosurgery for cervical cancer and tells the nurse, "I am not exactly sure what the health care provider is going to do." Which is the best response by the nurse?
   a. "You will have medication injected in the area."
   b. "You will have liquid nitrogen to freeze the area."
   c. "You will have a laser remove the area."
   d. "You will have radiofrequency to ablate the area."

7. The nurse at the clinic explains to the patient that the surgeon will be removing a mole on the patient's back that has the potential to develop into cancer. Which type of procedure does the nurse educate the patient regarding?
   a. Diagnostic
   b. Palliative
   c. Prophylactic
   d. Reconstructive

8. A patient will be receiving radiation for 6 weeks for the treatment of breast cancer and asks the nurse why it takes so long. Which is the best response by the nurse?
   a. "It allows time for you to cope with the treatment."
   b. "It will allow time for the repair of healthy tissue."
   c. "It will decrease the incidence of leukopenia and thrombocytopenia."
   d. "It is not really understood why you have to go for 6 weeks of treatment."

9. A patient with uterine cancer is being treated with internal radiation therapy. Which is the nurse's priority action when caring for this patient?
   a. Explain to the patient that she will continue to emit radiation for approximately 1 week after the implant is removed.
   b. Maintain as much distance as possible from the patient while in the room.
   c. Alert family members that they should restrict their visiting to 5 minutes at any one time.
   d. Wear a lead apron when providing direct patient care.

10. The nurse is caring for a patient that will be receiving chemotherapy for the treatment of cancer. Which information related to chemotherapy should the nurse discuss with the patient?
   a. It attacks cancer cells during their vulnerable phase.
   b. It functions against disseminated disease.
   c. It causes a systemic reaction.
   d. It targets normal body cells as well as cancer cells.

11. A patient is taking vincristine, for the treatment of cancer. Which system should the nurse be sure to assess for symptoms of toxicity?
   a. Gastrointestinal system
   b. Nervous system
   c. Pulmonary system
   d. Urinary system

12. The nurse assesses that extravasation of a chemotherapy agent has occurred. Which will the initial action of the nurse be?
   a. Apply a warm compress to the area.
   b. Discontinue the infusion.
   c. Inject an antidote, if required.
   d. Place ice over the site of infiltration.

13. Which intervention should the nurse provide to reduce the incidence of renal damage when a patient is taking a chemotherapy regimen?
    a. Encourage fluid intake to dilute the urine.
    b. Take measures to acidify the urine and prevent uric acid crystallization.
    c. Withhold medication when the blood urea nitrogen level exceeds 20 mg/dL.
    d. Limit fluids to 1000 mL daily to prevent accumulation of the drug's end products after cell lysis.

14. A patient is receiving chemotherapy and receiving allopurinol. Which response is appropriate when the patient asks why they have to take this medication?
    a. It stimulates the immune system against the tumor cells.
    b. It treats drug-related anemia.
    c. It prevents alopecia.
    d. It lowers serum and uric acid levels.

15. A patient is to receive Bacille Calmette–Guerin (BCG). For which condition will the patient be required to take this medication?
    a. For cancer of the bladder
    b. For cancer of the breast
    c. For cancer of the lungs
    d. For skin cancer

16. Which is the best way for the nurse to assess the nutritional status of a patient with cancer?
    a. Weigh the patient daily.
    b. Monitor daily caloric intake.
    c. Observe for proper wound healing.
    d. Assess BUN and creatinine levels.

CHAPTER 13

Palliative and End-of-Life Care

Learning Outcomes

1. Compare and contrast the settings where palliative care and end-of-life care are provided.
2. Describe the principles and components of hospice care in the United States, including the Medicare hospice benefit.
3. Apply skills for communicating with patients who are seriously ill and their families in order to provide culturally and spiritually sensitive care.
4. Identify components of uncomplicated grief and mourning and implement nursing measures to support patients and families.

SECTION I: ASSESSING YOUR UNDERSTANDING

Activity A *Fill in the blanks.*

1. Dr. _____, who spearheaded a movement to increase an awareness of the dying process among health care practitioners, published a landmark book, _____, in 1969.

2. _____ is a type of palliative care, focusing on comfort at the end of life.

3. _____ is an essential component that is rooted in communication and cooperation among the various disciplines, with each member of the team contributing to a single integrated care plan that addresses the needs of the patient and the family.

4. The _____ is based on ambulation, activity, outward evidence of disease, self-care, intake, and level of consciousness.

5. Two types of medications routinely used to treat the underlying obstructed pathology associated with dyspnea are _____ and _____, improving overall lung function.

6. _____ is an intense response after a loss where profound emotions persist (usually >1 year).

Activity B *Briefly answer the following.*

1. Name the eight key domains underlying a more comprehensive and humane approach to care of the dying as identified by the National Consensus Project for Quality Palliative Care (NCP, 2013).

   _____

   _____

2. Define the terms *palliative care* and *hospice care*.

   _____

   _____

3. What are the common end-of-life symptoms for those patients that are diagnosed with severe COVID-19?

   _____

   _____

4. What is the difference between the living will and durable power of attorney?

_____

_____

5. According to the National Palliative Care Registry in 2017, what are the most common primary diagnoses seen by palliative care specialists?

_____

_____

SECTION II: APPLYING YOUR KNOWLEDGE

Activity C *Consider the scenario and answer the questions.*

Mrs. Betty Smith is accompanied to the clinic by her daughter for follow-up care related to advanced uterine cancer. Her daughter reports that although she prepares her favorite foods, Betty is not interested in eating anything. The daughter states, "With Mom's declining health, I am going to need help with her care."

1. What education will the nurse provide regarding oral intake and end-of-life care?

_____

_____

2. What suggestions could the nurse make to help the patient and family receive assistance with Betty's care?

_____

_____

SECTION III: PRACTICING FOR NCLEX

Activity D *Answer the following questions.*

1. A patient is diagnosed with a terminal illness and has been given less than 6 months to live. Which type of referral will the nurse make to assist this patient and family at home?

a. A rehabilitation center

b. Hospice

c. Adult day care

d. Physical therapy

2. A patient diagnosed with terminal pancreatic cancer is unaware of the diagnosis, and the family has requested that the patient not be told. Which is the best response to the family by the nurse?

a. "It is unfair for the patient to be unaware of the diagnosis and should be immediately told."

b. "I refuse to lie to a patient that I am taking care of and will answer honestly if asked."

c. "Would it be easier to inform the patient if a member of the clergy went with you?"

d. "I don't blame you for not saying anything. Let them enjoy the rest of their life."

3. A patient with terminal cancer is admitted into hospice care. When performing the admission, the nurse observes the patient exhibiting signs of depression. Which intervention by the nurse is most appropriate?

a. Inform the patient that although they are depressed, it takes too long for antidepressants to start working.

b. Refer the patient to an inpatient psychiatric unit for treatment of depression.

c. Notify the health care provider of the need to prescribe an antidepressant to address the patient's depression.

d. Notify family members to maintain a one-on-one vigilant observation of the patient to prevent suicide.

4. A patient with end-stage chronic obstructive pulmonary disease is admitted to a hospice facility and asks the admitting nurse, "How long will I be allowed to stay here?" Which is the **best** response by the nurse?

a. "You will be able to stay only for approximately 1 month and then you will be discharged."

b. "You will be able to stay for 2 months before being discharged."

c. "There is no time limit for your stay. You can stay until you die."

d. "When your stay reaches 6 months, you will be re-certified for a continued stay."

5. A patient authorizes an adult child to make medical decisions and brings the completed forms for the nurse to place on the chart. Which form does the nurse identify this as?

   a. An advance directive

   b. A living will

   c. A standard addendum to a will

   d. A proxy directive

6. A dying patient states to the nurse, "I know I'm dying, aren't I?" Which is the **best** response by the nurse?

   a. "This must be very difficult for you."

   b. "Tell me more about what's on your mind."

   c. "I'm so sorry. I know how you must feel."

   d. "You know you're dying?"

7. A terminally ill patient in pain asks the nurse to administer enough pain medication to end the suffering forever. Which is the **best** response by the nurse?

   a. "I can't do that, I will go to jail."

   b. "I am surprised that you would ask me to do something like that."

   c. "I will see if the primary provider will order enough for that to occur."

   d. "I will notify the primary provider that the current dose of medication is not relieving your pain."

8. A patient's family member asks the nurse what the purpose of hospice is. Which is the **best** response by the nurse?

   a. "It will hasten the death of the patient."

   b. "It will prolong life in a dignified manner."

   c. "It will use artificial means of life support if the patient requests it."

   d. "It will enable the patient to remain home if that is what is desired."

9. A terminally ill patient is admitted to the hospital. The patient grabs the nurse's hand and asks, "Am I dying?" Which response is be **best** for the nurse to give?

   a. "Why do you think that?"

   b. "Did someone tell you that you are dying?"

   c. "Tell me more about what's on your mind."

   d. "I am not at liberty to disclose that information."

10. A patient near the end of life is experiencing anorexia–cachexia syndrome. Which characteristics of the syndrome does the nurse recognize? (Select all that apply.)

    a. Alterations in carbohydrate, fat, and protein metabolism

    b. Endocrine dysfunction

    c. Anemia

    d. Neurologic dysfunction

    e. Bladder incontinence

Perioperative Concepts and Nursing Management

CHAPTER 14

Preoperative Nursing Management

Learning Outcomes

1. Define the phases of perioperative patient care.
2. Perform a comprehensive preoperative assessment to identify pertinent health and surgical risk factors.
3. Describe considerations related to preoperative nursing care of older adult patients, patients with obesity, and people with disability.
4. Identify the regulatory documents that are required prior to a patient entering surgery.
5. Initiate the immediate preoperative preparation and education of the patient.

SECTION I: ASSESSING YOUR UNDERSTANDING

Activity A *Fill in the blanks.*

1. The preoperative phase begins _____ and ends when the patient _____.

2. The intraoperative phase begins when the patient _____ and ends when _____.

3. The hazards of surgery for the older adult are directly proportional to _____ and _____.

4. The leading causes of postoperative morbidity and mortality in older adults are _____ and _____ complications.

5. Patients with diabetes that undergo surgical procedures are at risk for four complications: _____, _____, _____, and _____.

6. Aspirin is withheld _____ days prior to surgery, if possible, because it acts by _____.

Activity B *Briefly answer the following.*

1. Informed consent for a surgical procedure is necessary when a procedure meets any of the following: _____, _____, _____, _____.

2. List three significant nutritional concerns for the older adult surgical patient: _____, _____, and _____.

3. Name three primary goals necessary to promote postoperative mobility: _____, _____, and _____.

4. What are 10 potential risk factors related to surgery?

_____ _____

_____ _____

_____ _____

_____ _____

_____ _____

Activity C *Match the nutrient in Column II with its associated rationale for use in Column I.*

Column I

_____ 1. Essential for normal blood clotting

_____ 2. Allows collagen deposition to occur

_____ 3. Necessary for DNA synthesis

_____ 4. Increases inflammatory response in wounds

_____ 5. Vital for capillary formation

Column II

a. Protein

b. Vitamin C

c. Vitamin A

d. Vitamin K

e. Zinc

Activity D

Medication Administration

For each drug classification, list the potential effects of interaction with anesthetics.

1. Anticoagulants _____

2. Anticonvulsant agents _____

3. Corticosteroids _____

4. Diuretics _____

5. Insulin _____

6. Phenothiazines _____

7. Tranquilizers _____

8. Monoamine oxidase inhibitors (MAOIs)

_____

Preoperative Nursing

For each essential preoperative nursing activity, write an appropriate nursing goal. An example is provided.

1. (Example) Restriction of nutrition and fluids
   <u>Prevent aspiration</u>

2. Intestinal preparation _____

3. Preoperative skin preparation (cleansing)

_____

4. Urinary catheterization _____

5. Administration of preoperative medications

_____

6. Transportation of patient to presurgical suite

_____

SECTION II: APPLYING YOUR KNOWLEDGE

Activity E *Consider the scenario and answer the questions.*

The nurse is caring for a patient who is scheduled for an inguinal hernia repair with general anesthesia. While performing a preoperative history and physical assessment, the nurse suspects that the patient has a history of substance abuse. The patient does admit to smoking a pack of cigarettes daily for 15 years.

1. What priority interventions should the nurse instruct the patient to do in order to prevent complications postoperatively?

_____

_____

2. What is the best method for the nurse to obtain information about the patient's possible use of substances?

_____

_____

3. What education regarding smoking should the nurse provide to the patient prior to scheduling the patient for the surgical procedure?

_____

_____

SECTION III: PRACTICING FOR NCLEX

Activity F *Answer the following questions.*

1. The on-call perioperative team is called for an emergent surgery to be performed as soon as they arrive. Which surgical procedure is considered urgent?

   a. An appendectomy

   b. An exploratory laparotomy

   c. A repair of multiple stab wounds

   d. A face-lift

2. A patient is scheduled for a reduction mammoplasty. Which classification of surgery does the nurse document on the perioperative document?

a. Urgent

b. Optional

c. Required

d. Reconstructive

3. A patient is scheduled for a surgical procedure. For which surgical procedure will the nurse prepare an informed consent form for the surgeon to sign?

a. An open reduction of a fracture

b. An insertion of an intravenous catheter

c. Irrigation of the external ear canal

d. Urethral catheterization

4. The nurse is caring for a patient with alcoholism. When will the nurse assess for symptoms of alcoholic withdrawal?

a. Within the first 12 hours

b. About 24 hours postoperatively

c. On the second or third day

d. Four days after a surgical procedure

5. The health care provider schedules an elective surgical procedure for a patient who smokes cigarettes. When will the nurse recommend that the patient cease smoking before the surgical procedure to minimize risks associate with cigarette smoking?

a. 4 to 8 weeks

b. 3 to 4 months

c. 2 weeks

d. 3 weeks

6. The nurse is caring for a patient with cirrhosis of the liver who has undergone a surgical procedure. Which laboratory results should immediately be reported to the health care provider?

a. When the patient's blood ammonia concentration reaches 180 mg/dL

b. When a lactate dehydrogenase concentration is 300 units

c. When a serum albumin concentration is 5.0 g/dL

d. When a serum globulin concentration reaches 2.8 g/dL

7. A patient with kidney injury is scheduled for a surgical procedure. Which laboratory results reported to the health care provider may result in cancellation of the procedure?

a. A blood urea nitrogen level of 42 mg/dL

b. A creatine kinase level of 120 U/L

c. A serum creatinine level of 0.9 mg/dL

d. A urine creatinine level of 1.2 mg/dL

8. A patient with uncontrolled diabetes is scheduled for a surgical procedure. Which chief life-threatening hazard will the nurse monitor for?

a. Dehydration

b. Hypertension

c. Hypoglycemia

d. Glucosuria

9. A patient with diabetes is scheduled for a surgical procedure. Which blood glucose level goal demonstrates strict glycemic control?

a. 80 to 110 mg/dL

b. 150 to 240 mg/dL

c. 250 to 300 mg/dL

d. 300 to 350 mg/dL

10. The nurse is monitoring a presurgical patient for electrolyte imbalance. Which classification of medication may cause electrolyte imbalance?

a. Corticosteroids

b. Diuretics

c. Phenothiazines

d. Insulin

11. The nurse assesses an older adult patient who reports dimmed vision. Which will the nurse include in the plan of care to meet this patient's immediate needs?

a. A safe environment

b. Restrictions of the patient's unassisted mobility activities

c. Preparation for probable cataract extractions

d. Referral to an ophthalmologist

12. The nurse is caring for a patient with obesity prior to a surgical procedure. Which surgical complications that correlate with obesity should the nurse monitor for? (Select all that apply.)

    a. Cardiovascular system

    b. Gastrointestinal system

    c. Pulmonary system

    d. Renal system

    e. Nervous system

13. A patient informs the nurse that they are experiencing some anxiety about their scheduled procedure. Which cognitive strategy could the nurse implement to assist with alleviating the anxiety?

    a. Administer antianxiety medication.

    b. Cancel the scheduled procedure.

    c. Inform the patient that there is nothing to be nervous about.

    d. Have the patient inhale aromatic essential oils.

14. The patient asks the nurse why food is withheld before surgery. Which is the best response by the nurse?

    a. "Aspiration is a concern and can be a complication if food or fluid is taken close to the surgery time."

    b. "Distention is a severe complication if food or fluid is taken close to the surgery time."

    c. "Infection may occur if food or fluid is taken prior to surgery."

    d. "Obstruction will occur if food or fluid is taken prior to surgery."

15. A patient is scheduled for a surgical procedure. Which indication does the nurse have that the patient understands the impending procedure?

    a. The patient participates willingly in the preoperative preparation.

    b. The patient discusses stress factors causing the patient to feel depressed.

    c. The patient expresses concern about postoperative pain.

    d. The patient verbalizes fears to family.

16. Which behaviors exhibited by a patient scheduled for surgery demonstrate hidden fears regarding the procedure? (Select all that apply.)

    a. The patient tells the nurse of concerns with the outcome of the procedure.

    b. The patient informs the nurse of problems with postoperative nausea in the past and that it was a bad experience.

    c. The patient avoids communication with the nurse.

    d. The patient repeatedly asks questions that have previously been answered.

    e. The patient talks incessantly.

17. A patient is preparing for a surgical procedure and states to the nurse, "I'm so nervous about my surgery." Which is the best response by the nurse?

    a. "Relax. Your recovery period will be shorter if you're less nervous."

    b. "Stop worrying. It only makes you more nervous."

    c. "You needn't worry. Your surgeon has done this surgery many times before."

    d. "Would you like to discuss the concerns that you have?"

18. Why is assessment of dentition important in the patient preparing to have a surgical procedure with general anesthesia?

    a. The patient may require referral to the dentist.

    b. Oral hygiene is important for all patients.

    c. Decayed teeth or dental prosthesis can become dislodged during intubation.

    d. The patient can sue if a tooth falls out during surgery.

19. A patient preparing for a surgical procedure is taking corticosteroids for Crohn's disease. Which will the patient be monitored for?

    a. Obstruction

    b. Infection

    c. Hypoglycemia

    d. Adrenal insufficiency

20. A patient having a surgical procedure takes aspirin 325 mg daily for prevention of platelet aggregation. When will the patient stop taking the aspirin before the surgery?

    a. 2 weeks

    b. 4 weeks

    c. 7 to 10 days

    d. 2 to 3 days

Intraoperative Nursing Management

1. Describe the roles of the surgical team members during the intraoperative phase of care.
2. Identify adverse effects of surgery and anesthesia.
3. Describe ways to decrease the risk of surgical site infections.
4. Compare types of anesthesia with regard to uses, advantages, disadvantages, and nursing responsibilities.
5. Use the nursing process to optimize patient outcomes during the intraoperative period.

SECTION I: ASSESSING YOUR UNDERSTANDING

Activity A *Fill in the blanks.*

1. When lasers are being used in the perioperative setting, _____ should be clearly posted to alert personnel.

2. A _____ should be used during surgical procedures to remove generalized smoke plume generated by standard electric cautery units.

3. Spinal anesthesia is a conduction nerve block that occurs when a local anesthetic is injected into _____.

4. The conduction block anesthesia commonly used for pain relief in labor is the _____.

5. With malignant hyperthermia, the core body temperature can increase 1° to 2°C every 5 minutes, reaching or exceeding a body temperature of _____ degrees in a short amount of time.

6. A patient is in stage I: beginning anesthesia. The circulating nurse should be sure that a _____ is provided.

7. Patients may be given _____, a clear, nonparticulate antacid to increase gastric fluid pH.

Activity B *Briefly answer the following.*

1. Differentiate between the restricted zone, semirestricted zone, and the unrestricted zone.

_____

_____

_____

2. Explain why anesthesia dosage is reduced with the older adult patient.

_____

_____

3. List four primary responsibilities of a Registered Nurse First Assistant (RNFA).

_____   _____

_____   _____

4. List five health hazards associated with the surgical environment: _____, _____, _____, _____, and _____.

5. Which nursing assessment indicates that a patient has recovered from the effects of spinal anesthesia?

_____

6. List five potential intraoperative complications: _____, _____, _____, _____, and _____.

7. Distinguish between the purposes for three types of anesthesia: epidural, general, and local.

_____

_____

8. List 10 potential adverse effects of surgery and anesthesia and their associated causes.

_____

_____

_____

_____

9. Why are older adults at a higher risk of complications from anesthesia?

_____

_____

10. What risks are to be avoided when lasers are used in the surgical environment?

_____

_____

11. What is meant by *anesthesia awareness*, and which patients are at the greatest risk for this phenomenon?

_____

_____

Activity C

Inhalation Anesthetic Agents

Match the inhalation anesthetic agent in Column II with its associated nursing implication found in Column I.

Column I

____ 1. Monitor blood pressure frequently

____ 2. Trigger for malignant hyperthermia, laryngospasm

____ 3. Observe malignant hyperthermia and arrhythmias

____ 4. Monitor chest pain, nausea, vomiting, hypertension, stroke

____ 5. Monitor for possible respiratory depression

Column II

a. Desflurane

b. Sevoflurane

c. Nitrous oxide

d. Halothane

e. Enflurane

Common Intravenous Medications

Match the commonly used intravenous medication in Column II with its associated common usage in Column I.

Column I

____ 1. Sedation with regional anesthesia

____ 2. Hypnotic and anxiolytic; adjunct to induction

____ 3. Epidural infusion for postoperative analgesia

____ 4. Maintenance of relaxation

____ 5. Skeletal muscle relaxation for orthopedic surgery

Column II

a. Fentanyl

b. Midazolam

c. Pancuronium

d. Propofol

e. Succinylcholine

SECTION II: APPLYING YOUR KNOWLEDGE

Activity D *Consider the scenarios and answer the questions.*

CASE STUDY: General Anesthesia

Ms. Anne Barmer, age 34, is in excellent health and is scheduled for open reduction of a fractured femur after sustaining a fall while skiing. The general anesthetic drugs to be used include sevoflurane and nitrous oxide.

1. What does the nurse understand are the advantages of sevoflurane?

2. What should the nurse make it a priority to monitor for when nitrous oxide is used?

3. After the patient has been given sevoflurane, what is it important for the nurse to monitor for?

CASE STUDY: Moderate Sedation

Mr. Jim Barnes, age 22, has dislocated his right shoulder while playing basketball. He will be having a closed reduction of his shoulder with moderate sedation in the emergency department.

1. What does moderate sedation involve?

2. What should the nurse continually assess while performing moderate sedation?

3. What is the goal of moderate sedation?

SECTION III: PRACTICING FOR NCLEX

Activity E *Answer the following questions.*

1. Which are the circulating nurse's responsibilities, in contrast to the scrub nurse's responsibilities?
   a. Assisting the surgeon
   b. Coordinating the surgical team
   c. Setting up the sterile tables
   d. Passing instruments

2. The circulating nurse is preparing a patient for a surgical procedure. Which primary responsibility does the circulating nurse have in the perioperative experience?
   a. Discussing the complications of the surgical procedure with the patient
   b. Coordinating the efforts of the surgical team
   c. Marking the operative site
   d. Passing instruments during the intraoperative phase

3. An unconscious patient with normal pulse and respirations would be considered to be in what stage of general anesthesia?
   a. Beginning anesthesia
   b. Excitement
   c. Surgical anesthesia
   d. Medullary depression

4. Why will the nurse be vigilant with assessment of perioperative risks on the older adult patient? (Select all that apply.)
   a. Ciliary action decreases, reducing the cough reflex.
   b. Fatty tissue increases, prolonging the effects of anesthesia.
   c. Liver size decreases, reducing the metabolism of anesthetics.
   d. Peristalsis increases.
   e. The elasticity of skin increases and decreases the risk of shearing.

5. The nurse identifies that, postoperatively, a general anesthetic is primarily eliminated via what organ(s)?
   a. The kidneys
   b. The lungs
   c. The skin
   d. The liver

6. The anesthesiologist is administering a stable and safe nondepolarizing muscle relaxant. Which medication does the nurse identify will be given?
   a. Succinylcholine chloride
   b. Vecuronium bromide
   c. Pancuronium bromide
   d. Decamethonium

7. Which intravenous anesthetic given by the anesthesiologist has a powerful respiratory depressant effect sufficient to cause apnea and cardiovascular depression?

   a. Etomidate

   b. Ketamine

   c. Sodium thiopental

   d. Midazolam

8. The nurse is completing a postoperative assessment for a patient who has received a depolarizing neuromuscular blocking agent. The nursing assessment includes careful monitoring of which body system?

   a. Cardiovascular system

   b. Endocrine system

   c. Gastrointestinal system

   d. Genitourinary system

9. A patient reports a headache after receiving spinal anesthesia. Which does the nurse determine is the cause of the headache related to the spinal anesthesia? (Select all that apply.)

   a. The patient lying in the supine position

   b. Leakage of spinal fluid from the subarachnoid space

   c. Size of the spinal needle used

   d. Degree of patient hydration

   e. An allergic reaction to the medication used

10. The surgeon requests lidocaine 2% with epinephrine for use in local infiltration anesthesia. Which does the nurse identify is the purpose of adding epinephrine to the lidocaine? (Select all that apply.)

    a. The epinephrine causes vasoconstriction.

    b. The epinephrine prevents rapid absorption of the anesthetic drug.

    c. The epinephrine prolongs the local action of the anesthetic agent.

    d. The lidocaine will not anesthetize the area locally without the epinephrine.

    e. The epinephrine will prevent the patient from having an allergic reaction to the lidocaine.

11. The patient asks the nurse how long the local infiltration anesthetic will last. Which is the nurse's **best** response?

    a. "The anesthetic may last for 1 hour."

    b. "The anesthetic may last for 3 hours."

    c. "The anesthetic may last for 5 hours."

    d. "The anesthetic may last for 7 hours."

12. A patient is scheduled to have a heart valve replacement with a porcine valve. Which patient does the nurse understand may refuse the use of any porcine-based product?

    a. A patient of Catholic faith

    b. A patient of Jewish faith

    c. A patient of Baptist faith

    d. A patient of Lutheran faith

13. The nurse is caring for a patient who is at risk for malignant hyperthermia subsequent to general anesthesia. Which is the most common early sign that the nurse will assess for?

    a. Hypertension

    b. Muscle rigidity

    c. Oliguria

    d. Tachycardia

14. The nurse is placing a patient in the Trendelenburg position for a surgical procedure. Which is the best way for the nurse to perform the proper positioning for the patient?

    a. Flat on the back with arms next to the sides

    b. On the back with head lowered so that the plane of the body meets the horizontal on an angle

    c. On the back with legs and thighs flexed at right angles

    d. On the side with uppermost leg adducted and flexed at the knee

15. The patient received ketamine during a surgical procedure. Which intervention by the nurse will assist with an optimal recovery period?

    a. Make sure that the patient is stimulated frequently.

    b. Place the patient in a darkened, quiet part of the recovery area.

    c. The patient does not require a recovery period and may go back to the hospital room.

    d. Speak to the patient in a loud, clear voice.

16. A patient is having a surgical procedure that requires the patient to be in the prone position. Which is an expected patient outcome?

    a. The patient will not experience anxiety during the preoperative phase

    b. The patient will not experience signs of an allergic reaction

    c. The patient remains free of perioperative positioning injury

    d. The patient will not experience signs and symptoms of infection

17. The circulating nurse is performing a skin preparation for a patient who is unconscious from general anesthesia when the scrub nurse states, "I know her, she sure has gotten fat!" Which is the best response by the circulating nurse?

    a. "It is inappropriate to make comments even when patients appear to be unconscious from anesthesia."

    b. "She sure has gained weight. I hope that she will heal after the surgery."

    c. "Be sure you don't say anything like that when she is coming out of the anesthesia in case she hears you."

    d. "If you say anything like that again, I will report you to the nurse manager."

18. The patient is having a repair of a vaginal prolapse. Which position will the nurse place the patient in?

    a. Left lateral Sims'

    b. Prone position

    c. Lithotomy position

    d. Trendelenburg

19. The anesthesiologist informs the circulating nurse that the patient is experiencing malignant hyperthermia. Which medication will the nurse immediately prepare to administer?

    a. Dantrolene sodium

    b. Fentanyl citrate

    c. Naloxone

    d. Sodium thiopental

CHAPTER 16

Postoperative Nursing Management

Learning Outcomes

1. Describe the responsibilities of the postanesthesia care nurse in the prevention of immediate postoperative complications.
2. Identify common postoperative problems and their management.
3. Explain variables that affect wound healing and surgical site infections.
4. Implement nursing care to enhance recovery in the postoperative phase.
5. Use the nursing process as a framework for care of the hospitalized patient recovering from surgery.

SECTION I: ASSESSING YOUR UNDERSTANDING

Activity A *Fill in the blanks.*

1. The primary nursing objective during the immediate postoperative assessment is to maintain _____ and prevent _____.

2. The primary cardiovascular complications seen in the PACU include _____, _____, _____, _____, and _____.

3. The *most serious* and *most frequent* postoperative complications involve the _____ system.

4. Two potential postoperative complications following abdominal surgery are _____ and _____.

5. The return of peristalsis in the postoperative period can be determined by the presence of _____ and _____, both of which are assessed by the nurse.

6. Pain stimulates _____, which increases _____ and _____.

7. Noxious impulses stimulate _____, which increases _____ and _____.

8. Hypothalamic stress responses increase _____ and _____, which can lead to _____ and _____.

Activity B *Briefly answer the following.*

1. List five areas of concern for a postanesthesia care unit (PACU) nurse who has just received a patient from the operating room: _____, _____, _____, _____, and _____.

2. How will the nurse monitor for cardiovascular stability?

_____

_____

3. Explain patient-controlled analgesia (PCA).

_____

_____

4. Explain why the postoperative complications of atelectasis and hypostatic pneumonia are reduced as a result of early ambulation.

_____

_____

5. Distinguish between wound *dehiscence* and *evisceration*.

_____

_____

6. What are the eight classic signs of hypovolemic shock?

_____

_____

7. What nursing assessment activities and interventions may detect postoperative deep vein thrombosis and pulmonary embolism?

_____

_____

8. How does the nurse know when the patient is ready for discharge from the PACU?

_____

_____

9. What three postoperative conditions put a patient at risk for common respiratory complications?

_____

_____

_____

10. How do these factors affect the progress of wound healing?

Age _____

Edema _____

Nutritional deficits _____

Oxygen deficits _____

Medications _____

Systemic disorders _____

SECTION II: APPLYING YOUR KNOWLEDGE

Activity C *Consider the scenarios and answer the questions.*

CASE STUDY: Hypopharyngeal Obstruction

Mrs. Dean is unconscious when she is transferred to the PACU after a prolonged surgical procedure with general anesthesia.

1. What is the primary objective in the immediate postoperative period?

_____

2. What signs would the nurse recognize as indicative of a hypopharyngeal obstruction?

_____

3. What intervention does the nurse provide to treat hypopharyngeal airway obstruction?

_____

CASE STUDY: Wound Healing

Mrs. Carter is returned from the PACU to a patient care area after a routine laparoscopic cholecystectomy.

1. What are the three phases of wound healing for this surgical patient?

_____

2. What should the ongoing assessment of the surgical site involve?

_____

3. What clinical manifestations does the nurse observe in the inflammatory phase of wound healing in the postoperative patient?

_____

4. What interventions can the nurse provide to promote adequate tissue oxygenation during the inflammatory phase of wound healing?

_____

SECTION III: PRACTICING FOR NCLEX

Activity D *Answer the following questions.*

1. The nurse is caring for a patient in the immediate postoperative period. Which complication requiring early intervention will the nurse carefully monitor for?

   a. Laryngospasm

   b. Hyperventilation

   c. Hypoxemia and hypercapnia

   d. Pulmonary edema and embolism

2. A patient arrives in the PACU unconscious. Which position will the nurse place the patient in unless otherwise contraindicated?

   a. Flat on the back, without elevation of the head, to facilitate frequent turning and minimize pulmonary complications

   b. In semi-Fowler position, to promote respiratory function and reduce the incidence of orthostatic hypotension when the patient can eventually stand

   c. In Fowler position, which most closely simulates a sitting position, thus facilitating respiratory as well as gastrointestinal functioning

   d. On the side with a pillow at the patient's back and the chin extended, to minimize the dangers of aspiration

3. The nurse is monitoring cardiovascular function in a postoperative patient. Which method will the nurse use to measure cardiovascular function?

   a. Complete blood count

   b. Central venous pressure

   c. Upper endoscopy

   d. Chest x-ray

4. The nurse is monitoring a patient immediately after a surgical procedure. Which measurement will the nurse immediately report to the surgeon?

   a. A systolic blood pressure lower than 90 mm Hg

   b. A temperature reading between 97° and 98°F

   c. Respirations between 20 and 25 breaths/min

   d. A hemoglobin of 13.6

5. The nurse is preparing a patient for discharge from the postanesthesia care unit (PACU). Which evidence indicates that the patient is ready for discharge from the PACU? (Select all that apply.)

   a. The patient has been extubated but still has an oropharyngeal airway inside.

   b. The patient is arousable but falls back to sleep rapidly.

   c. The patient has a blood pressure within 10 mm Hg of the baseline.

   d. The patient has sonorous respirations and occasionally requires chin lift.

   e. The patient rates pain a 9 out of 10 on a 0 to 10 scale after receiving morphine sulfate.

6. The nurse is preparing to discharge a patient from the PACU using the Aldrete scoring system. With which score can the patient be transferred out of the recovery room?

   a. 2

   b. 4

   c. 6

   d. 7

7. Using the Aldrete score, a nurse would give a patient an admission cardiovascular score of 2 if the patient's blood pressure is which percentage of their preanesthetic level?

   a. 20%

   b. 30% to 40%

   c. 40% to 50%

   d. Greater than 50%

8. A patient is experiencing postoperative vomiting. Which is the priority nursing action?

   a. Measure the amount of vomitus to estimate fluid loss, in order to accurately monitor fluid balance.

   b. Offer tepid water and juices to replace lost fluids and electrolytes.

   c. Support the wound area so that unnecessary strain will not disrupt the integrity of the incision.

   d. Turn the patient's head completely to one side to prevent aspiration of vomitus into the lungs.

9. The nurse measures the postoperative urinary output for a patient. Which results will the nurse report to the surgeon for a 2-hour period?

   a. <30 mL

   b. Between 75 and 100 mL

   c. Between 100 and 200 mL

   d. >200 mL

10. When will the nurse encourage the postoperative patient to get out of bed?

    a. Within 6 to 8 hours after surgery

    b. Between 10 and 12 hours after surgery

    c. As soon as it is indicated

    d. On the second postoperative day

11. The nurse is caring for an older adult patient after a surgical procedure. Which common postoperative complication will the nurse monitor the patient for?

    a. Pleurisy

    b. Pneumonia

    c. Hypoxemia

    d. Pulmonary edema

12. The nurse documents the presence of granulation tissue in a healing wound. Which is the **best** way for the nurse to describe the tissue?

    a. Necrotic and hard

    b. Pale yet able to blanch with digital pressure

    c. Pink to red and soft, bleeding easily

    d. White with long, thin areas of scar tissue

13. A health care provider's admitting note lists a wound as healing by second intention. Which condition of the wound does the nurse expect to find?

    a. A deep, open wound that was previously sutured

    b. A sutured incision with a little tissue reaction

    c. A wound with a deep, wide scar that was previously resutured

    d. A wound in which the edges were not approximated

14. A patient has a wound that has hemorrhaged. Which does the nurse identify is the cause of the patient's increased risk of infection?

    a. Reduced amount of oxygen and nutrients are available.

    b. The tissue becomes less resilient.

    c. Retrograde bacterial contamination may occur.

    d. Dead space and dead cells provide a culture medium.

15. The nurse assesses postoperative abdominal distention in a patient. Which does the nurse determine that the distention may be directly related to?

    a. A temporary loss of peristalsis and gas accumulation in the intestines

    b. Beginning food intake in the immediate postoperative period

    c. Improper body positioning during the recovery period

    d. The type of anesthetic administered

16. The nurse is concerned that a postoperative patient may have a paralytic ileus. Which assessment data correlates with the nurse's suspicion?

    a. Abdominal tightness

    b. Abdominal distention

    c. Absence of bowel sounds

    d. Increased abdominal girth

17. The nurse determines that a patient is at risk for the development of thrombophlebitis. Which preventative actions will the nurse take? (Select all that apply.)

    a. Assisting the patient with leg exercises

    b. Encouraging early ambulation

    c. Massaging the legs every 4 hours

    d. Avoiding placement of pillows or blanket rolls under the patient's knees

    e. Applying compression stockings only at night

18. A patient has developed a postoperative deep vein thrombosis (DVT). Which complication related to the DVT will the nurse closely monitor for?

    a. Pulmonary embolism

    b. Immobility because of calf pain

    c. Marked tenderness over the anteromedial surface of the thigh

    d. Swelling of the entire leg owing to edema

19. Which intervention by the nurse is most effective for reducing hospital-acquired infections?

    a. Administration of prophylactic antibiotics

    b. Aseptic wound care

    c. Control of upper respiratory tract infections

    d. Proper handwashing techniques

20. The nurse is assessing a postoperative patient's abdominal wound and observes a portion of intestines protruding through the wound. Which is the priority action by the nurse?

    a. Apply an abdominal binder snugly so that the intestines can be slowly pushed back into the abdominal cavity.

    b. Approximate the wound edges with adhesive tape so that the intestines can be gently pushed back into the abdomen.

    c. Carefully push the exposed intestines back into the abdominal cavity.

    d. Cover the protruding coils of intestines with sterile dressings moistened with sterile saline solution.

Gas Exchange and Respiratory Function

CHAPTER 17

Assessment of Respiratory Function

Learning Outcomes

1. Describe the structures and functions of the upper and lower respiratory tracts and concepts of ventilation, diffusion, perfusion, and ventilation–perfusion imbalances.
2. Explain and demonstrate proper techniques utilized to perform a comprehensive respiratory assessment.
3. Discriminate between normal and abnormal assessment findings of the respiratory system identified by inspection, palpation, percussion, and auscultation.
4. Recognize and evaluate the major symptoms of respiratory dysfunction by applying concepts from the patient's health history and physical assessment findings.
5. Identify the diagnostic tests used to evaluate respiratory function and related nursing implications.

SECTION I: ASSESSING YOUR UNDERSTANDING

Activity A *Fill in the blanks.*

1. The two centers in the brain that are responsible for the neurologic control of ventilation are _____ and _____.

2. The alveoli begin to lose elasticity at about age ____ years, resulting in decreased gas diffusion.

3. The lungs are enclosed in a serous membrane called the _____.

4. The left lung, in contrast to the right lung, has _____.

5. The divisions of the lung proceed in the following order, beginning at the mainstem bronchi: _____, _____, _____, and _____.

6. _____ are the alveolar cells that secrete surfactant.

7. Gas exchange between the lungs and blood and between the blood and tissues is called _____.

8. The maximum volume of air that can be inhaled after a normal inhalation is known as _____.

9. Tidal volume, which may not significantly change with disease, has a normal value of approximately _____ mL.

10. The exchange of oxygen and carbon dioxide from the alveoli into the blood occurs by _____.

11. The pulmonary circulation is considered a _____.

12. The symbol used to identify the partial pressure of oxygen is _____.

Activity B *Briefly answer the following.*

1. Distinguish between the terms *ventilation* and *respiration*.

   _____

   _____

2. Describe the function of the epiglottis.

   _____

   _____

3. List four conditions that cause low compliance or distensibility of the lungs:

   _____, _____,

   _____, and _____.

4. Define the term *partial pressure*.

   _____

   _____

5. List six major signs and symptoms of respiratory disease.

   _____   _____

   _____   _____

   _____   _____

6. _____ is a high-pitched, musical sound that is continuous, meaning it is heard on either expiration (asthma) or inspiration (bronchitis).

7. Explain the breathing pattern characterized as Cheyne–Stokes respirations.

   _____

   _____

8. What is the purpose of cilia?_____

   _____

9. What are four common phenomena that can alter bronchial diameter?

   _____, _____,

   _____, _____.

10. Compare and contrast the concepts of diffusion and pulmonary perfusion. _____

    _____

SECTION II: APPLYING YOUR KNOWLEDGE

Activity C *Consider the scenarios and answer the questions.*

CASE STUDY: Bronchoscopy

Mr. Kecklin is scheduled for a diagnostic bronchoscopy and possible biopsy after a CT scan located a suspicious nodule on the left lung.

1. The nurse is preparing the patient for the bronchoscopy. What interventions by the nurse are required prior to the procedure?

   _____

   _____

2. What complications will the nurse be aware may occur during a bronchoscopy?

   _____

   _____

3. After the bronchoscopy, what will the nurse assess Mr. Kecklin for?

   _____

   _____

4. What nursing actions are appropriate in the care of Mr. Kecklin after his bronchoscopy?

   _____

   _____

CASE STUDY: Thoracentesis

Mrs. Lomar is admitted to the clinical area for a thoracentesis. The health care provider will be removing excess air from the pleural cavity.

1. What interventions by the nurse are required prior to the thoracentesis?

   _____

   _____

2. Into which position will the nurse assist the patient prior to the thoracentesis?

   _____

   _____

3. What anatomic site will the health care provider use for the thoracentesis?

   _____

   _____

4. What will the nurse assess for after the patient has a thoracentesis?

_____

_____

SECTION III: PRACTICING FOR NCLEX

Activity D *Answer the following questions.*

1. A patient with sinus congestion reports discomfort when the nurse is palpating the supraorbital ridges. The nurse is aware that the patient is referring to which sinus?

   a. Frontal
   b. Ethmoidal
   c. Maxillary
   d. Sphenoidal

2. When the nurse is assessing the older adult patient, which gerontologic changes in the respiratory system will the nurse be aware of? (Select all that apply.)

   a. Decreased alveolar duct diameter
   b. Increased presence of mucus
   c. Decreased gag reflex
   d. Increased presence of collagen in alveolar walls
   e. Decreased presence of mucus

3. A nurse caring for a patient with a pulmonary embolism understands that high ventilation–perfusion ratio may exist. What does this mean for the patient?

   a. Perfusion exceeds ventilation
   b. There is an absence of perfusion and ventilation
   c. Ventilation exceeds perfusion
   d. Ventilation matches perfusion

4. The nurse is measuring a patient pulse oximetry reading after the patient reports slight shortness of breath when ambulating. Which oxygen saturation reading will the nurse identify as acceptable?

   a. 40 mm Hg
   b. 75 mm Hg
   c. 80 mm Hg
   d. 95 mm Hg

5. The nurse is taking a respiratory history for a patient who has come into the clinic with a chronic cough. Which information will the nurse obtain from this patient? (Select all that apply.)

   a. Financial ability to pay the bill
   b. Social support
   c. Previous history of lung disease in the patient or family
   d. Occupational and environmental influences
   e. Previous history of smoking

6. A patient comes to the emergency department reporting a knifelike pain when taking a deep breath. What does this type of pain likely indicate to the nurse?

   a. Bacterial pneumonia
   b. Bronchogenic carcinoma
   c. Lung infarction
   d. Pleurisy

7. The nurse is caring for a patient with a pulmonary disorder. Which observation by the nurse is indicative of a very late symptom of hypoxia?

   a. Cyanosis
   b. Dyspnea
   c. Restlessness
   d. Confusion

8. The nurse inspects the thorax of a patient with advanced emphysema. How does the nurse document the chest configuration for this patient?

   a. Barrel chest
   b. Funnel chest
   c. Kyphoscoliosis
   d. Pigeon chest

9. The nurse is performing chest auscultation for a patient with asthma. How does the nurse describe the high-pitched, sibilant, musical sounds that are heard?

   a. Rales
   b. Crackles
   c. Wheezes
   d. Rhonchi

10. The nurse auscultates crackles in a patient with a respiratory disorder. Which condition does the nurse identify correlates with this assessment finding?

    a. Asthma

    b. Bronchospasm

    c. Collapsed alveoli

    d. Pulmonary fibrosis

11. When performing an assessment for a patient, the nurse percusses tactile fremitus with hyperresonant sounds. Which diagnosis does the nurse correlate these assessment findings with?

    a. Bronchitis

    b. Emphysema

    c. Atelectasis

    d. Pulmonary edema

12. The nurse is reviewing the blood gas results for a patient with pneumonia. Which arterial blood gas measurement best reflects the adequacy of alveolar ventilation?

    a. PaO_2

    b. $PaCO_2$

    c. pH

    d. SaO_2

13. The nurse is instructing the patient on the collection of a sputum specimen. Which will be included in the instructions? (Select all that apply.)

    a. Initially, clear the nose and throat.

    b. Spit surface mucus and saliva into a sterile specimen container.

    c. Take a few deep breaths before coughing.

    d. Use diaphragmatic contractions to aid in the expulsion of sputum.

    e. Rinse with mouthwash prior to providing the specimen.

14. A health care provider requests a study of diaphragmatic motion because of suspected pathology. Which diagnostic test will the nurse prepare the patient for?

    a. Barium swallow

    b. Bronchogram

    c. Fluoroscopy

    d. Tomogram

15. The nurse is educating a patient who is scheduled for a perfusion lung scan. Which will be included in the information related to the procedure? (Select all that apply.)

    a. A mask will be placed over the nose and mouth during the test.

    b. The patient will be expected to lie under the camera.

    c. The imaging time will amount to 20 to 40 minutes.

    d. The patient will be expected to be NPO for 12 hours prior to the procedure.

    e. An injection will be placed into the lung during the procedure.

16. The nurse is performing an assessment for a patient with congestive heart failure and asks if the patient has difficulty breathing in any position other than upright. How will the nurse document this finding when the patient confirms that they do have difficulty?

    a. Dyspnea

    b. Orthopnea

    c. Tachypnea

    d. Bradypnea

17. The nurse is interviewing a patient who reports a dry, irritating cough that is not "bringing anything up." Which medication will the nurse question the patient about taking?

    a. Angiotensin-converting enzyme (ACE) inhibitors

    b. Aspirin

    c. Bronchodilators

    d. Cardiac glycosides

18. Which assessment finding by the nurse indicates that the patient has chronic hypoxia?

    a. Crackles

    b. Peripheral edema

    c. Clubbing of the fingers

    d. Cyanosis

19. When observing the chest wall of a patient, the nurse detects a depression in the lower portion of the sternum. Which assessment finding will the nurse anticipate detecting due to this condition?

a. Clubbing of fingers

b. Cyanosis

c. Crackles

d. Murmurs

20. The nurse is performing an assessment of a patient who arrived in the emergency department with a barbiturate overdose. The respirations are normal for 3 to 4 breaths followed by a 60-second period of apnea. How will the nurse document the respirations?

a. Cheyne–Stokes

b. Tachypnea

c. Bradypnea

d. Biot respirations

Management of Patients with Upper Respiratory Tract Disorders

Learning Outcomes

1. Describe nursing management of patients with upper airway disorders and of patients with epistaxis.
2. Compare and contrast the upper respiratory tract infections according to cause, incidence, clinical manifestations, management, and the significance of preventive health care.
3. Use the nursing process as a framework for care of the patient with upper airway infection and the patient undergoing laryngectomy.

SECTION I: ASSESSING YOUR UNDERSTANDING

Activity A *Fill in the blanks.*

1. The most common cause of laryngitis is _____, with symptoms including _____, _____, and _____.
2. Medication therapy for allergic and nonallergic rhinitis focuses on _____.
3. _____ remain the most common treatment for rhinitis and are administered for sneezing, pruritus, and rhinorrhea.

4. Rhinosinusitis is classified by duration of symptoms as _____, _____, and _____.
5. _____ is the most common major suppurative complication of sore throat.
6. The most serious complication of a tonsillectomy is _____.

Activity B *Briefly answer the following.*

1. Explain how rhinitis can lead to rhinosinusitis.

   _____

   _____

   _____

2. Name four bacterial organisms that account for more than 60% of all cases of acute rhinosinusitis: _____, _____, _____, and _____.
3. If untreated, chronic rhinosinusitis can lead to severe complications. List four: _____, _____, _____, and _____.

4. List four possible nursing diagnoses for a patient with an upper airway infection: _____, _____, _____, and _____.

5. List five potential complications of an upper airway infection: _____, _____, _____, _____, and _____.

6. List the clinical manifestations that are used to diagnose obstructive sleep apnea.

_____

_____

_____

7. List three types of alaryngeal communication: _____, _____, and _____.

Activity C *Match the term listed in Column II with its associated definition for surgical options for laryngeal cancer listed in Column I.*

Column I

_____ **1.** Removal of the mucosa on the edge of the vocal cord

_____ **2.** Excision of the vocal cord for lesions in the middle third of the vocal cord

_____ **3.** Complete removal of the larynx

_____ **4.** Portion of the larynx is removed, along with one vocal cord, and the tumor

_____ **5.** Microelectrodes are used for surgical resection of smaller laryngeal tumors

Column II

a. Partial laryngectomy

b. Vocal cord stripping

c. Total laryngectomy

d. Laser surgery

e. Cordectomy

SECTION II: APPLYING YOUR KNOWLEDGE

Activity D *Consider the scenarios and answer the questions.*

CASE STUDY: Tonsillectomy and Adenoidectomy

Isabel, a 14-year-old girl, has just undergone a tonsillectomy and adenoidectomy. The staff nurse assists her with transport from the recovery area to her room.

1. The nurse observes Isabel swallowing frequently. What may this assessment finding indicate to the nurse?

_____

2. What specific postoperative complication should the nurse monitor for?

_____

3. What recommended postoperative position should the nurse ensure that Isabel maintains?

_____

_____

4. Isabel is to be discharged the same day of her tonsillectomy. What education should the nurse provide to Isabel and her family?

_____

CASE STUDY: Epistaxis

Gilberta, a 16-year-old high school student, is being sent by the school nurse with her parents to the emergency department of a local hospital for uncontrolled epistaxis.

1. What should the school nurse instruct Gilberta and her parents to do to control the bleeding during transport to the hospital?

_____

_____

_____

2. What emergency medication will be provided to act as a vasoconstrictor and stop the bleeding in the Emergency Department?

_____

3. Gilberta had nasal packing with a compressed nasal sponge inserted to control the epistaxis. What education will be provided related to the packing upon discharge from the Emergency Department?

CASE STUDY: Cancer of the Larynx

Mrs. Carlyle, a 64 year old with a 40-year history of smoking 1½ packs of cigarettes per day, recently retired from the chemical laboratory department of a large company. After months of reporting a persistent cough, sore throat, pain, and burning in the throat, Mrs. Carlyle is being evaluated for possible cancer of the larynx.

1. The nurse is assessing Mrs. Carlyle upon admission. Which physical assessment technique should the nurse use to assess for laryngeal carcinoma?

2. Mrs. Carlyle asks the nurse what her treatment will be for stage I cancer of the larynx. What is the best response by the nurse?

3. The health care provider determines that radiation and chemotherapy will need to be done prior to surgery. What will the patient need to do prior to beginning any treatment regimen?

CASE STUDY: Laryngectomy

Mr. Jerome, a 52-year-old patient, is scheduled for a total laryngectomy due to a stage IV laryngeal cancer.

1. Before developing the perioperative plan of care, the nurse needs to know whether Jerome's voice will be preserved. What surgical procedure will preserve the voice box?

2. Jerome is scheduled for a total laryngectomy. What education should the nurse provide to the patient in the preoperative phase of surgery?

3. The nurse is educating Jerome about the presence of a nasogastric catheter after surgery. The nurse should inform him that he will begin receiving oral feedings approximately how long after the surgery?

4. Jerome asks the nurse when the laryngectomy tube will be removed. What is the best response by the nurse?

SECTION III: PRACTICING FOR NCLEX

Activity E *Answer the following questions.*

1. A patient comes to the clinic reporting symptoms of the common cold and wants something to help relieve the symptoms. Which will the nurse include in educating the patient about the uncomplicated common cold? (Select all that apply.)

   a. Tell the patient to take prescribed antibiotics to decrease the severity of symptoms.

   b. Inform the patient about the symptoms of secondary infection.

   c. Suggest that the patient take adequate fluids and get plenty of rest.

   d. Inform the patient that the virus is contagious for 2 days before symptoms appear and during the first part of the symptomatic phase.

   e. Inform the patient that taking an antihistamine will help to decrease the duration of the cold.

2. A patient has herpes simplex infection that developed after having the common cold. Which prescribed medication will the nurse educate the patient about regarding treatment of the herpes simplex?

   a. An antiviral agent such as acyclovir

   b. An antibiotic such as amoxicillin

   c. An antihistamine such as diphenhydramine

   d. An ointment such as bacitracin

3. A patient has been diagnosed with acute rhinosinusitis caused by a bacterial organism. Which antibiotic of choice for treatment of this disorder will the nurse educate the patient about?

    a. Amoxicillin–clavulanate

    b. Cephalexin

    c. Azithromycin

    d. Clarithromycin

4. The nurse is educating a patient diagnosed with acute bacterial rhinosinusitis about interventions that may assist with symptom control. Which will the nurse include in this information? (Select all that apply.)

    a. Take an over-the-counter nasal decongestant.

    b. Take an over-the-counter antihistamine.

    c. Ensure an adequate fluid intake.

    d. Increase the humidity in the home.

    e. Apply local heat to promote drainage.

5. A patient comes to the clinic reporting a sore throat and is diagnosed with acute pharyngitis. Which causative bacteria does the nurse identify was the likely cause of the acute pharyngitis?

    a. Group A, beta-hemolytic streptococci

    b. Gram-negative *Klebsiella*

    c. *Pseudomonas aeruginosa*

    d. *Staphylococcus aureus*

6. A patient diagnosed 2 weeks ago with acute pharyngitis comes to the clinic stating that the sore throat got better for a couple of days and is now back along with an earache. Which complications should the patient be assessed for related to the acute pharyngitis? (Select all that apply.)

    a. Mastoiditis

    b. Otitis media

    c. Peritonsillar abscess

    d. Pericarditis

    e. Encephalitis

7. The nurse is educating the patient diagnosed with acute pharyngitis on methods to alleviate discomfort. Which interventions should the nurse include in the information? (Select all that apply.)

    a. Apply an ice collar.

    b. Stay on bed rest during the febrile stage of the illness.

    c. Gargle with an alcohol-based mouthwash.

    d. Try a liquid or soft diet during the acute stage of the disease.

    e. Drink warm or hot liquids during the acute stage of the disease.

8. A patient comes to the clinic and is diagnosed with tonsillitis and adenoiditis. Which bacterial pathogen does the nurse identify is commonly associated with tonsillitis and adenoiditis?

    a. Gram-negative *Klebsiella*

    b. *Pseudomonas aeruginosa*

    c. Group A, beta-hemolytic streptococcus

    d. *Staphylococcus aureus*

9. A patient comes to the clinic reporting a possible upper respiratory infection. Which will the nurse assess that would indicate that an upper respiratory infection may be present?

    a. The nasal mucosa

    b. The buccal mucosa

    c. The frontal sinuses

    d. The tracheal mucosa

10. A patient playing softball was hit in the nose by the ball and has been determined to have an uncomplicated fractured nose with epistaxis. Which task will the nurse prepare to assist the health care provider with?

    a. Preparing the patient for a septoplasty

    b. Applying nasal packing

    c. Administering nasal lavage

    d. Applying steroidal nasal spray

11. A patient arrives in the emergency department with an edematous face, tongue, and difficulty breathing after starting a new medication for hypertension. When reviewing medication, which antihypertensive would the nurse suspect as the likely causative factor?

    a. Metoprolol succinate
    b. Amlodipine
    c. Enalapril
    d. Valsartan

12. The nurse is assessing a patient who smokes two packs of cigarettes per day and has a strong family history of cancer. Which early sign of cancer of the larynx does the nurse assess for in this patient?

    a. Burning of the throat when hot liquids are ingested
    b. Enlarged cervical nodes
    c. Dysphagia
    d. Affected voice sounds

13. A patient is diagnosed as being in the early stage of laryngeal cancer of the glottis with only one vocal cord involved. For which type of surgical intervention will the nurse plan to provide education?

    a. Total laryngectomy
    b. Cordectomy
    c. Vocal cord stripping
    d. Partial laryngectomy

14. A patient with an advanced laryngeal tumor is to have radiation therapy. The patient tells the nurse, "If I am going to have radiation, I won't need surgery." Which is the best response by the nurse?

    a. "That is correct. The radiation will eradicate the tumor and you won't have to have further treatment."
    b. "Radiation is used to shrink the tumor size and is an adjunct to surgery."
    c. "All patients have to have radiation before they have surgery. It is protocol."
    d. "You really don't have to have radiation but you won't have to have such invasive surgery if you have the radiation first."

15. The nurse is caring for a patient who had a total laryngectomy and has drains in place. When does the nurse understand that the drains will most likely be removed?

    a. When the patient has less than 30 mL for 2 consecutive days
    b. When the patient states that there is discomfort and requests removal
    c. When the drainage tube comes out
    d. In 1 week when the patient no longer has serous drainage

Management of Patients with Chest and Lower Respiratory Tract Disorders

Learning Outcomes

1. Identify patients at risk for atelectasis and the nursing interventions related to its prevention and management.
2. Compare the various pulmonary infections with regard to causes, clinical manifestations, nursing management, complications, and prevention.
3. Identify the nursing care of a patient with an endotracheal tube, with mechanical ventilation, or with a tracheostomy.
4. Relate the therapeutic management of acute respiratory distress syndrome to the underlying pathophysiology of the syndrome.
5. Describe preventive measures appropriate for controlling and eliminating occupational lung disease.
6. Discuss the modes of therapy and related nursing management of patients with lung cancer.
7. Use the nursing process as a framework for care of the patient with pneumonia, receiving mechanical ventilation, or with a thoracotomy.
8. Describe the complications of chest trauma and their clinical manifestations and nursing management.
9. Explain the principles of chest drainage and the nursing responsibilities related to the care of the patient with a chest drainage system.

SECTION I: ASSESSING YOUR UNDERSTANDING

Activity A *Fill in the blanks.*

1. Hospital-acquired pneumonia develops _____ hours or more after admission and does not appear to be incubating at the time of admission.

2. In current tuberculosis (TB) treatment, four first-line medications are used: _____, _____, _____, and _____.

3. A(n) _____ is an accumulation of thick, purulent fluid within the pleural space, often with fibrin development and a loculated area where infection is located.

4. _____, _____, and _____ are hallmarks of the severity of atelectasis.

5. When a nonfunctioning nasogastric tube allows the gastric contents to accumulate in the stomach, a condition known as _____ may result.

6. Three common pathogens that cause aspiration pneumonia are _____, _____, and _____

7. Pneumonia tends to occur in patients with one or more of these five underlying disorders: _____, _____, _____, _____, and _____.

8. Three severe complications of pneumonia are _____, _____, and _____.

9. Four respiratory system mechanisms that can lead to acute respiratory failure (ARF) are _____, _____, _____, and _____.

10. The most serious complication and most frequent cause of death among patients with COVID-19 is _____.

Activity B *Briefly answer the following.*

1. Atelectasis, which refers to closure or collapse of alveoli, may be chronic or acute in nature. What are some of the possible causes of atelectasis in the postoperative patient?

_____ _____

_____ _____

_____ _____

_____ _____

_____

2. Name seven possible clinical manifestations of atelectasis.

_____ _____

_____ _____

_____ _____

_____

3. Identify eight nursing interventions that are used to prevent atelectasis.

_____ _____

_____ _____

_____ _____

_____ _____

4. Explain the meaning of the term *superinfection*.

_____ _____

_____ _____

5. Describe the characteristic and diagnostic feature of ARDS.

_____

6. Define the etiology of cor pulmonale.

_____

_____

7. List at least six etiologic factors and nursing assessments for patients with ARDS.

_____ _____

_____ _____

_____ _____

Activity C *Match the classification of tuberculosis in Column II with its associated definition listed in Column I.*

Column I

____ 1. Disease; not clinically active

____ 2. Latent infection; no disease (e.g., positive PPD)

____ 3. Suspected disease; diagnosis pending

____ 4. Exposure; no evidence of infection

____ 5. No exposure; no infection

____ 6. Disease; clinically active

Column II

a. Class 0

b. Class 1

c. Class 2

d. Class 3

e. Class 4

f. Class 5

SECTION II: APPLYING YOUR KNOWLEDGE

Activity D *Consider the scenarios and answer the questions.*

CASE STUDY: Community-Acquired Pneumonia

Theresa, a 20-year-old college student, lives in a small dormitory with 30 other students. Four weeks into the spring semester, she was diagnosed as having bacterial pneumonia and was admitted to the hospital.

1. Which intervention will be important to encourage to decrease the viscosity of the secretions?

_____

2. The nurse is assessing Theresa during the admission process. Which manifestations of bacterial pneumonia does the nurse identify?

_____

_____

3. The nurse assesses Theresa for arterial hypoxemia. What is the explanation for the development of this complication?

_____

_____

_____

4. The nurse is assessing vital signs and lung sounds every 4 hours. Which complications will the nurse monitor for?

_____

CASE STUDY: Tuberculosis

Mr. Carrera, a 67-year-old retired baker, is admitted to the clinical area for confirmation of suspected tuberculosis. He reports a lack of appetite, fatigue, and is experiencing "indigestion." He reports a temperature elevation in the afternoon hours of 100° to 100.4°F with chills.

1. Mr. Carrera's Mantoux tuberculin test yields an induration area of 6 to 10 mm. What does the nurse interpret these findings to indicate?

_____

2. Mr. Carrera has undergone a series of additional tests, and a diagnosis is confirmed. Which test provides confirmation that the patient has tuberculosis?

_____

3. Mr. Carrera is started on a multiple-drug regimen. Which medication does the nurse discuss with the health care provider that may interfere with the metabolism of the beta-blocker he is presently taking?

_____

CASE STUDY: Acute Respiratory Distress Syndrome

Mrs. Wray is admitted to the unit with a diagnosis of ARDS. She was receiving treatment at home for viral pneumonia and had appeared to be improving until yesterday.

1. The nurse is assessing Mrs. Wray for associated clinical manifestations with ARDS. Which symptoms identified by the nurse positively correlate with ARDS?

_____

_____

2. The nurse is performing a neurologic assessment. Which symptoms observed by the nurse indicate that Wray is developing cerebral hypoxia?

_____

3. The nurse observes that Wray is receiving oxygen by way of a nasal cannula at 6 L/min. What does the nurse determine Wray's FiO_2 would be?

_____

CASE STUDY: Pulmonary Embolism

Mrs. Sandy, a 37-year-old recovering from multiple fractures sustained in a car injury, is admitted to the intensive care unit for treatment of a pulmonary embolism. Before admission, she was short of breath after walking up a flight of stairs.

1. Mrs. Sandy asks the nurse what could have caused this, since she was getting better from the injury and getting plenty of rest. Which is the best response by the nurse?

_____

_____

2. Which symptom most frequently occurs in the presence of a pulmonary embolism?

_____

3. With a diagnosis of pulmonary embolism, what decrease in function should the nurse assess for?

_____

SECTION III: PRACTICING FOR NCLEX

Activity E *Answer the following questions.*

1. The nurse is developing a plan of care for a patient with acute tracheobronchitis. Which nursing interventions will be included in the plan of care? (Select all that apply.)

   a. Increasing fluid intake to remove secretions

   b. Encouraging the patient to remain in bed

   c. Using cool-vapor therapy to relieve laryngeal and tracheal irritation

   d. Giving 3-L fluid per day

   e. Administering a narcotic analgesic for pain

2. The nurse is collecting a sputum culture to identify the causative organism for a patient with acute tracheobronchitis. Which causative fungal organism does the nurse suspect?

   a. *Aspergillus*

   b. *Haemophilus*

   c. *Mycoplasma pneumoniae*

   d. *Streptococcus pneumoniae*

3. The nurse is conducting a community program about prevention of respiratory illness. Which illness does the nurse recognize is the most common cause of death in the United States?

   a. Atelectasis

   b. Pulmonary embolus

   c. Pneumonia

   d. Tracheobronchitis

4. A patient comes to the clinic reporting fever, cough, and chest discomfort. The nurse auscultates crackles in the left lower base of the lung and suspects that the patient may have pneumonia. Which does the nurse identify is the most common organism that causes community-acquired pneumonia?

   a. *Staphylococcus aureus*

   b. *Mycobacterium tuberculosis*

   c. *Pseudomonas aeruginosa*

   d. *Streptococcus pneumoniae*

5. A patient has a Mantoux skin test prior to being placed on a biologic medication for the treatment of Crohn's disease. Which results would determine that the medication may be administered as prescribed by the nurse?

   a. 0 to 4 mm

   b. 5 to 6 mm

   c. 7 to 8 mm

   d. 9 mm

6. The nurse is educating a patient who will be started on an antituberculosis medication regimen. The patient asks the nurse, "How long will I have to be on these medications?" Which statement by the nurse is **most** informative?

   a. "You will need to take the medication for 3 months."

   b. "Depending on your symptoms, 3 to 5 months is the most you will take them."

   c. "It is important that you take the medication as prescribed for 6 to 12 months."

   d. "Most patients have to take the medication for at least 13 to 18 months."

7. The nurse is caring for a patient with pleurisy. Which symptoms does the nurse identify correlate with the patient's illness?

   a. Dullness or flatness on percussion over areas of collected fluid

   b. Dyspnea and coughing

   c. Fever and chills

   d. Stabbing pain during respiratory movement

8. The nurse is auscultating the patient's lung sounds to determine if there is the presence of fluid overload. Which adventitious lung sounds are significant for pulmonary edema?

   a. Crackles in the lung bases

   b. Low-pitched rhonchi during expiration

   c. Pleural friction rub

   d. Sibilant wheezes

9. A patient is being educated by the nurse about the administration of isoniazid (INH) therapy for tuberculosis. Which statement made by the patient indicates that the education is understood?

   a. "I am going to have a tuna fish sandwich for lunch."

   b. "It is all right if I drink a glass of red wine with my dinner."

   c. "It is all right if I have a grilled cheese sandwich with American cheese."

   d. "It is fine if I eat sushi with a little bit of soy sauce."

10. A patient who wears contact lenses is to be placed on rifampin for tuberculosis therapy. Which information will the nurse provide to the patient?

    a. "Only wear your contact lenses during the day and take them out in the evening before bed."

    b. "You should switch to wearing your glasses while taking this medication."

    c. "The health care provider can give you eye drops to prevent any problems."

    d. "There are no significant problems with wearing contact lenses."

11. The nurse is caring for a patient with suspected acute respiratory distress syndrome (ARDS) with a PO_2 of 53. The patient is placed on oxygen via facemask and the PO_2 remains the same. Which key characteristic of ARDS does the nurse identify is occurring?

    a. Unresponsive arterial hypoxemia

    b. Diminished alveolar dilation

    c. Tachypnea

    d. Increased PaO_2

12. A patient is admitted to the hospital with pulmonary arterial hypertension. Which significant assessment finding by the nurse will be reported to the health care provider?

    a. Ascites

    b. Dyspnea

    c. Hypertension

    d. Syncope

13. The nurse is assessing a patient who has been admitted with possible acute respiratory distress syndrome (ARDS). Which findings would distinguish ARDS from cardiogenic pulmonary edema?

    a. Elevated white blood count

    b. Elevated troponin levels

    c. Elevated myoglobin levels

    d. Elevated B-type natriuretic peptide (BNP) levels

14. A patient with pulmonary hypertension has a positive vasoreactivity test. Which medication will the nurse administer to the patient as prescribed?

    a. Calcium channel blockers

    b. Angiotensin-converting enzyme inhibitor

    c. Beta-blockers

    d. Angiotensin receptor blockers

15. The nurse assesses a patient for a possible pulmonary embolism. Which frequent sign of pulmonary embolus does the nurse identify on assessment?

    a. Cough

    b. Hemoptysis

    c. Syncope

    d. Tachypnea

16. The nurse is administering anticoagulant therapy with heparin. Which international normalized ratio (INR) does the nurse identify as within therapeutic range and will continue administration of the heparin?

    a. 0.5 to 1.0

    b. 1.5 to 2.5

    c. 2.0 to 2.5

    d. 3.0 to 3.5

17. The nurse is planning the care for a patient at risk for the development of a pulmonary embolism. Which nursing actions will be included in the care plan? (Select all that apply.)

    a. Encourage a liberal fluid intake.

    b. Assist the patient to do leg elevations above the level of the heart.

    c. Instruct the patient to dangle the legs over the side of the bed for 30 minutes, four times a day.

    d. Use elastic stockings, especially when decreased mobility would promote venous stasis.

    e. Apply a sequential compression device.

18. The nurse is assisting with an endotracheal insertion for a patient in respiratory failure. Which nursing action will ensure that the endotracheal tube is placed in the appropriate position?

a. Obtain a chest x-ray for confirmation of tube placement.

b. Observe condensation in the endotracheal tube.

c. Listen to breath sounds on the anterior chest wall.

d. Observe the patient's oxygen saturation level.

19. The nurse is having an information session with a women's group at the YMCA about lung cancer. Which frequent and commonly experienced symptom will the nurse include in the session?

a. Copious sputum production

b. Coughing

c. Dyspnea

d. Severe pain

20. A patient arrives in the emergency department after being involved in a motor vehicle crash. The nurse observes paradoxical chest movement when removing the patient's shirt. What does the nurse know that this finding indicates?

a. Pneumothorax

b. Flail chest

c. ARDS

d. Tension pneumothorax

CHAPTER 20

Management of Patients with Chronic Pulmonary Disease

Learning Outcomes

1. Describe the pathophysiology, clinical manifestations, treatment, and medical and nursing management of chronic pulmonary diseases, including chronic obstructive pulmonary disease, bronchiectasis, asthma, and cystic fibrosis.
2. Discuss the major risk factors for developing chronic obstructive pulmonary disease and nursing interventions to minimize or prevent these risk factors.
3. Use the nursing process as a framework for care of the patient with chronic obstructive pulmonary disease.
4. Develop an education plan for patients with chronic obstructive pulmonary disease.
5. Discuss nursing management of and patient education and transitions in care considerations for patients receiving oxygen therapy.
6. Describe asthma self-management strategies.

SECTION I: ASSESSING YOUR UNDERSTANDING

Activity A *Fill in the blanks.*

1. _____, one of the complications of emphysema, is right-sided heart failure brought on by long-term high blood pressure in the pulmonary arteries.

2. _____ depresses the activity of scavenger cells and affects the respiratory tract's ciliary cleansing mechanism, which keeps breathing passages free of inhaled irritants, bacteria, and other foreign matter.

3. The most important environmental risk factor for COPD worldwide is _____.

4. _____ is used to evaluate airflow obstruction, which is determined by the ratio of FEV_1 to forced vital capacity (FVC).

5. A _____ is a surgical option for select patients with bullous emphysema.

6. The *single most cost-effective* intervention to reduce the risk of developing COPD or slow its progression is _____.

7. Primary causes for an acute exacerbation of COPD are _____ and _____.

8. To help prevent infections in patients with COPD, the nurse should recommend vaccination against two bacterial organisms: _____ and _____.

9. The strongest predisposing factor for asthma is _____; the three most common symptoms are _____, _____, and _____.

10. Complications of asthma may include
_____, _____,
_____, and _____.

11. _____ includes postural drainage, chest percussion and vibration, and breathing retraining.

Activity B *Briefly answer the following.*

1. Describe the results of chronic airway inflammation in COPD.

_____

_____

_____

2. Describe the two main types of *emphysema.*

_____

_____

3. What are the three primary goals of pulmonary rehabilitation?

_____

_____

_____

4. List the three *primary symptoms* associated with the progressive stage of COPD.

_____

_____

_____

5. List five of the nine major factors that determine the clinical course and survival of patients with COPD.

_____

_____

_____

6. Describe three ways that bronchodilators relieve bronchospasm.

_____

_____

_____

Activity C *Match the drug category listed in Column II with an associated medication in Column I.*

Column I

___ 1. Albuterol

___ 2. Ipratropium bromide

___ 3. Combivent

___ 4. Theophylline

___ 5. Montelukast

___ 6. Cromolyn sodium

Column II

a. Mast cell stabilizer

b. Leukotriene modifier

c. Anticholinergic agent

d. Methylxanthine

e. Combination short-acting beta-2 adrenergic agonist agent

f. Beta-2 adrenergic agonist agent

SECTION II: APPLYING YOUR KNOWLEDGE

Activity D *Consider the scenario and answer the questions.*

CASE STUDY: Emphysema

Mrs. Burch, who has had emphysema for 25 years, is admitted to the hospital with a diagnosis of bronchitis.

1. The nurse observes that she has an increase in anterior–posterior diameter, or "barrel chest." What is the cause of the alteration in the chest shape and size?

_____

_____

2. The nurse identifies the need to monitor for what major presenting symptom of emphysema?

_____

3. The nurse is assessing the results of Mrs. Burch's arterial blood gas. Which blood gas analysis will correlate with the diagnosis of emphysema?

_____

4. Mrs. Burch is administered a bronchodilator to reduce airway obstruction. What side effects from this medication should the nurse educate her about?

_____

_____

5. The nurse is educating Mrs. Burch about diaphragmatic breathing. How will this type of breathing help relieve her symptoms?

_____

_____

6. The health care provider prescribes oxygen therapy for Mrs. Burch. Which delivery system will be most effective?

_____

_____

SECTION III: PRACTICING FOR NCLEX

Activity E *Answer the following questions.*

1. A patient comes to the clinic for the third time in 2 months with chronic bronchitis. Which clinical symptoms does the nurse assess in this patient?

a. Chest pain during respiration

b. Sputum and a productive cough

c. Fever, chills, and diaphoresis

d. Tachypnea and tachycardia

2. The nurse is assigned to care for a patient with COPD experiencing hypoxemia and hypercapnia. When planning care for this patient, which outcome of treatment will the nurse evaluate?

a. The patient will demonstrate adequate oxygenation.

b. The patient will avoid the use of supplementary oxygen to decrease hypoxic drive.

c. Monitor pulse oximetry every 8 hours while awake.

d. Educate the patient about the use of diaphragmatic breathing techniques.

3. A nurse notes that the FEV_1/FVC ratio is less than 70% for a patient with COPD. Which stage should the nurse document the patient is in?

a. 0

b. I

c. II

d. III

4. Upon assessment, the nurse suspects that a patient with COPD may have bronchospasm. Which manifestations validate the nurse's concern? (Select all that apply.)

a. Compromised gas exchange

b. Decreased airflow

c. Wheezes

d. Jugular vein distention

e. Ascites

5. The health care provider prescribes a beta-2 adrenergic agonist agent that is short-acting and administered only by inhaler. Which medication does the nurse administer as prescribed?

a. Metaproterenol

b. Terbutaline

c. Formoterol

d. Isoproterenol

6. A patient with end-stage COPD and heart failure asks the nurse about lung reduction surgery. Which is the best response by the nurse?

a. "You are not a candidate because you have heart failure."

b. "You would have a difficult time recovering from the procedure."

c. "At this point, do you really want to go through something like that?"

d. "You and your primary provider should discuss the options that are available for treatment."

7. The nurse is monitoring a patient with bronchiectasis. Which complication should the nurse be alert for?

a. Atelectasis

b. Emphysema

c. Pleurisy

d. Pneumonia

8. A patient is prescribed a mast cell stabilizer for the treatment of asthma. Which commonly used medication will the nurse educate the patient about?

a. Albuterol

b. Budesonide

c. Cromolyn sodium

d. Theophylline

9. The nurse is caring for a patient with status asthmaticus in the intensive care unit (ICU). Which blood gas analysis related to hyperventilation does the nurse observe with this patient?

   a. Metabolic acidosis

   b. Metabolic alkalosis

   c. Respiratory acidosis

   d. Respiratory alkalosis

10. A child is having an asthma attack and the parent cannot remember which inhaler to use for quick relief. The nurse accesses the child's medication information and tells the parent to use which inhalant?

    a. Cromolyn sodium

    b. Theophylline

    c. Salmeterol

    d. Albuterol

11. The nurse is educating a patient with asthma about preventative measures to avoid having an asthma attack. Which preventative intervention will the nurse educate the patient about to prevent an asthma attack?

    a. Use a long-acting steroid inhaler when an attack is coming.

    b. Avoid exercise and any strenuous activity.

    c. Prepare a written action plan.

    d. Stay in the house if it is too cold or too hot.

12. The nurse is assigned to care for a patient in the intensive care unit (ICU) with status asthmaticus. Why does the nurse include fluid intake as being an important aspect of the plan of care? (Select all that apply.)

    a. To combat dehydration

    b. To assist with the effectiveness of the corticosteroids

    c. To loosen secretions

    d. To facilitate expectoration

    e. To relieve bronchospasm

13. A patient is being treated for status asthmaticus. Which arterial blood gas analysis does the nurse evaluate that can indicate impending respiratory failure?

    a. Respiratory acidosis

    b. Respiratory alkalosis

    c. Metabolic acidosis

    d. Metabolic alkalosis

14. A patient with cystic fibrosis is admitted to the hospital with pneumonia. When will the nurse administer the pancreatic enzymes that the patient has been prescribed?

    a. After meals and at bedtime

    b. One hour prior to mealtime in the morning

    c. With meals

    d. Three times a day regardless of meal time

15. The nurse is instructing the patient with asthma in the use of a newly prescribed leukotriene receptor antagonist. Which education will the nurse include?

    a. Take the medication with meals because it may cause nausea.

    b. Take the medication separately without other medications.

    c. Take the medication an hour before meals or 2 hours after a meal.

    d. Take the medication with a small amount of liquid.

Cardiovascular and Circulatory Function

CHAPTER 21

Assessment of Cardiovascular Function

Learning Outcomes

1. Describe the structure and function of the cardiovascular system as well as associated cardiac risk factors.
2. Explain and demonstrate the proper techniques to perform a comprehensive cardiovascular assessment.
3. Discriminate between normal and abnormal assessment findings identified by inspection, palpation, percussion, and auscultation of the cardiovascular system.
4. Recognize and evaluate the major manifestations of cardiovascular dysfunction by applying concepts from the patient's health history and physical assessment findings.
5. Identify diagnostic tests and methods of hemodynamic monitoring (e.g., central venous pressure, pulmonary artery pressure, and arterial pressure monitoring) of the cardiovascular system and related nursing implications.

SECTION I: ASSESSING YOUR UNDERSTANDING

Activity A *Fill in the blanks.*

1. Orthostatic hypotension is a sustained decrease of at least _____ mm Hg in systolic BP or _____ mm Hg in diastolic BP within 3 minutes of moving from a lying or sitting to a standing position.

2. _____, _____, and _____ are measured to evaluate a person's risk of developing coronary artery disease (CAD), especially if there is a family history of premature heart disease, or to diagnose a specific lipoprotein abnormality.

3. Homocysteine, an amino acid, is linked to the development of _____ because it can damage the endothelial lining of arteries and promote thrombus formation.

4. A chest x-ray is obtained to determine the _____, _____, and _____ of the heart.

5. After having a cardiac catheterization, the patient is to remain in the bed for _____ to _____ hours.

6. The three factors that determine stroke volume are _____, _____, and _____.

7. Three major cardiovascular risk factors are _____, _____, and _____.

8. If CAD is present, the American Heart Association (AHA) recommends the following laboratory measurements: low-density lipoprotein (LDL), _____; blood pressure (BP), _____; serum glucose concentration, _____; and a body mass index (BMI) of _____.

9. The two most specific enzymes traditionally used to analyze an acute myocardial infarction (MI) are _____ and _____; two biomarkers, _____ and _____, are early indicators of a myocardial infarction (MI).

Activity B *Briefly answer the following.*

1. List the five categories of cardiovascular disease (CVD).

_____ _____

_____ _____

_____

2. Distinguish between the functions of the atrioventricular and the semilunar valves.

_____

_____

_____

_____

3. Briefly explain depolarization as it relates to cardiac physiology.

_____

_____

_____

4. Estimate the cardiac output, per beat, for an adult heart rate of 76 beats per minute (bpm) with an average stroke volume of 70 mL per beat.

_____

5. Describe Starling law of the heart.

_____

_____

_____

6. List four physiologic effects on the cardiovascular system that are associated with the aging process.

_____ _____

_____ _____

7. To assess the apical pulse, the nurse would find the following location:

_____.

8. List several purposes of cardiac catheterization.

_____

_____

_____

9. Describe selective angiography.

_____

_____

_____

10. Discuss the implications of a low central venous pressure reading.

_____

_____

11. Identify four of seven possible complications of pulmonary artery monitoring: _____,

_____, _____,

and _____.

Activity C

PART I

Match the anatomic term in Column II with its associated function in Column I.

Column I

___ 1. Separates the right and left atria

___ 2. Is located at the juncture of the superior vena cava and the right atrium

___ 3. Supports the heart in the mediastinum

___ 4. Sits between the right ventricle and the pulmonary artery

___ 5. Distributes venous blood to the lungs

___ 6. Is embedded in the right atrial wall near the tricuspid valve

Column II

a. Parietal pericardium

b. Pulmonary artery

c. Bicuspid valve

d. Pulmonic valve

e. Sinoatrial node

f. Atrioventricular node

PART II

Match the terminology associated with coronary atherosclerosis in Column II with its function/characteristic listed in Column I.

Column I

_____ **1.** A principal blood lipid

_____ **2.** A risk factor that causes pulmonary damage

_____ **3.** The functional lesion of atherosclerosis

_____ **4.** Biochemical substances, soluble in fat, that accumulate within a blood vessel

_____ **5.** A risk factor that is endocrine in origin

_____ **6.** A risk factor associated with a type A personality

_____ **7.** A risk factor related to weight gain

_____ **8.** A recommended dietary restriction that is a risk factor for heart disease

_____ **9.** A symptom of myocardial ischemia

_____ **10.** Myocardial manifestation of coronary artery disease (CAD)

_____ **11.** A lifestyle habit that is considered a modifiable risk factor for heart disease

Column II

a. Atheroma

b. Obesity

c. Chest pain

d. Cholesterol

e. Inactivity

f. Lipids

g. Smoking

h. Arrhythmias

i. Diabetes

j. Fat

k. Stress

Activity D *Compare the following two figures found in Table 21-2, Assessing Chest Pain, in the textbook, depicting the pain pathway of musculoskeletal disorders and pericarditis. Fill in the blanks in the below table.*

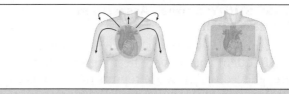

	Pericarditis	Musculoskeletal Disorders
Duration of pain:	_____	_____
Precipitating events and aggravating factors:	_____	_____
	_____	_____
	_____	_____
	_____	_____
	_____	_____
Alleviating factors:	_____	_____
	_____	_____
	_____	_____

SECTION II: APPLYING YOUR KNOWLEDGE

Activity E *Consider the scenario and answer the questions.*

CASE STUDY: Cardiac Assessment for Chest Pain

Mr. Anderson is a 45-year-old patient reporting frequent episodes of chest pressure that are relieved with rest. He reports that he has a stressful job that requires traveling and that he eats out often. He expresses concern that he has a heart condition and would like to get a "checkup."

1. The nurse observes a bluish tinge around his lips. What does the nurse determine that these assessment findings indicate?

2. The nurse takes a baseline blood pressure measurement after the patient has rested for 10 minutes in a supine position. Which reading reflects a reduced pulse pressure?
   a. 140/90 mm Hg
   b. 140/100 mm Hg
   c. 140/110 mm Hg
   d. 140/120 mm Hg

3. Five minutes after the initial blood pressure measurement is taken, the nurse assesses additional readings with the patient in a sitting and then in a standing position. Which reading is indicative of an abnormal postural response?
   a. lying, 140/110; sitting, 130/110; standing, 135/106 mm Hg
   b. lying, 140/110; sitting, 135/112; standing, 130/115 mm Hg
   c. lying, 140/110; sitting, 135/100; standing, 120/90 mm Hg
   d. lying, 140/110; sitting, 130/108; standing, 125/108 mm Hg

4. The nurse returns Mr. Anderson to the supine position and measures for jugular vein distention. The finding that would indicate an abnormal increase in the volume of the venous system would be obvious distention of the veins when the patient is positioned at what angle?

5. The nurse auscultates the apex of the heart. Over what area should the nurse place the stethoscope?

SECTION III: PRACTICING FOR NCLEX

Activity F *Answer the following questions.*

1. The nurse is caring for a patient with a diagnosis of pericarditis. Where does the nurse identify that the inflammation is located?
   a. The thin fibrous sac encasing the heart
   b. The inner lining of the heart and valves
   c. The heart's muscle fibers
   d. The exterior layer of the heart

2. The nurse is assessing heart sounds in a patient with heart failure. An abnormal heart sound is detected early in diastole. How will the nurse document this finding?
   a. S_1
   b. S_2
   c. S_3
   d. S_4

3. The nurse is performing an assessment of the patient's heart. Where will the nurse locate the apical pulse if the heart is in a normal position?
   a. Left second intercostal space at the midclavicular line
   b. Right second intercostal space at the midclavicular line
   c. Right third intercostal space at the midclavicular line
   d. Left fifth intercostal space at the midclavicular line

4. A patient's heart rate is observed to be 140 bpm on the monitor. Which complication should the nurse closely monitor the patient for?
   a. Myocardial ischemia
   b. A pulmonary embolism
   c. Right-sided heart failure
   d. A stroke

5. The nurse is administering a beta-blocker to a patient in order to decrease automaticity. Which medication will the nurse administer?

   a. Diltiazem

   b. Metoprolol

   c. Amiodarone

   d. Propafenone

6. The patient has a heart rate of 72 bpm with a regular rhythm. Where does the nurse identify that the impulse arises from?

   a. The AV node

   b. The Purkinje fibers

   c. The sinoatrial node

   d. The ventricles

7. The nurse is assessing a patient's electrocardiogram (ECG). Which phase does the nurse identify as the resting phase before the next depolarization?

   a. Phase 1

   b. Phase 2

   c. Phase 3

   d. Phase 4

8. The nurse is reviewing the results of the patient's echocardiogram and observes that the ejection fraction is 35%. The nurse anticipates that the patient will receive treatment for which condition?

   a. Pulmonary embolism

   b. Myocardial infarction

   c. Pericarditis

   d. Heart failure

9. The nurse is educating a patient at risk for atherosclerosis. Which nonmodifiable risk factors does the nurse identify for the patient?

   a. Stress

   b. Obesity

   c. Positive family history

   d. Hyperlipidemia

10. The nurse is assessing a patient's blood pressure. Which does the nurse document as the difference between the systolic and the diastolic pressures?

    a. Pulse pressure

    b. Auscultatory gap

    c. Pulse deficit

    d. Korotkoff sound

11. The nurse is assessing a patient who reports feeling "lightheaded." When obtaining orthostatic vital signs, which does the nurse report to the health care provider as a significant finding?

    a. A heart rate of 20 bpm above the resting rate

    b. An unchanged systolic pressure

    c. An increase of 10 mm Hg blood pressure reading

    d. An increase of 5 mm Hg in diastolic pressure

12. The nurse observes a certified nursing assistant (CNA) obtaining a blood pressure reading with a cuff that is too small for the patient. Which information should the nurse provide to the CNA about the use of a cuff that is too small for a patient?

    a. The results will be falsely decreased.

    b. The results will be falsely elevated.

    c. It will give an accurate reading.

    d. It will be significantly different with each reading.

13. A patient is going through menopause and asks the nurse about estrogen replacement for its cardioprotective benefits. Which is the best response by the nurse?

    a. "That's a great idea. You don't want to have a heart attack."

    b. "Replacement of estrogen will protect a woman after she goes into menopause."

    c. "Estrogen is actually potentially harmful and is no longer a recommended therapy."

    d. "You need to research it and determine what you want to do."

14. A patient tells the nurse, "I was straining to have a bowel movement and felt like I was going to faint. I took my pulse and it was so slow." Which does the nurse inform the patient about this occurrence?

    a. The patient may have had a myocardial infarction.

    b. The patient had a vagal response.

    c. The patient was anxious about being constipated.

    d. The patient may have an abdominal aortic aneurysm.

15. A patient had a cardiac catheterization and is now in the recovery area. Which nursing priority interventions should be included in the plan of care? (Select all that apply.)

    a. Assessing the peripheral pulses in the affected extremity

    b. Checking the insertion site for hematoma formation

    c. Evaluating temperature and color in the affected extremity

    d. Assisting the patient to the bathroom after the procedure

    e. Assessing vital signs every 8 hours

CHAPTER 22

Management of Patients with Arrhythmias and Conduction Problems

Learning Outcomes

1. Correlate the components of the normal electrocardiogram (ECG) with physiologic events of the heart.
2. Define the ECG as a waveform that represents the cardiac electrical event in relation to the lead (placement of electrodes).
3. Analyze elements of an ECG rhythm strip: ventricular and atrial rate, ventricular and atrial rhythm, QRS complex and shape, QRS duration, P wave and shape, PR interval, and P:QRS ratio.
4. Identify the ECG criteria, causes and management of arrhythmias, and use the nursing process as a framework for care of the patient with an arrhythmia, including conduction disturbances.
5. Compare the different types of pacemakers, their uses, possible complications, and nursing implications.
6. Describe the key points of using a defibrillator; identify the purpose of an implantable cardioverter defibrillator, the types available, and the nursing implications.
7. Describe the nursing management of patients with implantable cardiac devices.

SECTION I: ASSESSING YOUR UNDERSTANDING

Activity A *Fill in the blanks.*

1. The term _____ is used to describe an irregular or erratic heart rhythm.

2. The ability of the cardiac muscle to initiate an electrical impulse is called _____.

3. The ability of the cardiac muscle to transmit electrical impulses is called _____.

4. The term _____ is used to describe the electrical stimulation of the heart.

5. The ventricles relax in the _____ stage of conduction.

6. _____ treats arrhythmias by destroying causative cells.

7. The total time for ventricular depolarization and repolarization is represented on an electrocardiogram (ECG) reading as the _____.

8. The PR interval on an ECG strip that reflects normal sinus rhythm would be between _____ and _____.

9. An arrhythmia common in normal hearts and described by patients as "my heart skipped a beat" is _____.

10. A "sawtooth" P wave is seen on an ECG strip with _____.

11. Sinus tachycardia occurs when the ventricular and atrial rates are greater than _____.

Activity B *Briefly answer the following.*

1. What are the four sites of origin for impulses that are used to name arrhythmias?

_____
_____

2. Describe the normal electrical conduction through the heart.

_____
_____
_____

3. Name five causes of sinus tachycardia.

_____
_____

4. What rate and rhythm are characteristic of ventricular tachycardia?

_____
_____

5. List three potential collaborative problems that a nurse would choose for a patient with arrhythmias.

_____
_____
_____

6. What is the difference between cardioversion and defibrillation?

_____
_____
_____

7. How are the electrode paddles placed on the patient's chest for defibrillation?

_____
_____
_____

8. Describe the difference between on-demand and fixed-rate or asynchronous pacemaker.

_____
_____
_____

9. Describe the "maze procedure" used in cardiac conduction surgery.

_____
_____
_____

Activity C *Match the description in Column II with the key term in Column I.*

Column I
___ **1.** P wave
___ **2.** QRS complex
___ **3.** T wave
___ **4.** U wave
___ **5.** PR interval
___ **6.** ST segment
___ **7.** QT interval
___ **8.** TP interval

Column II
a. End of T wave to beginning of next P wave
b. Atrial depolarization
c. Normal range 0.32 to 0.40
d. Ventricular depolarization
e. Early ventricular depolarization
f. Ventricular repolarization
g. Normal range 0.12 to 0.20
h. Repolarization of the Purkinje fibers

SECTION II: APPLYING YOUR KNOWLEDGE

Graph Analysis

Analyze the following ECG graphs and answer the questions.

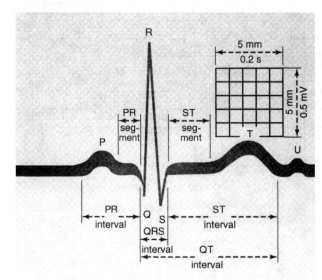

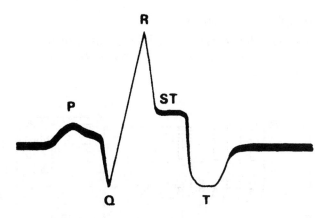

Each small box on the graph above represents 0.04 seconds on the horizontal axis and 1 mm or 0.1 mV on the vertical axis. The PR interval is measured from the beginning of the P wave to the beginning of the QRS complex; the QRS complex is measured from the beginning of the Q wave to the end of the S wave; the QT interval is measured from the beginning of the Q wave to the end of the T wave.

1. Look at the above graphic recording of cardiac electrical activity. For each action below, choose a wave deflection that corresponds to it, and write the appropriate letter or letters on the line provided:

   a. ____ ventricular muscle repolarization

   b. ____ time required for an impulse to travel through the atria and the conduction system to the Purkinje fibers

   c. ____ atrial muscle depolarization

   d. ____ ventricular muscle depolarization

   e. ____ early ventricular repolarization of the ventricles

2. Consider the above graphic recording, and identify three alterations that are consistent with myocardial ischemia and infarction hours to days after the attack:

   a. _____

   b. _____

   c. _____

Graphic Recordings

Analyze the graphic recording for each of the following arrhythmias and describe the altered deflection.

1.

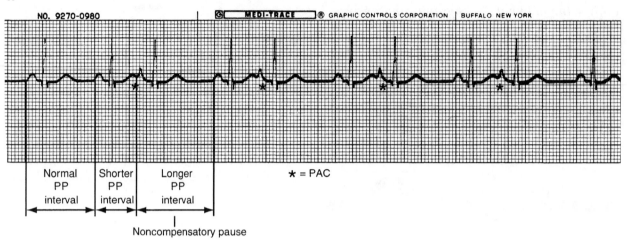

Premature atrial complexes (PACs)

_____

_____

_____

2.

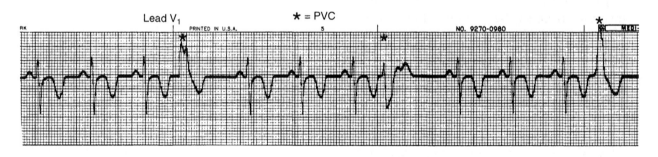

Multifocal PVCs in quadrigeminy

_____

_____

_____

3.

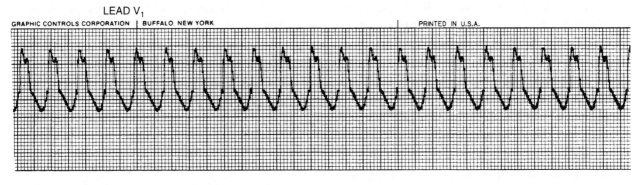

LEAD V₁

Ventricular tachycardia

_____

_____

_____

Activity E *Consider the scenario and answer the questions.*

CASE STUDY: Permanent Pacemaker

Mr. Woo, age 58, is scheduled for permanent pacemaker insertion as treatment for a tachyarrhythmia that does not respond to medication therapy. He is scheduled for an insertion of a permanent pacemaker.

1. Mr. Woo's pacemaker is set at 72 bpm. His heart rate is 76 bpm. Is this expected? Explain the rationale for your answer.

_____

_____

2. For which potential complications will the nurse monitor?

_____

3. What common initial postoperative complication will the nurse monitor for after Mr. Woo has an insertion of a permanent pacemaker?

_____

4. What will the nurse document about Mr. Woo's pacemaker on the EMR?

_____

_____

5. Which nursing interventions and expected patient outcomes will be used to meet the outcomes of patient care?

_____

_____

_____

_____

SECTION III: PRACTICING FOR NCLEX

Activity F *Answer the following questions.*

1. A patient comes to the emergency department reporting chest pain after using cocaine. The nurse assesses the patient and obtains vital signs with results as follows: blood pressure 140/92, heart rate 128, respiratory rate 26, and an oxygen saturation of 98%. Which rhythm on the monitor will the nurse view?

a. Sinus bradycardia

b. Ventricular tachycardia

c. Normal sinus rhythm

d. Sinus tachycardia

2. The nurse is attempting to determine the ventricular rate and rhythm of a patient's telemetry strip. Which will the nurse examine to determine this part of the analysis?
   a. PP interval
   b. QT interval
   c. RR interval
   d. TP interval

3. The nurse is monitoring a patient in the postanesthesia care unit (PACU) following a coronary artery bypass graft, observing a regular ventricular rate of 82 bpm and "sawtooth" P waves with an atrial rate of approximately 300 bpm. How does the nurse interpret this rhythm?
   a. Atrial fibrillation
   b. Atrial flutter
   c. Ventricular tachycardia
   d. Ventricular fibrillation

4. A patient with mitral valve stenosis and coronary artery disease (CAD) is in the telemetry unit diagnosed with pneumonia. The nurse assesses a 6-second rhythm strip and determines that the ventricular rhythm is highly irregular at 88, with no discernible P waves. Which is the nurse's analysis of this rhythm?
   a. Atrial flutter
   b. Ventricular flutter
   c. Sinus tachycardia
   d. Nonparoxysmal junctional tachycardia

5. A patient with hypertension has newly diagnosed atrial fibrillation. Which medication does the nurse anticipate administering to prevent the complication of atrial thrombi?
   a. Adenosine
   b. Amiodarone
   c. Warfarin
   d. Atropine

6. The nurse in the intensive care unit (ICU) hears an alarm sound in the patient's room. Arriving in the room, the patient is unresponsive, without a pulse, and a flat line on the monitor. Which is the first action by the nurse?
   a. Begin cardiopulmonary resuscitation (CPR).
   b. Administer epinephrine.
   c. Administer atropine 0.5 mg.
   d. Defibrillate with 360 J (monophasic defibrillator).

7. The nurse is defibrillating a patient in ventricular fibrillation with paddles on a monophasic defibrillator. How much paddle pressure should the nurse apply when defibrillating?
   a. 5 to 10 lb
   b. 10 to 15 lb
   c. 15 to 20 lb
   d. 20 to 25 lb

8. A patient with dilated cardiomyopathy is having frequent episodes of ventricular fibrillation. Which choice would be best to sense and terminate these episodes?
   a. Implantable cardioverter defibrillator (ICD)
   b. Pacemaker
   c. Atropine
   d. Epinephrine

9. The nurse is observing the monitor of a patient with a first-degree atrioventricular (AV) block. Which characteristics of this rhythm does the nurse identify?
   a. A variable heart rate, usually fewer than 60 bpm
   b. An irregular rhythm
   c. Delayed conduction, producing a prolonged PR interval
   d. P waves hidden with the QRS complex

10. The nurse is assessing vital signs in a patient with a permanent pacemaker. Which will the nurse document about the pacemaker?

    a. Date and time of insertion

    b. Location of the generator

    c. Model number

    d. Pacer rate

11. A patient has had an ICD inserted. Which will the nurse be sure to include in the education of this patient prior to discharge? (Select all that apply.)

    a. Avoid magnetic fields such as metal detection booths.

    b. Call for emergency assistance if feeling dizzy.

    c. Record events that trigger a shock sensation.

    d. The patient may have a throbbing pain that is normal.

    e. The patient will have to schedule monthly chest x-rays to make sure the device is patent.

12. A patient is 2 days postoperative after having a permanent pacemaker inserted. The nurse observes that the patient is having continuous hiccups as the patient states, "I thought this was normal." Which does the nurse identify is occurring with this patient?

    a. Fracture of the lead wire

    b. Lead wire dislodgment

    c. Faulty generator

    d. Sensitivity is too low

13. A patient who had a myocardial infarction is experiencing severe chest pain and alerts the nurse. The nurse begins the assessment but suddenly the patient becomes unresponsive, no pulse, with the monitor showing a rapid, disorganized ventricular rhythm. Which will the nurse interpret this rhythm to be?

    a. Ventricular tachycardia

    b. Atrial fibrillation

    c. Third-degree heart block

    d. Ventricular fibrillation

14. A patient has a persistent third-degree heart block and has had several periods of syncope. Which priority treatment will the nurse prepare for the patient?

    a. Insertion of a pacemaker

    b. Administration of atropine

    c. Administration of epinephrine

    d. Insertion of an ICD

15. A patient has had several episodes of recurrent tachyarrhythmias over the last 5 months and medication therapy has not been effective. Which procedure will the nurse prepare the patient for?

    a. Insertion of an ICD

    b. Insertion of a permanent pacemaker

    c. Catheter ablation therapy

    d. Maze procedure

CHAPTER 23

Management of Patients with Coronary Vascular Disorders

Learning Outcomes

1. Describe the pathophysiology, clinical manifestations, and treatment of coronary vascular disorders including coronary atherosclerosis, angina pectoris, and myocardial infarction.
2. Use the nursing process as a framework for care of the patient with angina pectoris, with acute coronary syndrome, or who has undergone cardiac surgery.
3. Describe percutaneous coronary interventional and coronary artery revascularization procedures.
4. Identify the nursing care of a patient who has had a percutaneous coronary interventional procedure for treatment of coronary artery disease.

SECTION I: ASSESSING YOUR UNDERSTANDING

Activity A *Fill in the blanks.*

1. A thrombus is a dangerous complication of atherosclerosis because it can lead to _____ and _____.

2. A person at increased risk for heart disease is encouraged to stop _____ through any means possible.

3. _____ use by women who smoke is inadvisable because these medications significantly increase the risk for CAD and sudden cardiac death.

4. Hypertension is defined as blood pressure measurements _____ mm Hg on an average of two to three measurements obtained on two to three separate occasions.

5. The patient with suspected myocardial infarction (MI) should immediately receive _____, _____, _____, and _____.

6. The leading cause of death in the United States for men and women of all ethnic and racial groups is _____.

7. The most common cause of cardiovascular disease is _____.

8. The most frequently occurring sign of myocardial ischemia is _____.

9. _____ is known to be an inflammatory marker for cardiovascular risk, including acute coronary events and stroke.

10. Management of coronary heart disease requires a therapeutic range of cholesterol and lipoproteins. An acceptable blood level of total cholesterol is _____ with an LDL/HDL ratio of _____. The desired level of LDL should be _____, and the HDL level should be greater than _____. Triglycerides should be less than _____.

11. A _____ physical assessment is critical to detect complications and any change in patient status.

12. The key, diagnostic indicator for MI seen on an electrocardiogram (ECG) is _____.

13. The vessel most commonly used for coronary artery bypass grafting (CABG) is the _____.

14. A possible complication of rupture or hemorrhage of the lipid core into the plaque is _____.

Activity B *Briefly answer the following.*

1. List four modifiable risk factors that are considered major causes of coronary artery disease.

_____ _____

_____ _____

2. A positive diagnosis of metabolic syndrome occurs when three of the following six conditions are met:

_____ _____

_____ _____

_____ _____

3. List three collaborative problems for a patient with angina.

_____ _____

_____

4. List four symptoms seen in postpericardiotomy syndrome.

_____ _____

_____ _____

5. Describe an atheroma:

_____

_____

_____

6. What is the purpose of a percutaneous transluminal coronary angioplasty?

_____

_____

Activity C *Match the medication affecting lipoprotein metabolism in Column II with the associated classification in Column I.*

Column I

_____ 1. HMG-CoA reductase inhibitor

_____ 2. Nicotinic acid

_____ 3. Fibric acids

_____ 4. Bile acid sequestrants

_____ 5. Cholesterol absorption inhibitor

_____ 6. Omega-3 acid ethyl esters

Column II

a. Fish oil capsule

b. Fenofibrate

c. Colestipol

d. Ezetimibe

e. Niacin

f. Pravastatin

SECTION II: APPLYING YOUR KNOWLEDGE

Activity D *Consider the scenarios and answer the questions.*

CASE STUDY: Angina Pectoris

Mrs. Jones, a 64-year-old retired secretary, is admitted to the acute care unit for management of chest pain caused by angina pectoris.

1. The patient asks the nurse, "What is causing this pain?" What is the best response by the nurse?

_____

_____

2. The patient is diagnosed with chronic stable angina. The nurse can identify that her pain may follow what type of pattern?

_____

3. Mrs. Jones is prescribed nitroglycerin PRN for the treatment of chest pain. What is it important for the nurse to include when educating her regarding the action of nitroglycerin?

_____

_____

_____

4. Mrs. Jones was administered a nitroglycerin tablet at 10:00 AM, after her morning care without relief of chest pain. Another dose was administered 5 minutes later. Ten minutes later and still in pain, she calls the nurse and states that she is still having chest pain. What is the priority intervention by the nurse?

_____

_____

CASE STUDY: Decreased Myocardial Tissue Perfusion

Mr. Lillis, a 46-year-old bricklayer, is brought to the ED by ambulance with a suspected diagnosis of MI. He appears ashen, is diaphoretic, has a heart rate of 110 beats per minute (bpm), and reports severe chest pain.

1. The nurse is aware that there is a critical time period for this patient. When should the nurse be most vigilant in monitoring this patient?

_____

2. The nurse is interpreting the results of the ECG. What findings does the nurse understand are indicative of initial myocardial injury?

_____

3. The nurse evaluates a series of laboratory tests within the first few hours. What laboratory results are positive indicators of myocardial infarction (MI)?

_____

4. The nurse should closely monitor the patient for a complication of an MI that leads to sudden death during the first 48 hours. Which complication should the nurse monitor for?

_____

SECTION III: PREPARING FOR NCLEX

Activity E *Answer the following questions.*

1. The nurse is reviewing the results of a total cholesterol level for a patient who has been taking simvastatin. Which results indicate the medication is having the desired outcome?
   a. 160 to 190 mg/dL
   b. 210 to 240 mg/dL
   c. 250 to 275 mg/dL
   d. 280 to 300 mg/dL

2. The nurse is discussing risk factors for developing coronary artery disease (CAD) with a patient in the clinic. Which results would indicate that the patient is not at significant risk for the development of CAD?
   a. Cholesterol, 280 mg/dL
   b. Low-density lipoprotein (LDL), 160 mg/dL
   c. High-density lipoprotein (HDL), 80 mg/dL
   d. A ratio of LDL to HDL, 4.5 to 1.0

3. The nurse is educating a patient regarding a new prescription for propranolol. Which statement made by the patient indicates that further education is needed?
   a. "If I am not experiencing chest pain, I can discontinue the use of the propranolol."
   b. "Since I am diabetic, I need to monitor my glucose levels as prescribed."
   c. "This will help decrease the incidence of chest pain prior to exercises."
   d. "I may experience an increase in tiredness and dizziness when first starting the medication."

4. The nurse is educating the patient about the administration of nitroglycerin prior to being discharged from the hospital. Which information should the nurse include in the instructions?

   a. Take a nitroglycerin tablet and if the pain is not relieved, drive to the nearest emergency department.

   b. Take two nitroglycerin tablets, and if the pain is not relieved, go to the emergency department.

   c. Take a nitroglycerin tablet and repeat every 5 minutes if the pain is not relieved until a total of three are taken. If pain is not relieved, activate the emergency medical system.

   d. Take two nitroglycerin tablets every 10 minutes until a total of six tablets are taken. If pain is not relieved, activate the emergency medical system.

5. The nurse administers propranolol hydrochloride to a patient with a heart rate of 64 bpm. One hour later, the nurse observes the heart rate on the monitor to be 36 bpm. Which medication should the nurse prepare to administer to elevate the heart rate?

   a. Digoxin

   b. Atropine sulfate

   c. Protamine sulfate

   d. Sodium nitroprusside

6. The nurse is administering diltiazem to a patient who has symptomatic sinus tachycardia at a rate of 132 bpm. Which is the anticipated action of the drug for this patient?

   a. Decreases the sinoatrial node automaticity.

   b. Increases the atrioventricular node conduction.

   c. Increases the heart rate.

   d. Creates a positive inotropic effect.

7. Which ECG finding(s) does the nurse observe in a patient who has had a myocardial infarction (MI)? (Select all that apply.)

   a. An absent P wave

   b. An abnormal Q wave

   c. T-wave inversion

   d. ST-segment elevation

   e. Prolonged PR interval

8. The nurse is educating a patient diagnosed with angina pectoris about the difference between the pain of angina and a myocardial infarction (MI). How will the nurse describe the pain that may be experienced during an MI? (Select all that apply.)

   a. It is relieved by rest and inactivity.

   b. It is substernal in location.

   c. It is sudden in onset and prolonged in duration.

   d. It is viselike and radiates to the shoulders and arms.

   e. It subsides after taking nitroglycerin.

9. The nurse is reviewing the laboratory results for a patient having a suspected myocardial infarction (MI). Which cardiac-specific isoenzyme does the nurse observe for myocardial cell damage?

   a. Alkaline phosphatase

   b. Creatine kinase (CK-MB)

   c. Myoglobin

   d. Troponin

10. The nurse is caring for a patient who is experiencing chest pain associated with a myocardial infarction (MI). Which medication will the nurse administer intravenously to reduce pain and anxiety?

    a. Meperidine hydrochloride

    b. Hydromorphone hydrochloride

    c. Morphine sulfate

    d. Codeine sulfate

11. A patient with coronary artery disease (CAD) is having a cardiac catheterization. Which indicator is present for the patient to have a percutaneous transluminal coronary angioplasty (PTCA)?

    a. The patient has compromised left ventricular function.

    b. The patient has had angina longer than 3 years.

    c. The patient has at least a 70% occlusion of a major coronary artery.

    d. The patient has an ejection fraction of 65%.

12. The nurse is assessing a postoperative patient who had a percutaneous transluminal coronary angioplasty (PTCA). Which potential complications should the nurse monitor for? (Select all that apply.)

    a. Abrupt closure of the artery

    b. Arterial dissection

    c. Coronary artery vasospasm

    d. Aortic dissection

    e. Nerve root pressure

13. A patient in the recovery room after cardiac surgery begins to have extremity paresthesia, peaked T waves, and mental confusion. Which type of electrolyte imbalance should the nurse assess the patient for?

    a. Calcium

    b. Magnesium

    c. Potassium

    d. Sodium

14. A patient has had cardiac surgery and is being monitored in the intensive care unit (ICU). Which complication should the nurse monitor for that is associated with an alteration in preload?

    a. Cardiac tamponade

    b. Elevated central venous pressure

    c. Hypertension

    d. Hypothermia

15. A patient who had coronary artery bypass graft (CABG) is exhibiting signs of cardiac failure. Which nursing actions would be appropriate for this patient? (Select all that apply.)

    a. Administration of furosemide

    b. Administration of digoxin

    c. Administration of milrinone

    d. Preparation of the patient for dialysis

    e. Administration of nitroprusside

Management of Patients with Structural, Infectious, and Inflammatory Cardiac Disorders

Learning Outcomes

1. Define valvular disorders of the heart and describe the pathophysiology, clinical manifestations, as well as the medical and nursing management of patients with mitral and aortic disorders.
2. Differentiate between the different types of cardiac valve repair and replacement procedures used to treat valvular problems and the care needed by patients who undergo these procedures.
3. Identify the pathophysiology, clinical manifestations, as well as the medical and nursing management of patients with cardiomyopathies.
4. Describe the pathophysiology, clinical manifestations, as well as the medical and nursing management of patients with infections of the heart.
5. Use the nursing process as a framework for care of the patient with a cardiomyopathy and the patient with pericarditis.

SECTION I: ASSESSING YOUR UNDERSTANDING

Activity A *Fill in the blanks.*

1. Often the first and only sign of mitral valve prolapse is an extra heart sound, referred to as a _____.

2. Mitral regurgitation involves blood flowing back from the _____ into the _____ during systole.

3. When valves do not open completely, a condition called _____ occurs, and blood flow through the valve is reduced.

4. _____ is beneficial for mitral valve stenosis in younger patients, for aortic valve stenosis in older patients, and for patients with complex medical conditions that place them at high risk for complications of more extensive surgical procedures.

5. Surgical repair of chordae tendineae is called _____.

6. If arrhythmias occur with mitral valve prolapse, the nurse advises the patient to avoid _____, _____, and _____.

7. A nurse, using auscultation to identify aortic regurgitation, would place the stethoscope _____ and would expect to hear _____.

8. With aortic stenosis, the patient should receive _____ to prevent endocarditis.

9. Prompt treatment of streptococcal pharyngitis with _____ can prevent almost all attacks of _____.

10. Infective endocarditis is usually caused by the following bacteria: _____, _____, _____, and _____.

11. Patients with myocarditis may be extremely sensitive to _____ (medication) and should therefore be monitored for serum levels to prevent _____.

Activity B *Briefly answer the following.*

1. Describe the basic dysfunction of mitral valve prolapse.

_____

_____

_____

2. List four potential complications or collaborative problems for patients with cardiomyopathy.

_____

_____

3. Identify five common indicators for heart transplantation.

_____

_____

4. Briefly describe the pathophysiology of infective endocarditis, beginning with the formation of vegetation.

_____

_____

_____

5. Briefly describe the pathophysiology of myocarditis.

_____

_____

_____

_____

6. Identify the anatomic landmark for auscultation of a pericardial friction rub.

_____

_____

7. List six underlying causes of pericarditis.

_____

_____

Activity C *Match the pathophysiology listed in Column II with the valvular disorder listed in Column I.*

Column I

_____ **1.** Mitral valve prolapse

_____ **2.** Mitral stenosis

_____ **3.** Mitral regurgitation

_____ **4.** Aortic valve stenosis

_____ **5.** Aortic regurgitation

Column II

a. Leaflet malformation prevents complete closure during systole.

b. Can be caused by rheumatic endocarditis.

c. Characterized by a significantly widened pulse pressure.

d. Blood flows back from the left ventricle into the left atrium during systole.

e. Thickening and contracture of mitral valve cusps.

SECTION II: APPLYING YOUR KNOWLEDGE

Activity D *Consider the scenarios and answer the questions.*

CASE STUDY: Infective Endocarditis

Mr. Fontana, a 60-year-old account executive, is admitted to the hospital with a diagnosis of infective endocarditis and a history of mitral valve prolapse. When performing an assessment, the patient reports to the nurse a loss of appetite, joint pain, intermittent fever, and a 4.54-kg weight loss in the past 2 months.

1. While examining Mr. Fontana's eyes during the admission assessment, the nurse assesses conjunctival hemorrhages with pale centers. How will the nurse document this finding?

   _____

2. The nurse is assessing the patient for central nervous system (CNS) manifestations of the infectious disease. What symptoms should the nurse report as significant?

   _____

   _____

   _____

3. The nurse receives the blood culture results and notes that the *Streptococcus viridans* organism has been identified. How long does the nurse anticipate that the patient will remain on antibiotic intravenous infusion?

   _____

CASE STUDY: Acute Pericarditis

Mr. Russell is a 46-year-old construction worker who developed symptoms of acute pericarditis secondary to a viral infection. The patient reports pain in the pericardium as demonstrated by pointing to the site. The nurse auscultates a friction rub when performing the physical assessment.

1. The patient is experiencing pericardial pain. To alleviate this discomfort, what position will the nurse assist the patient with maintaining?

   _____

   _____

2. When planning Mr. Russell's care, what are the patient outcomes that will be developed for the management of the patient's pericarditis?

   _____

   _____

   _____

3. The nurse is auscultating Mr. Russell's chest for a pericardial friction rub. Where will the nurse auscultate in order to locate the rub?

   _____

SECTION III: PRACTICING FOR NCLEX

Activity E *Answer the following questions.*

1. A patient at the clinic describes shortness of breath, periods of feeling "lightheaded," and feeling fatigued despite a full night's sleep. The nurse obtains vital signs and auscultates a systolic click. Which will the nurse suspect from the assessment findings?

   a. Mitral valve prolapse

   b. Mitral regurgitation

   c. Aortic stenosis

   d. Aortic regurgitation

2. The nurse is educating a patient about the care related to a new diagnosis of mitral valve prolapse. Which statement made by the patient demonstrates understanding of the education?

   a. "I will avoid caffeine, alcohol, and smoking."

   b. "I will take antibiotics before getting my teeth cleaned."

   c. "I shouldn't get a tattoo but I can get my tongue pierced."

   d. "This disorder will progress and I will need a heart transplant."

3. The nurse is auscultating the heart sounds of a patient with mitral stenosis. The pulse rhythm is weak and irregular. Which rhythm does the nurse identify on the electrocardiogram (ECG)?

   a. First-degree atrioventricular block

   b. Ventricular tachycardia

   c. Atrial fibrillation

   d. Sinus arrhythmia

4. The nurse is performing an assessment for a patient with suspected mitral valve regurgitation. Which type of murmur does the nurse correlate with this diagnosis?

   a. Mitral click

   b. High-pitched blowing sound at the apex

   c. Low-pitched diastolic murmur at the apex

   d. Diastolic murmur at the left sternal border

5. The nurse is assessing a patient and palpates a pulse with quick, sharp strokes that suddenly collapse. The nurse determines that this type of pulse is diagnostic for which disorder?

   a. Mitral insufficiency

   b. Tricuspid insufficiency

   c. Tricuspid stenosis

   d. Aortic regurgitation

6. A patient has been diagnosed with fused mitral leaflets, causing a backward flow of blood. Which type of procedure will the nurse prepare the patient for that is commonly performed for this issue?

   a. Annuloplasty

   b. Commissurotomy

   c. Valve replacement

   d. Chordoplasty

7. A patient has received a heterograft or a tricuspid valve replacement. Which statement made by the patient demonstrates understanding of the valve replacement?

   a. "The xenograft will last for the rest of my life, at least 20 years."

   b. "I will have to take an antirejection drug for the duration of the xenograft."

   c. "I will not take long-term anticoagulation because I want to get pregnant."

   d. "My valve comes from a cadaver."

8. A patient is admitted with suspected cardiomyopathy. Which diagnostic test would be most helpful with the identification of this disorder?

   a. Serial enzyme studies

   b. Cardiac catheterization

   c. Echocardiogram

   d. Phonocardiogram

9. A patient has had a successful heart transplant for end-stage heart disease. Which immunosuppressant will be necessary for this patient to take to prevent rejection?

   a. Nifedipine

   b. Cyclosporine

   c. Verapamil

   d. Vancomycin

10. A patient is diagnosed with rheumatic endocarditis. Which bacterium is the nurse aware causes this inflammatory response?

    a. Group A, beta-hemolytic streptococcus

    b. *Pseudomonas aeruginosa*

    c. *Serratia marcescens*

    d. *Staphylococcus aureus*

11. A patient admitted to the hospital is suspected to have rheumatic endocarditis. Which diagnostic test does the nurse prepare the patient for?

    a. Throat culture

    b. Echocardiogram

    c. Electrocardiogram

    d. Complete blood count

12. The nurse identifies that a patient has a characteristic symptom of pericarditis. Which symptom does the nurse recognize as significant for this diagnosis?

    a. Dyspnea

    b. Constant chest pain

    c. Fatigue lasting more than 1 month

    d. Uncontrolled restlessness

13. A patient is admitted with a diagnosis of pericarditis. When reviewing the prescriptions for the patient, which medication will the nurse question and discuss with the health care provider?

    a. Colchicine

    b. Indomethacin

    c. Ibuprofen

    d. Prednisone

14. The nurse is caring for a patient diagnosed with pericarditis. Which serious complication should this patient be monitored for?

a. Cardiac tamponade

b. Decreased venous pressure

c. Hypertension

d. Left ventricular hypertrophy

15. The nurse is obtaining a history from a patient diagnosed with hypertrophic cardiomyopathy. Which information obtained from the patient is indicative of this form of cardiomyopathy?

a. A history of alcoholism

b. A history of amyloidosis

c. A parent has the same disorder

d. A long-standing history of hypertension

CHAPTER 25

Management of Patients with Complications from Heart Disease

Learning Outcomes

1. Recognize the etiology, pathophysiology, and clinical manifestations of the different classifications of heart failure.
2. Describe the medical management, including recommended pharmacologic treatments, for patients with heart failure.
3. Use the nursing process as a framework for care of the patient with heart failure.
4. Identify additional heart disease disorders and medical and nursing management of patients with complications from heart disease.

SECTION I: ASSESSING YOUR UNDERSTANDING

Activity A *Fill in the blanks.*

1. Two factors that determine preload are
   _____ and _____.
   Two factors that determine afterload are
   _____ and _____.

2. Three noninvasive tests are used to assess cardiac hemodynamics: _____ for right ventricular preload, _____ for left ventricular afterload, and _____ for left ventricular preload.

3. The most common thromboembolitic problem among patients with heart failure is
   _____

4. The cough associated with left ventricular failure is initially _____ and
   _____.

5. Four common etiologic factors that cause myocardial dysfunction include
   _____, _____,
   _____, and _____.

6. Name three types of cardiomyopathy:
   _____, _____,
   and _____. Of these,
   _____ is the most common.

7. The primary clinical manifestations of pulmonary congestion in left-sided heart failure are
   _____, _____,
   _____, _____,
   and a probable _____.

8. The primary systemic clinical manifestations of right-sided heart failure are _____, _____, _____, _____, _____, and _____.

9. _____, _____, and _____ are three types of drugs that are the cornerstone therapy for systolic heart failure.

10. Coronary atherosclerosis results in tissue ischemia, which causes myocardial dysfunction, because _____ and _____ result from _____.

Activity B *Briefly answer the following.*

1. Decipher the formula CO = HR × SV.

_____

_____

2. Compare and contrast *preload* and *afterload*.

_____

_____

_____

_____

3. What four common side effects of diuretics should the nurse discuss with a patient?

_____   _____

_____   _____

4. What are some of the reasons that older adult patients are hospitalized with heart failure?

_____   _____

_____   _____

_____   _____

5. Which medication administered will block parasympathetic action, increase SA node automaticity and AV node conduction?

_____

Activity C *Match the type of ventricular heart failure listed in Column II with its associated pathophysiology in Column I.*

Column I	Column II
___ 1. Fatigability	a. Left-sided heart failure
___ 2. Dependent edema	b. Right-sided heart failure
___ 3. Pulmonary congestion predominates	
___ 4. Distended neck veins	
___ 5. Ascites	
___ 6. Dyspnea from fluid in alveoli	
___ 7. Orthopnea	
___ 8. Hepatomegaly	
___ 9. Cough that may be blood tinged	
___ 10. Nocturia	

SECTION II: APPLYING YOUR KNOWLEDGE

Activity D *Consider the scenario and answer the questions.*

CASE STUDY: Pulmonary Edema

Mr. Wolman is to be discharged from the hospital to home. He is 79 years old, lives with his wife, and has just recovered from mild pulmonary edema secondary to congestive heart failure.

1. What would the rationale be for the nurse advising Mr. Wolman to rest frequently at home?

_____

_____

2. What position will the nurse inform the patient to sleep in when he goes home? Why?

_____

_____

3. Mr. Wolman will be discharged with a prescription of digoxin 0.25 mg once daily. What education will the nurse include regarding symptoms of toxicity?

_____

_____

4. Mr. Wolman also takes furosemide (40 mg) twice a day. What foods will the nurse suggest that are supplements for potassium?

_____

SECTION III: PRACTICING FOR NCLEX

Activity E *Answer the following questions.*

1. The nurse is assessing a patient who reports no symptoms of heart failure at rest but is symptomatic with increased physical activity. Under which New York Heart Association classification does the nurse understand this patient is categorized?

   a. I

   b. II

   c. III

   d. IV

2. The nurse observes that a patient has 2+ pitting edema in the lower extremities. Which will this indicate to the nurse regarding fluid retention?

   a. A weight gain of 4 lb

   b. A weight gain of 6 lb

   c. A weight gain of 8 lb

   d. A weight gain of 10 lb

3. A patient has been experiencing an increase in shortness of breath and fatigue. The health care provider has prescribed a diagnostic test in order to determine which type of heart failure the patient is having. Which diagnostic test does the nurse prepare the patient for?

   a. A chest x-ray

   b. An echocardiogram

   c. An electrocardiogram

   d. A ventriculogram

4. A patient is seen in the emergency department (ED) with heart failure secondary to dilated cardiomyopathy. Which key diagnostic test does the nurse assess to determine the severity of the patient's heart failure?

   a. Blood urea nitrogen (BUN)

   b. Complete blood count (CBC)

   c. B-type natriuretic peptide (BNP)

   d. Serum electrolytes

5. A patient has missed two doses of digitalis. Which laboratory results would indicate to the nurse that the patient is within therapeutic range?

   a. 0.25 mg/mL

   b. 4.0 mg/mL

   c. 2.0 mg/mL

   d. 3.2 mg/mL

6. A patient is admitted to the intensive care unit (ICU) with left-sided heart failure. Which clinical manifestations correlate with the left-sided heart failure identified by the nurse when performing an assessment? (Select all that apply.)

   a. Jugular vein distention

   b. Ascites

   c. Pulmonary crackles

   d. Dyspnea

   e. Cough

7. The nurse is assigned to care for a patient with heart failure. Which classification of medication does the nurse administer that will improve symptoms as well as increase survival?

   a. Angiotensin-converting enzyme inhibitor (ACE)

   b. Calcium channel blocker

   c. Diuretic

   d. Bile acid sequestrants

8. A patient taking an ACE inhibitor has developed a dry, hacking cough. Because of this side effect, the patient no longer wants to take that medication. Which medication having similar hemodynamic effects does the nurse identify the health care provider will likely prescribe?

   a. Valsartan

   b. Furosemide

   c. Metoprolol

   d. Isosorbide dinitrate

9. A patient with severe pulmonary edema is intubated by the respiratory therapist. Which priority action by the nurse will assist in the confirmation of tube placement in the proper position in the trachea?

   a. Observe for mist in the endotracheal tube.

   b. Listen for breath sounds over the epigastrium.

   c. Call for a chest x-ray.

   d. Attach a pulse oximeter probe and obtain values.

10. A patient is prescribed an aldosterone antagonist for the treatment of heart failure. Which finding by the nurse indicates that the medication will be withheld and the health care provider notified?

    a. A BUN of 9 mg/dL

    b. A hemoglobin level of 14.6 g/dL

    c. A potassium level of 3.8 mEq/L

    d. A creatinine level of 3.2 mg/dL

11. The nurse hears the alarm sound on the telemetry monitor and observes a flat line. The patient is found unresponsive, without a pulse, and no respiratory effort. Which action will the nurse perform first?

    a. Administer epinephrine 1:10,000 10-mL IV push.

    b. Deliver breaths with a bag-valve mask.

    c. Defibrillate the patient with 360 J.

    d. Call for help and begin chest compressions.

12. The nurse is preparing to administer furosemide to a patient with heart failure. Which action(s) will the nurse perform prior to administering the medication? (Select all that apply.)

    a. Check the potassium level.

    b. Assess for signs of volume depletion.

    c. Monitor the creatinine level.

    d. Assess lung sounds.

    e. Check the AST and ALT levels.

13. The nurse is preparing to administer hydralazine and isosorbide dinitrate. When obtaining vital signs, the nurse notes that the blood pressure is 90/60 mm Hg. Which is the priority action by the nurse?

    a. Hold the medication and call the health care provider.

    b. Administer the medication and check the blood pressure in 30 minutes.

    c. Administer a saline bolus of 250 mL and then administer the medication.

    d. Administer the hydralazine and hold the isosorbide dinitrate.

14. A patient seen in the clinic has been diagnosed with stage A heart failure (according to the staging classification of the American College of Cardiology [ACC]). Which education will the nurse provide to this patient?

    a. Information about ACE inhibitors and risk factor reduction

    b. Information about diuretic therapy and risk factor reduction

    c. Information about beta-blockers, ACE inhibitors, and diuretics

    d. Information about implantable cardioverter/defibrillators

15. The health care provider writes orders for a patient to receive an angiotensin II receptor blocker for treatment of heart failure. Which medication does the nurse administer?

    a. Digoxin

    b. Valsartan

    c. Metolazone

    d. Carvedilol

Assessment and Management of Patients with Vascular Disorders and Problems of Peripheral Circulation

Learning Outcomes

1. Identify anatomic and physiologic factors that affect peripheral blood flow and tissue oxygenation.
2. Apply assessment parameters appropriate for determining the status of peripheral circulation.
3. Use the nursing process as a framework for care of the patient with arterial and venous disorders.
4. Compare the pathophysiology, clinical manifestations, management, and prevention of diseases of the arteries.
5. Describe the pathophysiology, clinical manifestations, management, and prevention of venous thromboembolism, venous insufficiency, leg ulcers, and varicose veins.
6. Describe the pathophysiology, clinical manifestations, and management of lymphatic disorders, and cellulitis.

SECTION I: ASSESSING YOUR UNDERSTANDING

Activity A *Fill in the blanks.*

1. Arterioles resist blood flow by altering their diameter, and are often referred to as _____.

2. The hallmark symptom of peripheral arterial occlusive disease is _____.

3. _____ is a sensitive marker of cardiovascular inflammation, both systemically and locally.

4. Venous stasis, postthrombotic syndrome, is characterized by _____, _____, _____, and _____.

5. The strongest risk factor for the development of atherosclerotic lesions is _____.

143

Activity B *Briefly answer the following.*

1. Which six clinical symptoms are associated with acute arterial embolism, known as the six Ps?

    _____ _____

    _____ _____

    _____ _____

2. List the classic triad (Virchow's) of factors associated with the development of venous thromboembolism.

    _____

    _____

3. What is the most important factor in regulating the caliber of blood vessels, which determines resistance to flow?

    _____

    _____

    _____

4. Describe the etiology of pain associated with the condition known as *intermittent claudication*.

    _____

    _____

    _____

5. Describe the clinical picture of a patient presenting with a dissecting thoracic aortic aneurysm.

    _____

    _____

6. In what ways can patients with peripheral vascular disease maintain foot and leg care?

    _____

    _____

7. Identify four major complications of venous thrombosis.

    _____

    _____

Activity C *Match the type of vessel insufficiency listed in Column II with its associated symptom listed in Column I.*

Column I

____ **1.** Intermittent claudication

____ **2.** Paresthesia

____ **3.** Dependent rubor

____ **4.** Cold, pale extremity

____ **5.** Ulcers of lower legs and ankles

____ **6.** Muscle fatigue and cramping

____ **7.** Diminished or absent pulses

____ **8.** Reddish-blue discoloration with dependency

Column II

a. Arterial insufficiency

b. Venous insufficiency

SECTION II: APPLYING YOUR KNOWLEDGE

Activity D *Consider the scenario and answer the questions.*

CASE STUDY: Peripheral Arterial Occlusive Disease

Fred Dunst, a 43-year-old construction worker, has a history of hypertension. He smokes two packs of cigarettes a day, is concerned about the possibility of being unemployed due to recent company layoffs, and has difficulty coping with stress. His current concern is calf pain during minimal exercise, which decreases with rest and has occurred for 1 month.

1. What is the hallmark symptom of peripheral arterial occlusion disease?

    _____

2. Which is the priority for preparing the patient for an ankle-brachial index (ABI) test?

    _____

3. The nurse is educating the patient about managing his condition. Which methods can the nurse suggest to increase arterial blood supply?

_____

_____

_____

4. What is the best method for the nurse to assess Fred's peripheral pulses to obtain consistent results with other health care practitioners?

_____

_____

_____

SECTION III: PRACTICING FOR NCLEX

Activity E *Answer the following questions.*

1. Which factor is most important in regulating the caliber of blood vessels, determining the resistance to flow?
   a. Hormonal secretion
   b. Independent arterial wall activity
   c. The influence of circulating chemicals
   d. The sympathetic nervous system

2. The nurse assesses a patient with suspected acute venous insufficiency. Which clinical manifestations indicates this condition to the nurse? (Select all that apply.)
   a. Cool and cyanotic skin
   b. Initial absence of edema
   c. Sharp pain that may be relieved by the elevation of the extremity
   d. Full superficial veins
   e. Brisk capillary refill of the toes

3. The nurse is caring for a patient with peripheral arterial insufficiency. Which interventions will the nurse suggest to help relieve leg pain during rest?
   a. Elevating the limb above heart level
   b. Lowering the limb so that it is dependent
   c. Massaging the limb after application of cold compresses
   d. Placing the limb in a plane horizontal to the body

4. A patient is exhibiting signs of a thoracic aortic aneurysm. Which diagnostic test(s) will the nurse prepare the patient for? (Select all that apply.)
   a. Computed tomography
   b. Transesophageal echocardiography
   c. X-ray
   d. Electroencephalogram
   e. Electrocardiogram (ECG)

5. A client is exhibiting signs of an abdominal aortic aneurysm. Which assessment data will the nurse correlate with a diagnosis of abdominal aortic aneurysm? (Select all that apply.)
   a. A pulsatile abdominal mass
   b. Low back pain
   c. Lower abdominal pain
   d. Decreased bowel sounds
   e. Diarrhea

6. A patient with impaired renal function is scheduled for a multidetector computer tomography (MDCT) scan. Which preprocedural medication will the nurse administer to this patient?
   a. Oral N-acetylcysteine
   b. Oral iodine
   c. Dipyridamole
   d. Epinephrine

7. A patient is having an angiography to detect the presence of an aneurysm. After the contrast is administered by the interventionist, the patient reports nausea and difficulty breathing. Which medication is a priority to administer at this time?
   a. Metoprolol
   b. Epinephrine
   c. Hydrocortisone
   d. Cimetidine

8. The nurse is assisting a patient with peripheral arterial disease to ambulate in the hallway. Which will the nurse include in the education of the patient during ambulation?

   a. "As soon as you feel pain, we will go back and elevate your legs."

   b. "If you feel pain during the walk, keep walking until the end of the hallway is reached."

   c. "Walk to the point of pain, rest until the pain subsides, then resume ambulation."

   d. "If you feel any discomfort, stop and we will use a wheelchair to take you back to your room."

9. The nurse is assessing a patient 2 days postoperatively, who is suspected of having deep vein obstruction. The patient reports pain in the left lower extremity and there is a 2-cm difference in the right and left leg circumference. Which intervention will the nurse provide to promote arterial flow to the lower extremities?

   a. Administer a diuretic to decrease the edema in the left lower extremity.

   b. Assist with active range of motion (ROM) exercises to the left lower extremity.

   c. Apply cool compresses to the left lower extremity.

   d. Apply a heating pad to the patient's abdomen.

10. The nurse is monitoring a patient taking anticoagulation therapy. Which therapeutic range of the international normalized ratio (INR) indicates that the medication is having the desired effect?

    a. 2.0 to 3.0

    b. 4.0 to 5.0

    c. 5.0 to 6.0

    d. 7.0 to 8.0

11. The nurse is caring for a patient who has started anticoagulant therapy with warfarin. When does the nurse determine that therapeutic benefits will begin?

    a. Within 12 hours

    b. Within the first 24 hours

    c. In 2 days

    d. In 3 to 5 days

12. The nurse is caring for a patient with venous insufficiency. Which will the nurse assess the patient's lower extremities for?

    a. Rubor

    b. Cellulitis

    c. Dermatitis

    d. Ulceration

13. The nurse is educating a patient with chronic venous insufficiency about prevention of complications related to the disorder. Which will the nurse include in the information given to the patient? (Select all that apply.)

    a. Avoid constricting garments.

    b. Elevate the legs above the heart level for 30 minutes every 2 hours.

    c. Sit as much as possible to rest the valves in the legs.

    d. Sleep with the foot of the bed elevated about 6 inches.

    e. Sit on the side of the bed and dangle the feet.

14. The health care provider prescribed a Tegapore dressing to treat a venous ulcer. Which will the nurse determine the ABI will be if the circulatory status is adequate?

    a. 0.10

    b. 0.25

    c. 0.35

    d. 0.50

15. A patient with diabetes is being treated for a wound on the lower extremity that has been present for 30 days. Which option for treatment is available to increase diffusion of oxygen to the hypoxic wound?

    a. Surgical debridement

    b. Enzymatic debridement

    c. Hyperbaric oxygen

    d. Vacuum-assisted closure device

16. The nurse is performing wound care for a patient with a necrotic sacral wound. The prescribed treatment is isotonic saline solution with fine mesh gauze and a dry dressing to cover. Which type of debridement is the nurse performing?

    a. Surgical debridement

    b. Nonselective debridement

    c. Enzymatic debridement

    d. Selective debridement

CHAPTER 27

Assessment and Management of Patients with Hypertension

Learning Outcomes

1. Compare and contrast normal blood pressure and various stages of hypertension.
2. Identify pathophysiologic processes implicated in the progression of hypertension.
3. Demonstrate the proper techniques to perform an assessment and discriminate between normal and abnormal findings identified in the patient with hypertension.
4. Discuss risk factors and treatment approaches for hypertension, including lifestyle modifications and medication therapy.
5. Use the nursing process as a framework for care of the patient with hypertension.
6. Describe hypertensive crises and their treatments.

SECTION I: ASSESSING YOUR UNDERSTANDING

Activity A *Fill in the blanks.*

1. Blood pressure is the product of _____ multiplied by _____.

2. Cardiac output is the product of _____ multiplied by _____.

3. Patients with _____ have blood pressure readings that would suggest a diagnosis of hypertension when they are in health care settings (e.g., clinics) but are within the normal ranges in other settings.

4. The target blood pressure for all adults with hypertension is less than _____ mm Hg, regardless of age, including older adults.

5. Angiotensin II causes _____, _____, _____, _____, and _____.

6. Patients and caregivers should be cautioned that antihypertensive medications might cause _____.

7. Patients may experience _____ if antihypertensive medications are suddenly stopped.

8. _____ and _____ are the two classes of hypertensive crisis that require immediate intervention.

Activity B *Briefly answer the following.*

1. What is the correlation between cigarette smoking and high blood pressure?

_____

_____

_____

2. What is a major concern for medical and nursing management of hypertension?

_____

3. What conditions may trigger a hypertensive emergency or urgency?

_____

_____

_____

4. For a patient diagnosed with hypertension, what lifestyle modifications will assist with the management of the disease process?

_____

_____

_____

5. A patient is instructed to adhere to a DASH diet. What does the diet recommend?

_____

_____

_____

Activity C *Match the hypertension medication listed in Column II with its associated action listed in Column I.*

Column I

___ **1.** Blocks reabsorption of sodium and water in kidneys

___ **2.** Stimulates alpha-2 adrenergic receptors

___ **3.** Stimulates dopamine and alpha-2 adrenergic receptors

___ **4.** Blocks beta-adrenergic receptors

___ **5.** Inhibits aldosterone

___ **6.** Displaces norepinephrine from storage sites

Column II

a. Propranolol

b. Guanfacine

c. Spironolactone

d. Furosemide

e. Methyldopa

f. Fenoldopam

SECTION II: APPLYING YOUR KNOWLEDGE

Activity D *Consider the scenario and answer the questions.*

CASE STUDY: Secondary Hypertension

Mrs. Georgia, a 30-year-old woman, is diagnosed as having secondary hypertension when serial blood pressure recordings show her average reading to be 170/100 mm Hg. Her hypertension is the result of renal dysfunction.

1. How will Mrs. Georgia's kidneys help maintain her hypertensive state?

_____

_____

2. The nurse informs Mrs. Georgia that she should make an appointment to see her ophthalmologist. Why is it important that she adhere to follow up with an ophthalmologist?

_____

_____

_____

3. Mrs. Georgia is prescribed furosemide 20 mg once every day. What education will the nurse provide her regarding the action of furosemide?

_____

_____

4. What health promotion strategies can the nurse suggest to Mrs. Georgia to reduce complications and improve disease outcomes?

_____

_____

_____

SECTION III: PRACTICING FOR NCLEX

Activity E *Answer the following questions.*

1. A patient is being seen at the clinic on a monthly basis for assessment of blood pressure. The patient has been checking the blood pressure at home and has reported a systolic pressure of 158 and a diastolic pressure of 64. Which do these findings indicate to the nurse?
   a. Isolated systolic hypertension
   b. Secondary hypertension
   c. Primary hypertension
   d. Hypertensive urgency

2. The nurse is assessing a patient with severe hypertension. When performing a focused assessment of the eyes, which may be observed related to the hypertension?
   a. Cataracts
   b. Glaucoma
   c. Retinal detachment
   d. Papilledema

3. A patient with hypertension is waking up several times a night to urinate. Which laboratory studies will the nurse assess that may indicate pathologic changes in the kidneys due to the hypertension? (Select all that apply.)
   a. Creatinine
   b. Blood urea nitrogen (BUN)
   c. Complete blood count (CBC)
   d. Urine for culture and sensitivity
   e. AST and ALT

4. A patient with long-standing hypertension is admitted to the hospital with hypertensive urgency. The health care provider orders a chest x-ray, which reveals an enlarged heart. Which diagnostic test does the nurse prepare the patient for to determine left ventricular enlargement?
   a. Cardiac catheterization
   b. Echocardiography
   c. Stress test
   d. Tilt table test

5. A patient with hypertension has maintained a blood pressure of 130/70 mm Hg for 1 year while reducing dietary sodium and taking hydrochlorothiazide and atenolol. Which treatment plan will the nurse educate the patient about?
   a. Continue the medication and reduce dietary sodium.
   b. Discontinue the hydrochlorothiazide and atenolol and continue to reduce sodium intake.
   c. Gradually reduce the hydrochlorothiazide and atenolol and continue reduction of sodium intake.
   d. Gradually reduce the atenolol and continue the hydrochlorothiazide.

6. A patient is taking amiloride and lisinopril for the treatment of hypertension. Which laboratory studies should the nurse monitor while the patient is taking these two medications together?
   a. Magnesium level
   b. Potassium level
   c. Calcium level
   d. Sodium level

7. A patient has severe coronary artery disease (CAD) and hypertension. Which medication prescription should the nurse consult with the health care provider about that is contraindicated for a patient with severe CAD?
   a. Clonidine
   b. Amiloride
   c. Bumetanide
   d. Methyldopa

8. A patient has been diagnosed with prehypertension and is encouraged to exercise regularly and begin a weight loss program. After which period of time does the nurse inform the patient to return for a follow-up visit?
   a. 2 months
   b. 6 months
   c. 1 year
   d. 2 years

9. The nurse is assessing the blood pressure for a patient with hypertension and does not hear an auscultatory gap. Which outcome may be documented in this circumstance?

   a. A low diastolic reading

   b. A high systolic pressure reading

   c. A normal reading

   d. A high diastolic or low systolic reading

10. The nurse is performing an assessment for a patient to determine the effects of hypertension on the heart and blood vessels. Which specific assessment data will assist in determining this complication? (Select all that apply.)

    a. Heart rate

    b. Respiratory rate

    c. Heart rhythm

    d. Character of apical and peripheral pulses

    e. Lung sounds

11. The nurse is planning the care of a patient admitted to the hospital with hypertension. Which objective will help to meet the needs of this patient?

    a. Lower and control the blood pressure without adverse effects and undue cost.

    b. Make sure that the patient adheres to the therapeutic medication regimen.

    c. Instruct the patient to enter a weight loss program and begin an exercise regimen.

    d. Schedule the patient for all follow-up visits and make phone calls to the home to ensure adherence.

12. A patient informs the nurse, "I can't adhere to the dietary sodium decrease that is required for the treatment of my hypertension." Which education will the nurse provide to the patient regarding this statement?

    a. If dietary sodium isn't restricted, the patient will be unable to control the blood pressure and will be at risk for stroke.

    b. The patient can speak to the health care provider about increasing the dosage of medication instead of reducing the added salt.

    c. It takes 2 to 3 months for the taste buds to adapt to changes in salt intake.

    d. The patient should use other methods of flavoring foods.

13. A patient is flying overseas for 1 week for business and packed antihypertensive medications in a suitcase. After arriving at the intended destination, the patient found that the luggage had been stolen. If the patient cannot take the medication, which condition becomes a concern?

    a. Isolated systolic hypertension

    b. Rebound hypertension

    c. Angina

    d. Left ventricular hypertrophy

14. A patient is brought to the emergency department reporting a "bad headache" and an increase in blood pressure. The blood pressure reading obtained by the nurse is 260/180 mm Hg. Which is the therapeutic goal for reduction of the mean blood pressure?

    a. Reduce the blood pressure by 20% to 25% within the first hour of treatment.

    b. Reduce the blood pressure to about 140/80 mm Hg.

    c. Rapidly reduce the blood pressure so the patient will not suffer a stroke.

    d. Reduce the blood pressure by 50% within the first hour of treatment.

15. A patient arrives at the clinic for a follow-up visit for treatment of hypertension. The nurse obtains a blood pressure reading of 180/110 mm Hg but finds no evidence of impending or progressive organ damage when performing the assessment on the patient. Which situation does the nurse identify this patient is experiencing?

    a. Hypertensive emergency

    b. Primary hypertension

    c. Secondary hypertension

    d. Hypertensive urgency

Hematologic Function

CHAPTER 28

Assessment of Hematologic Function and Treatment Modalities

Learning Outcomes

1. Describe hematopoiesis and the processes involved in maintaining hemostasis.
2. Discuss the significance of the health history to the assessment of hematologic health and specify the appropriate techniques utilized to perform a comprehensive physical assessment of hematologic function.
3. Explain the diagnostic tests and related nursing implications used to evaluate hematologic function.
4. Identify therapies for blood disorders, including nursing implications for the administration of blood components.

SECTION I: ASSESSING YOUR UNDERSTANDING

Activity A *Fill in the blanks.*

1. The volume of blood in humans is about _____ L.

2. Blood cell formation (hematopoiesis) occurs in the _____.

3. Red bone marrow activity is confined in adults to the _____, _____, _____, and _____.

4. The principal function of the erythrocyte, which is composed primarily of _____, is to _____.

5. Each 100 mL of blood should normally contain _____ g of hemoglobin.

6. Women of childbearing years need an additional _____ daily of iron to replace that loss during menstruation.

7. The nurse advises a patient who is iron deficient to take extra vitamin _____, which is known for increasing iron absorption.

8. Plasma proteins consist primarily of _____ and _____.

9. The two most common areas used for bone marrow aspirations in an adult are _____ and _____.

Activity B *Briefly answer the following.*

1. A patient sustaining a trauma is at risk for excess blood loss. Which protective mechanism is activated to prevent excess blood loss?

_____

_____

_____

2. Describe why the stroma of the bone marrow is important.

_____

_____

_____

3. Name five substances that the bone marrow requires for normal erythrocyte production, and describe what can result if any of these factors are deficient.

_____

_____

_____

_____

4. When the health care provider informs the nurse that the patient has a "shift to the left," what does this mean?

_____

_____

_____

5. Describe how natural killer (NK) cells serve as an important part of the body's immune defense system.

_____

_____

_____

_____

6. When the nurse must administer blood or blood components, what knowledge is required?

_____

_____

_____

Activity C *Match the key term listed in Column II with its associated definition listed in Column I.*

Column I

____ 1. The fluid portion of blood

____ 2. Another term for platelets

Column II

a. Bone marrow

b. Monocytes

c. Hemostasis

d. RES

Column I

____ 3. The mature form of white blood cells (WBCs)

____ 4. The process of continually replacing blood cells

____ 5. The site of blood cell formation

____ 6. Makes up 95% of the mass of the red blood cell (RBC)

____ 7. The ingestion and digestion of bacteria by neutrophils

____ 8. The largest classification of leukocytes

____ 9. A clotting factor present in plasma

____10. A plasma protein primarily responsible for the maintenance of fluid balance

____11. The site of activity for most macrophages

____12. The process of stopping bleeding from a severed blood vessel

____13. A protein that forms the basis of blood clotting

____14. Integral component of the immune system

____15. The term for red blood cell

____16. The letters used for the term reticuloendothelial system

____17. The balance between clot formation and clot dissolution

____18. A term used to describe T lymphocytes

Column II

e. Plasma

f. Phagocytosis

g. Lymphocytes

h. Albumin

i. T cells

j. Thrombocytes

k. Spleen

l. Neutrophils

m. Hemostasis

n. Erythrocyte

o. Hematopoiesis

p. Hemoglobin

q. Fibrinogen

r. Plasminogen

SECTION II: APPLYING YOUR KNOWLEDGE

Activity D *Consider the scenario and answer the questions.*

CASE STUDY: Blood Transfusion

Mr. Jerry has been admitted to the hospital with a diagnosis of gastrointestinal bleeding and has a hemoglobin of 8 g/dL. He has been type- and cross-matched for two units of packed RBCs and is to receive his first unit.

1. The nurse is performing a pretransfusion history. Which information will be obtained prior to the transfusion?

   _____

   _____

   _____

2. The nurse is preparing to administer one unit of packed RBCs to Mr. Jerry. What assessment will the nurse make prior to initiating the transfusion?

   _____

   _____

   _____

3. The nurse begins the transfusion of packed cells after obtaining vital signs. Fifteen minutes after the infusion begins, he informs the nurse that he is itching all over. How does the nurse respond?

   _____

   _____

SECTION III: PRACTICING FOR NCLEX

Activity E *Answer the following questions.*

1. The patient has a deficiency in the leukocyte responsible for cell-mediated immunity. Which findings in the white blood cell count will the nurse identify that correlate with this deficiency?
   a. Basophils
   b. Monocytes
   c. Plasma cells
   d. T lymphocytes

2. An older adult patient presents to the clinic reporting feeling "exhausted all the time." The nurse will assess which laboratory values that commonly associate with this patient's symptoms?
   a. WBC count
   b. RBC count
   c. Thrombocyte count
   d. Levels of plasma proteins

3. A nurse is caring for a patient having a bone marrow aspiration with biopsy. Which complication will the nurse monitor for?
   a. Hemorrhage
   b. Infection
   c. Shock
   d. Splintering of bone fragments

4. A patient with chronic kidney disease is identified as having anemia. Which laboratory test results will the nurse likely observe?
   a. Decreased level of erythropoietin
   b. Decreased total iron-binding capacity
   c. Increased mean corpuscular volume
   d. Increased reticulocyte count

5. A female patient has a hemoglobin of 6.4 g/dL and is preparing to have a blood transfusion. Why would it be important for the nurse to obtain information about the patient's history of pregnancy prior to the transfusion?
   a. A high number of pregnancies can increase the risk of reaction.
   b. If the patient has never been pregnant, it increases the risk of reaction.
   c. Obtaining information about gravidity and parity is routine information for all female patients.
   d. If the patient has been pregnant, she may have developed allergies.

6. A patient will need a blood transfusion for the replacement of blood loss from the gastrointestinal tract. The patient states, "That stuff isn't safe!" Which response by the nurse will be the best?

   a. "I agree that you should be concerned with the safety of the blood, but it is important that you have this transfusion."

   b. "The blood is carefully screened, so there is no possibility of you contracting any illness or disease from the blood."

   c. "I understand your concern. The blood is carefully screened but is not completely risk free."

   d. "You will have to decide if refusing the blood transfusion is worth the risk to your health."

7. A patient with chronic anemia has had many blood transfusions over the last 3 years. Which type of transfusion reaction will the nurse monitor for that is commonly found in patients who frequently receive blood transfusions?

   a. Allergic reactions

   b. Acute hemolytic reaction

   c. Circulatory overload

   d. Febrile nonhemolytic reactions

8. The nurse is administering a blood transfusion to a patient over 4 hours. After 2 hours, the patient reports chills and has a fever of 101°F, an increase from a previous temperature of 99.2°F. Which does the nurse identify the patient is experiencing?

   a. The patient is having an allergic reaction to the blood.

   b. The patient is experiencing vascular collapse.

   c. The patient is having decrease in tissue perfusion from a shock state.

   d. The patient is having a febrile nonhemolytic reaction.

9. The nurse is administering two units of packed RBCs to an older adult patient with a bleeding duodenal ulcer. The patient begins to experience difficulty breathing and the nurse assesses crackles in the lung bases, jugular vein distention, and an increase in blood pressure. Which action by the nurse is a priority? (Select all that apply.)

   a. Continue the infusion but slow the rate down.

   b. Place the patient in an upright position with the feet dependent.

   c. Administer diuretics as prescribed.

   d. Discontinue the transfusion.

   e. Administer oxygen.

10. A patient receiving plasma develops transfusion-related acute lung injury (TRALI) 4 hours after the transfusion. Which type of aggressive therapy will the patient receive to prevent death from the injury? (Select all that apply.)

    a. Performance of serial chest x-rays

    b. Supplemental oxygen

    c. Provision of intravenous fluid support

    d. Intubation and mechanical ventilation

    e. Intra-aortic balloon pump

11. A patient who has long-term packed RBC transfusions develops symptoms of iron toxicity that affect liver function. Which immediate treatment will the nurse prepare the patient for that may help prevent organ damage?

    a. Iron chelation therapy

    b. Oxygen therapy

    c. Therapeutic phlebotomy

    d. Anticoagulation therapy

12. A patient develops a hemolytic reaction to a blood transfusion. Which priority actions will the nurse perform? (Select all that apply.)
    a. Administer diphenhydramine.
    b. Begin iron chelation therapy.
    c. Obtain appropriate blood specimens.
    d. Collect a urine sample to detect hemoglobin.
    e. Document the reaction according to policy.

13. The nurse is preparing a patient for a bone marrow aspiration and biopsy from the site of the posterior superior iliac crest. Which position will the nurse place the patient in?
    a. Lateral position with one leg flexed
    b. Lithotomy position
    c. Supine with head of the bed elevated 30 degrees
    d. Jackknife position

14. A patient with chronic kidney disease has chronic anemia. Which pharmacologic alternative to blood transfusion may be used for this patient?
    a. GM-CSF
    b. Erythropoietin
    c. Eltrombopag
    d. Thrombopoietin

15. A patient is undergoing plateletpheresis at the outpatient clinic. Which does the nurse identify as the most likely clinical disorder the patient is being treated for?
    a. Essential thrombocythemia
    b. Extreme leukocytosis
    c. Sickle cell disease
    d. Renal transplantation

Management of Patients with Nonmalignant Hematologic Disorders

Learning Outcomes

1. Differentiate between hypoproliferative and hemolytic anemias and compare the physiologic mechanisms, clinical manifestations, medical management, and nursing interventions for each.
2. Describe the processes involved in neutropenia and lymphopenia and the principles involved in medical and nursing management of patients with these disorders.
3. Specify the etiologies and the medical and nursing management of patients with secondary polycythemias and bleeding and thrombotic disorders.
4. Use the nursing process as a framework for care of the patient with anemia, with sickle cell disease, or with disseminated intravascular coagulation.

SECTION I: ASSESSING YOUR UNDERSTANDING

Activity A *Fill in the blanks.*

1. _____ is a condition in which the hemoglobin concentration is lower than normal, reflecting the presence of fewer than the normal number of erythrocytes within the circulatory system.

2. A healthy person can often tolerate as much as a _____% gradual reduction in hemoglobin without pronounced symptoms or significant incapacity.

3. Complications of severe anemia include _____, _____, and _____.

4. The overall prevalence of anemia increases with age, from _____% in people aged 65 to 69, to _____% in people over age 85.

5. A _____ assessment should be performed for patients with known megaloblastic anemia.

6. _____ and _____ should not be taken with iron preparations, because they greatly diminish the absorption of iron.

7. _____ is a rare disease caused by a decrease in or damage to marrow stem cells, damage to the microenvironment within the marrow, or replacement of the marrow with fat.

8. Chronic use of _____ to reduce gastric acid production can inhibit B_{12} absorption, as can the use of _____ in managing diabetes.

9. Assessment of patients who have or are at risk for megaloblastic anemia includes inspection of the _____, _____, and _____.

10. _____ is a severe hemolytic anemia that results from inheritance of the sickle hemoglobin gene, which causes the hemoglobin molecule to be defective.

11. _____ is a controversial treatment strategy that treats DIC by interrupting the thrombosis process.

Activity B *Briefly answer the following.*

1. Name five factors that influence the development of anemia-associated symptoms.

_____

_____

_____

2. When the patient has anemia, what medical management goal will the nurse assist the patient and health care team in achieving?

_____

3. Describe how anemia impacts the older adult patient.

_____

_____

_____

4. When the nurse is educating the patient and family about a healthy diet for the treatment of iron deficiency anemia, what should be included?

_____

_____

_____

5. List the four most common causes of iron deficiency anemia in men and postmenopausal women.

_____

_____

6. What chemical agents may be responsible for producing bone marrow aplasia?

_____

_____

_____

7. What diagnostic findings are present in patients who have sickle cell trait versus those present in patients who have sickle cell disease?

_____

_____

_____

_____

8. Describe at least five types of situations in which the transfusion of red blood cells (RBCs) is highly effective.

_____

_____

_____

9. Which triggers may lead to the development of disseminated intravascular coagulation (DIC)?

_____

_____

_____

Activity C *Match the type of anemia in Column I with the classification in Column II. Answers will be used more than once.*

Column I

____ 1. Aplastic anemia

____ 2. Sickle cell disease

____ 3. Folic acid deficiency

____ 4. Thalassemia major

____ 5. Iron deficiency

____ 6. B$_{12}$ deficiency

Column II

a. Hypoproliferative anemias

b. Megaloblastic anemias

c. Hemolytic anemias

SECTION II: APPLYING YOUR KNOWLEDGE

Activity D *Consider the scenario and answer the questions.*

George is a 75-year-old patient with urosepsis being treated in the intensive care unit (ICU). The nurse assesses George and finds that he has blood in his urine and stool, and is oozing blood from his central line site and his gums.

1. What does the nurse suspect may be occurring with George?

   _____

2. What medications should the nurse avoid administering to George?

   _____

   _____

   _____

3. The nurse is monitoring George's vital signs every 15 minutes. What other monitoring is essential to include along with the vital signs?

   _____

   _____

4. What medication does the nurse anticipate infusing?

   _____

SECTION III: PRACTICING FOR NCLEX

Activity E *Answer the following questions.*

1. The nurse is assessing a patient who reports feeling "constantly tired and very weak." The patient reports a very sore tongue, and upon observing the patient's oral cavity, the nurse notices the tongue is beefy red. Which type of anemia do these findings correlate with?
   a. Iron deficiency anemia
   b. Megaloblastic anemia
   c. Sickle cell disease
   d. Aplastic anemia

2. The nurse observes a coworker eating ice frequently. The nurse encourages the coworker to have an examination and diagnostic workup with the health care provider because frequently eating ice may indicate which type of anemia?
   a. Iron deficiency anemia
   b. Megaloblastic anemia
   c. Sickle cell disease
   d. Aplastic anemia

3. The nurse is performing an assessment for a patient with anemia admitted to the hospital for the administration of blood transfusions. Why would the nurse need to include a nutritional assessment for this patient?
   a. It is part of the required assessment information.
   b. It is important for the nurse to determine what type of foods the patient will eat.
   c. It may indicate deficiencies in essential nutrients.
   d. It will determine what type of anemia the patient has.

4. The nurse is assessing a patient who is a strict vegetarian. Which type of anemia is this patient at greatest risk for?
   a. Iron deficiency anemia
   b. Aplastic anemia
   c. Megaloblastic anemia
   d. Sickle cell disease

5. A patient describes numbness in the arms and hands with a tingling sensation and frequent stumbling when walking. Which vitamin deficiency does the nurse identify may contribute to some of these symptoms?
   a. Thiamine
   b. Folate
   c. B_{12}
   d. Iron

6. The nurse is educating a patient with iron deficiency anemia about food sources high in iron and how to enhance the absorption of iron when eating these foods. Which can the nurse inform the patient will enhance the absorption?

   a. Eating calf's liver with a glass of orange juice

   b. Eating leafy green vegetables with a glass of water

   c. Eating apple slices with carrots

   d. Eating a steak with mushrooms

7. A patient with end-stage kidney disease (ESKD) develops anemia. When reviewing the laboratory studies, which finding is significant in this stage of anemia?

   a. Potassium level of 5.2 mEq/L

   b. Magnesium level of 2.5 mg/dL

   c. Calcium level of 9.4 mg/dL

   d. Creatinine level of 6 mg/100 mL

8. A patient with end-stage kidney disease (ESKD) is taking recombinant erythropoietin for the treatment of anemia. Which laboratory study will be obtained at least monthly related to this medication?

   a. Potassium level

   b. Creatinine level

   c. Hemoglobin level

   d. Folate levels

9. A patient who had gastric bypass surgery 3 years ago is experiencing fatigue. The patient takes pantoprazole for the treatment of frequent heartburn. Which type of anemia is this patient at risk for?

   a. Aplastic anemia

   b. Iron deficiency anemia

   c. Sickle cell disease

   d. Pernicious anemia

10. The nurse is preparing the patient for a test to determine the cause of vitamin B_{12} deficiency. The patient will receive a small oral dose of radioactive vitamin B_{12} followed by a large parenteral dose of nonradioactive B_{12}. Which test is the patient being prepared for?

    a. Bone marrow aspiration

    b. Schilling test

    c. Bone marrow biopsy

    d. Magnetic resonance imaging (MRI) study

11. Which patient assessed by the nurse is identified as most likely to be affected by sickle cell disease?

    a. A 14-year-old African American boy

    b. A 26-year-old Eastern European Jewish woman

    c. An 18-year-old Chinese woman

    d. A 28-year-old Israeli man

12. A patient with sickle cell disease, brought to the emergency department by a parent, has a fever of 101.6°F, heart rate of 116, a respiratory rate of 32, and bilateral wheezes. Which do these findings indicate to the nurse?

    a. Pneumocystis pneumonia

    b. Acute chest syndrome

    c. An exacerbation of asthma

    d. Pulmonary edema

13. A patient with sickle cell disease is to begin treatment with hydroxyurea. Which education does the nurse provide about the benefits of treatment with this medication? (Select all that apply.)

    a. Fewer painful episodes of sickle cell crisis

    b. Lower incidence of acute chest syndrome

    c. Decreased need for blood transfusions

    d. Decreased need for other analgesic medications

    e. Ability to reverse the damage done from sickling of cells

14. A patient with sickle cell disease comes to the emergency department reporting severe pain in the back, right hip, and right arm. Which action is important for the nurse to perform?

    a. Administer aspirin.

    b. Administer ibuprofen.

    c. Start an intravenous line with dextrose 5% in 0.24 normal saline.

    d. Begin oxygen at 2 L/min.

15. A patient is taking prednisone 60 mg/day for the treatment of an acute exacerbation of Crohn's disease. The patient has developed lymphopenia with a lymphocyte count of less than 1500 mm³. Which will the nurse monitor the patient for?

    a. The onset of a bacterial infection

    b. Bleeding

    c. Abdominal pain

    d. Diarrhea

Management of Patients with Hematologic Neoplasms

Learning Outcomes

1. Compare and contrast the different types of leukemias in terms of their incidence, physiologic alterations, clinical manifestations, complications, and medical and nursing management.
2. Use the nursing process as a framework for care of the patient with acute leukemia.
3. Explain the differences between the various myeloproliferative disorders in terms of their incidence, physiologic alterations, clinical manifestations, complications, and medical and nursing management.
4. Compare and contrast Hodgkin and non-Hodgkin lymphomas in terms of their incidence, physiologic alterations, clinical manifestations, complications, and medical and nursing management.
5. Discuss medical and nursing care of the patient with multiple myeloma.

SECTION I: ASSESSING YOUR UNDERSTANDING

Activity A *Fill in the blanks.*

1. The development of hematologic neoplasms is complex. Understanding the processes and the rationale for treatments is important so that nurses may appropriately _____, _____, _____, and _____ with patients who have hematologic neoplasms.

2. Hematopoietic malignancies are often classified by the _____ involved.

3. Multiple myeloma is a malignancy of the most mature form of _____, the plasma cell.

4. The common feature of the _____ is an unregulated proliferation of leukocytes in the bone marrow.

5. The leukemias are commonly classified according to the stem cell line involved, either _____ or _____.

6. The leukemias are also classified as _____ or _____.

7. In acute myeloid leukemia (AML), any age group can be affected, although it infrequently occurs before the age of _____ and the incidence rises with age, with a peak incidence at the age of _____ years.

8. Complications of AML include _____ and _____, the major causes of death from this condition.

9. Chronic myeloid leukemia (CML) arises from a mutation in the myeloid _____.

10. Myelodysplastic syndromes (MDSs) are a group of clonal disorders of the myeloid stem cell that cause _____ in one or more types of cell lines.

Activity B *Briefly answer the following.*

1. What do the signs and symptoms of AML result from?

   _____

   _____

2. If a bone marrow analysis is performed on a patient with AML, what results are seen?

   _____

   _____

3. What is the goal of treatment in acute lymphocytic leukemia (ALL)?

   _____

   _____

   _____

4. Why is caring for a patient with myelodysplastic syndromes (MDSs) such a challenge?

   _____

5. What are the potential long-term complications of therapy for a patient with Hodgkin lymphoma?

   _____

   _____

   _____

Activity C *Match the name of the clonal stem cell disorder in Column I with the characteristics of the disorder in Column II.*

Column I

____ 1. Acute myeloid leukemia

____ 2. Chronic myeloid leukemia

____ 3. Acute lymphocytic leukemia

____ 4. Chronic lymphocytic leukemia

____ 5. Polycythemia vera

____ 6. Essential thrombocythemia

____ 7. Hodgkin lymphoma

____ 8. Non-Hodgkin lymphoma

____ 9. Multiple myeloma

Column II

a. Proliferative disorder of the myeloid stem cells

b. Malignant disease of the most mature form of B lymphocyte, the plasma cell

c. Arises from a mutation in the myeloid stem cell

d. Results from an uncontrolled proliferation of immature cells derived from the lymphoid stem cell

e. Stem cell disease within the bone marrow

f. Unicentric in origin and is initiated in a single node

g. Derived from a malignant clone of B lymphocytes

h. Results from a defect in the hematopoietic stem cell that differentiates into all myeloid cells

i. Heterogeneous group of cancers that originate from the neoplastic growth of lymphoid tissue

SECTION II: APPLYING YOUR KNOWLEDGE

Activity D *Consider the scenario and answer the questions.*

CASE STUDY: Multiple Myeloma

Mr. White, a 67-year-old man, has been seeing his health care provider reporting back pain. He has been treated for low back strain without relief. The health care provider performs laboratory studies, revealing an elevated protein level. A bone marrow biopsy is performed, with results positive for multiple myeloma.

1. When discussing the characteristics of Mr. White's bone pain, what does the nurse determine is congruent with his diagnosis of multiple myeloma?

   _____

   _____

   _____

2. When the nurse is reviewing Mr. White's laboratory results, a hemoglobin of 7.4 g/dL and a hematocrit of 34% is noted. What does the nurse suspect is causing these blood levels?

   _____

   _____

   _____

3. Mr. White is not a candidate for autologous hematopoietic stem cell transplantation (HSCT). What would be a primary treatment for him?

   _____

   _____

4. Why would nonsteroidal anti-inflammatory drugs (NSAIDs) be used with caution to control his pain?

   _____

   _____

   _____

SECTION III: PRACTICING FOR NCLEX

Activity E *Answer the following questions.*

1. A patient with acute myeloid leukemia (AML) is having aggressive chemotherapy to attempt to achieve remission and is aware that hospitalization will be necessary for several weeks. Which type of therapy will the nurse educate the patient about?

   a. Induction therapy

   b. Supportive therapy

   c. Antimicrobial therapy

   d. Standard therapy

2. A patient with acute myeloid leukemia (AML) is having hematopoietic stem cell transplantation (HSCT) with radiation therapy. Which complication will recognize the donor's lymphocytes as foreign and set up reactions to attack the foreign host?

   a. Acute respiratory distress syndrome

   b. Graft-versus-host disease

   c. Remission

   d. Bone marrow depression

3. The nurse is performing an assessment for a patient with acute myeloid leukemia (AML) and observes multiple areas of ecchymosis and petechiae. Which laboratory study will the nurse be most concerned about?

   a. WBC count of 4200 cells/mcL

   b. Hematocrit of 38%

   c. Platelet count of 9000/mm^3

   d. Creatinine level of 1.0 mg/dL

4. A patient with acute myeloid leukemia (AML) has a neutrophil count that persists at less than 100/mm^3. Which will the nurse cautiously monitor this patient for?

   a. Abdominal cramps

   b. Hypotension

   c. Seizure activity

   d. Infection

5. The nurse is caring for a patient with acute myeloid leukemia (AML) with high uric acid levels. Which medication administered by the nurse will prevent crystallization of uric acid and stone formation?

   a. Allopurinol

   b. Filgrastim

   c. Hydroxyurea

   d. Asparaginase

6. The nurse is caring for a patient with chronic myeloid leukemia (CML) taking imatinib mesylate. In which phase of the leukemia is this medication most useful to induce remission?

   a. Chronic

   b. Transformation

   c. Accelerated

   d. Blast crisis

7. The nurse is educating a patient taking imatinib mesylate for treatment of leukemia. Which will the nurse be sure to include when educating the patient about the best way to take the medication that will optimize absorption?

   a. Take the medication with a source of vitamin C to enhance absorption.

   b. Take antacids if needed for gastrointestinal (GI) upset 2 hours after taking the medication.

   c. Take the medication with food to enhance absorption.

   d. Take the medication with acetaminophen to prevent decreased absorption and GI upset.

8. Which patient assessed by the nurse is at greatest risk for the development of myelodysplastic syndromes (MDSs)?

   a. A 24-year-old female taking oral contraceptives

   b. A 40-year-old patient with a history of hypertension

   c. A 52-year-old patient with acute kidney injury

   d. A 72-year-old patient with a history of cancer

9. The nurse is administering packed RBC transfusions for a patient with MDS. The patient has had several transfusions and is likely to receive several more. Which is a priority for the nurse to monitor related to the transfusions?

   a. Creatinine and blood urea nitrogen (BUN) levels

   b. Iron levels

   c. Magnesium levels

   d. Potassium levels

10. The nurse is assessing a patient with polycythemia vera. Which skin assessment data will the nurse identify as a normal finding for this patient?

    a. Pale skin and mucous membranes

    b. Bronze skin tone

    c. Ruddy complexion

    d. Jaundice skin and sclera

11. A patient with polycythemia vera has a high RBC count and is at risk for the development of thrombosis. Which treatment is important to reduce blood viscosity and to deplete the patient's iron stores?

    a. Blood transfusions

    b. Radiation

    c. Chelation therapy

    d. Phlebotomy

12. A patient with polycythemia vera reports severe itching. Which triggers does the nurse know can cause this symptom? (Select all that apply.)

    a. Temperature change

    b. Allergic reaction to the RBC increase

    c. Alcohol consumption

    d. Exposure to water of any temperature

    e. Aspirin

13. The nurse is caring for a patient with Hodgkin lymphoma in the hospital and preparing discharge planning education. Because this patient is at risk for the development of a second malignancy, which education is beneficial for the nurse to discuss to reduce the risk factors? (Select all that apply.)

   a. Reduce exposure to excessive sunlight.

   b. Smoking cessation.

   c. Decrease alcohol intake.

   d. Decrease intake of antipyretic medications such as acetaminophen.

   e. Decrease fat intake.

14. A patient is taking hydroxyurea for the treatment of primary myelofibrosis. While the patient is taking this medication, which laboratory studies will the nurse monitor to determine effectiveness?

   a. Leukocyte and platelet count

   b. BUN and creatinine levels

   c. Aspartate aminotransferase (AST) and alanine transaminase (ALT) levels

   d. Hemoglobin and hematocrit

15. The nurse is caring for a patient who will begin taking long-term bisphosphonate therapy. Why is it important for the nurse to encourage the patient to receive a thorough evaluation of dentition, including panoramic dental x-rays?

   a. The patient is at risk for tooth decay.

   b. The patient will develop gingival hyperplasia.

   c. The patient can develop osteonecrosis of the jaw.

   d. The patient can develop loosening of the teeth.

Immunologic Function

CHAPTER 31

Assessment of Immune Function

Learning Outcomes

1. Describe the body's general immune responses and the stages of the immune response.
2. Differentiate between cellular and humoral immune responses.
3. Specify the effects of select variables on function of the immune system.
4. Use assessment parameters for determining the status of patients' immune function.

SECTION I: ASSESSING YOUR UNDERSTANDING

Activity A *Fill in the blanks.*

1. The immune system is essentially composed of _____, _____, and _____.

2. White blood cells (WBCs) involved in immunity are primarily produced in the _____.

3. T lymphocytes, descendants of stem cells, mature in the _____.

4. Granulocytes, which fight invasion by releasing histamine, do not include _____.

5. The leukocytes that arrive first at a site where inflammation occurs are _____.

6. WBCs that function as phagocytes are called _____.

7. The body's first line of defense is the _____.

8. The primary cells responsible for recognition of foreign antigens are _____.

9. Antibodies are believed to be a type of _____.

10. A deficient immune system response that is congenital in origin would be classified as a _____ disorder.

11. During the _____ stage of an immune response, lymphocytes interfere with disease by picking up specific antigens from organisms to alter their function.

Activity B *Briefly answer the following.*

1. What does cellular membrane damage result from?

   _____

   _____

2. Describe how effector T cells destroy foreign organisms.

   _____

   _____

3. Describe four ways that disorders of the immune system occur.

   _____

   _____

4. Distinguish between natural and acquired (active and passive) immunity.

_____

_____

5. What is complement, how is it formed, and how does it function?

_____

_____

_____

6. How do biologic response modifiers (BRMs) affect the immune response?

_____

_____

7. What age-related changes affect immunologic function?

_____

_____

_____

8. What effects do adrenal corticosteroids, antimetabolites, and antibiotics have on the immune system?

_____

_____

_____

Activity C

Immunoglobulins

Match the immunoglobulin (Ig) listed in Column II with its associated Ig activity listed in Column I. An answer may be used more than once.

Column I

____ **1.** Enhances phagocytosis

____ **2.** Appears in intravascular serum

____ **3.** Helps defend against parasites

____ **4.** Activates complement system

____ **5.** Protects against respiratory infections

____ **6.** Possible influence on B-lymphocyte differentiation

____ **7.** Prevents absorption of antigens from food

Column II

a. IgA

b. IgD

c. IgE

d. IgG

e. IgM

Medications

Match the immune system effect listed in Column II with its corresponding medication listed in Column I. An answer may be used more than once.

Column I

____ **1.** Cyclosporine

____ **2.** Dactinomycin

____ **3.** Indomethacin

____ **4.** Methotrexate

____ **5.** Mechlorethamine

____ **6.** Propylthiouracil

____ **7.** Vancomycin

Column II

a. Agranulocytosis, leukopenia

b. Agranulocytosis, neutropenia

c. Leukopenia, aplastic bone marrow

d. Leukopenia, T-cell inhibition

e. Transient leukopenia

SECTION II: APPLYING YOUR KNOWLEDGE

Activity D *Consider the scenario and answer the questions.*

Mrs. Bartosh, age 63, develops an infection of the abdominal incision site after having an open colon resection. She has a temperature of 101°F, WBC count of 26,000, and a culture of the surgical wound is positive for methicillin-resistant *Staphylococcus aureus* (MRSA).

1. What does the first line of defense, or the *phagocytic immune response,* involve?

   _____

   _____

2. What is the second protective response, or the *humoral immune response*?

   _____

   _____

3. What is the third mechanism of defense, or the *cellular immune response*?

   _____

   _____

SECTION III: PRACTICING FOR NCLEX

Activity E *Answer the following questions.*

1. A patient arrives at the clinic reporting a very sore throat and a fever of 100.8°F. A rapid strep test returns a positive result and the patient is given a prescription for an antibiotic. How did the streptococcal organism gain access to the patient to cause this infection?

   a. Through the mucous membranes of the throat

   b. Through the skin

   c. Breathing in airborne dust

   d. Being outside in the cold weather and decreasing resistance

2. A patient develops an infection while on vacation in Central America and is now taking the antibiotic chloramphenicol. Which complications of the medication will the patient be monitored for?

   a. Eosinophilia

   b. Neutropenia

   c. Aplastic anemia

   d. Hypoprothrombinemia

3. An older adult patient who is postmenopausal informs the nurse that she believes she has developed another urinary tract infection (UTI). Which risk factors do female patients in this age group have that increase the incidence of UTIs? (Select all that apply.)

   a. Residual urine

   b. Urinary incontinence

   c. Estrogen deficiency

   d. Decreased function of the thyroid gland

   e. Dry mucous membranes of the vagina

4. The nurse is caring for an older adult patient hospitalized with cellulitis of the right lower extremity. Why is it imperative that the nurse continually assess the physical and emotional status of this patient?

   a. Older patients are at risk for developing dementia.

   b. The patient will not respond to the antibiotic treatment as well as a younger patient would.

   c. Early recognition and management of factors influencing immune response may decrease morbidity and mortality.

   d. Older adult patients develop depression and suicidal tendencies when they are faced with chronic illness.

5. The nurse is caring for a patient in the hospital who is receiving a vitamin D supplement. Which education will the nurse provide to indicate the importance of this vitamin supplement? (Select all that apply.)
   a. Vitamin D deficiency is associated with increased risk of common cancers.
   b. Vitamin D deficiency is associated with increased risk of autoimmune disease.
   c. Vitamin D deficiency is associated with increased risk of congenital anomalies.
   d. Vitamin D deficiency is associated with increased risk of inflammatory disorders.
   e. Vitamin D deficiency is associated with increased risk of celiac disease.

6. An older adult patient develops a sacral pressure ulcer. Which will the nurse assess in order to ensure adequate wound healing and prevent poor outcomes for this patient? (Select all that apply.)
   a. The patient's ability to perform self-wound care
   b. Nutritional status
   c. Caloric intake
   d. Quality of food ingested
   e. The amount of carbohydrates the patient ingests

7. The nurse is caring for a female patient with an exacerbation of systemic lupus erythematosus. Which does the nurse determine is the reason that females tend to develop autoimmune disorders more frequently than men?
   a. Androgen tends to enhance immunity.
   b. Estrogen tends to enhance immunity.
   c. Testosterone tends to enhance immunity.
   d. Leukocytes are increased in females.

8. The nurse is obtaining a history from a patient with severe psoriasis. Which question is the most important to ask this patient to determine a genetic predisposition?
   a. "How did you know you developed this disease?"
   b. "Does anyone in your family have more than one autoimmune disease?"
   c. "How many children do you have?"
   d. "Does your spouse or significant other have an autoimmune disease?"

9. A patient has developed kidney failure and is discussing options with the health care provider for treatment. Which laboratory finding does the nurse identify that correlates with the kidney failure?
   a. A deficiency in circulating lymphocytes
   b. A deficiency in phosphorus
   c. Decreased amount of WBCs
   d. Increased amount of macrophages

10. A patient sustained severe partial-thickness burns to the face and trunk. The stressors associated with this patient's major injury have caused which immune process to occur?
    a. Cortisol is released from the adrenal cortex, which contributes to immunosuppression.
    b. Circulating lymphocytes will cause lymph node enlargement and altered lymph drainage.
    c. T lymphocytes are stimulated and produce antibodies.
    d. With the help of macrophages, B lymphocytes recognize the antigen of a foreign invader.

11. When obtaining a health history from a patient with possible abnormal immune function, which question will be a priority for the nurse to ask?
    a. "Have you ever been treated for a sexually transmitted infection?"
    b. "When was your last menstrual period?"
    c. "Do you have abdominal pain or discomfort?"
    d. "Have you ever received a blood transfusion?"

12. A patient tells the nurse, "I can't believe I have ineffective immune function and am getting sick again. I exercise rigorously and compete regularly." Which is the best response by the nurse?
    a. "Something must be seriously wrong. You should not be getting sick since you are so healthy."
    b. "Maybe you need to stop exercising so much. It can't be good for you."
    c. "It is possible that you are immunocompromised and may have HIV."
    d. "Rigorous exercise can cause negative effects on immune response."

13. The nurse is performing a physical assessment for a patient at the clinic and palpates enlarged inguinal lymph nodes on the left. Which assessment data will the nurse document? (Select all that apply.)

    a. Location

    b. Size

    c. Consistency

    d. Reports of tenderness

    e. Temperature

14. The nursing instructor is discussing the development of human immune deficiency virus (HIV) disease with the students. Which will the instructor inform the class about helper T cells?

    a. They are activated on recognition of antigens and stimulate the rest of the immune system.

    b. They attack the antigen directly by altering the cell membrane and causing cell lysis.

    c. They have the ability to decrease B-cell production.

    d. They are responsible for recognizing antigens from previous exposure and mounting an immune response.

15. A patient is being treated in the intensive care unit for sepsis related to ventilator-associated pneumonia. The patient is taking large doses of three different antibiotics. Which severe outcome will the nurse monitor for in the lab studies?

    a. Leukocytosis

    b. Bone marrow suppression

    c. Oral thrush

    d. Rash

Management of Patients with Immune Deficiency Disorders

Learning Outcomes

1. Identify the pathophysiology, clinical manifestations, and nursing management of patients with primary immune deficiency disorders.
2. Describe the modes of transmission of human immune deficiency virus infection and prevention strategies.
3. Explain the pathophysiology associated with the clinical manifestations of human immune deficiency virus and acquired immune deficiency syndrome and the purpose of antiretroviral therapy.
4. Use the nursing process as a framework for care of the patient with human immune deficiency virus/acquired immune deficiency syndrome.
5. Identify available resources for patients and support systems promote self-management of immune deficiency disorders.

SECTION I: ASSESSING YOUR UNDERSTANDING

Activity A *Fill in the blanks.*

1. Primary immunodeficiencies predispose people to three conditions: _____, _____, and _____.

2. Five disorders of common, primary immunode-ficiencies are _____, _____, _____, _____, and _____.

3. The _____ serves as the major laboratory indicator of immune function and prophylaxis for opportunistic infections, and is the strongest predictor of subsequent disease progression and survival (Panel, 2019).

4. The CDC estimates that only _____ people living with HIV in the United States are prescribed antiretroviral therapy (ART) and that among these individuals, only _____ have suppressed viral loads (Panel, 2019).

5. _____ results from rapid restoration of organism-specific immune responses to infections that cause either the deterioration of a treated infection or new presentation of a subclinical infection.

Activity B *Briefly answer the following.*

1. Which laboratory test will the nurse review first to identify antibody deficiencies?

   _____

2. Why are live vaccines contraindicated in patients with antibody deficiency disorders?

   _____

   _____

   _____

3. What are two major components of antiretroviral therapy (ART) resistance?

   _____

   _____

   _____

4. Patients who have neutropenia are at risk for what problem?

   _____

5. Discuss the assessment findings for a patient who has developed *Pneumocystis pneumonia (PCP).*

   _____

   _____

   _____

Activity C *Match the antiretroviral agent in Column I with the type of medication in Column II.*

Column I

____ 1. Maraviroc

____ 2. Enfuvirtide

____ 3. Dolutegravir

____ 4. Abacavir

____ 5. Atazanavir

____ 6. Efavirenz

Column II

a. Nucleoside reverse transcriptase inhibitors (NRTIs)

b. Nonnucleoside reverse transcriptase inhibitors

c. Protease inhibitors

d. Fusion inhibitor

e. Integrase inhibitors (INSTIs)

f. CCR5 antagonist

SECTION II: APPLYING YOUR KNOWLEDGE

Activity D *Consider the scenario and answer the questions.*

The nurse is conducting a community health and wellness seminar about human immune deficiency virus (HIV) and its prevalence in the community.

1. What should the nurse include in the educational program regarding the transmission of HIV?

   _____

   _____

   _____

2. What behavioral interventions can the nurse promote to prevent HIV infection?

   _____

   _____

   _____

3. What will the nurse encourage people to do if they believe there has been an exposure to HIV?

   _____

   _____

   _____

SECTION III: PRACTICING FOR NCLEX

Activity E *Answer the following questions.*

1. A patient is infected with HIV after sharing needles with another IV drug abuser. Upon infection with HIV, the immune system responds by making antibodies against the virus usually within how many weeks after infection?

   a. 1 to 2 weeks

   b. 3 to 6 weeks

   c. 3 to 12 weeks

   d. 6 to 18 weeks

2. An older adult female states to the nurse, "I am experiencing vaginal dryness since I have been sexually active again. I can't use barrier protection because it makes it worse." Which education will the nurse provide to the patient?

   a. Use a lamb skin condom instead of latex.

   b. This is common in postmenopausal women, and there are creams that can be used, and a latex condom should be used.

   c. Because the patient is older, it is not likely that she will acquire HIV.

   d. She should abstain from sex because she is at greatest risk for acquiring HIV.

3. A patient develops gastrointestinal (GI) bleeding from a gastric ulcer and requires blood transfusions. The patient states to the nurse, "I am not going to have a transfusion because I don't want to get AIDS." Which is the best response by the nurse?

   a. "I understand what you mean, you can never be sure if the blood is tainted."

   b. "I understand your concern. The blood is screened very carefully for different viruses as well as HIV."

   c. "If you don't have the blood transfusions, you may not make it through this episode of bleeding."

   d. "No one has gotten HIV from blood in a long time. You have to have the transfusion."

4. A new graduate is working at the hospital in the acute care unit. The preceptor observes the nurse emptying a patient's wound drain without gloves on. Which information will the preceptor discuss about standard precautions?

   a. Standard precautions should be used with all patients to reduce the risk of transmission of bloodborne pathogens.

   b. Standard precautions should be used only with patients who are HIV positive to reduce the risk of transmission of the HIV virus.

   c. It is only necessary to use gloves when you are emptying reservoirs that have body fluids in them.

   d. If you are careful and do not expose yourself to blood or body fluids, it is not necessary to use gloves all the time.

5. A patient with HIV has been on antiretroviral therapy (ART) for 6 months. The patient comes to the clinic with home medications, and the nurse observes that there are too many pills in the container. Which factors are associated with nonadherence to ART? (Select all that apply.)

   a. Lives alone

   b. Active substance abuse

   c. Taking other medication

   d. Depression

   e. Lack of social support

6. A patient is on ART for the treatment of HIV. Which does the nurse determine is an adequate CD4+ count to determine the effectiveness of treatment for a patient per year?

   a. 1 mm^3 to 10 mm^3

   b. 10 mm^3 to 20 mm^3

   c. 20 mm^3 to 45 mm^3

   d. 50 mm^3 to 150 mm^3

7. A patient who had unprotected sex with an HIV-infected partner arrives in the clinic requesting HIV testing. Results determine a negative HIV antibody test and an increased viral load. Which stage does the nurse identify the patient is in?

   a. Primary infection

   b. Secondary infection

   c. Tertiary infection

   d. Latent infection

8. A patient in the clinic states, "My boyfriend told me he went to the clinic and was treated for gonorrhea." While testing for this sexually transmitted infection (STI), which will be done for this patient?

   a. Test for HIV without informing the patient.

   b. Test for HIV, requiring the patient to sign a permit.

   c. Inform the patient that it would be beneficial to test for HIV.

   d. Administer treatment for the STI and discharge the patient.

9. A patient with HIV develops a nonproductive cough, shortness of breath, a fever of 101°F, and an O$_2$ saturation of 92%. Which infection caused by *Pneumocystis jirovecii* does the nurse monitor the patient for?

   a. *Mycobacterium avium* complex (MAC)

   b. *Pneumocystis pneumonia*

   c. Tuberculosis

   d. Community-acquired pneumonia

10. A patient with acquired immune deficiency syndrome (AIDS) informs the nurse of difficulty eating and swallowing, and shows the nurse white patches in the mouth. Which complication related to AIDS does the nurse identify has developed?

   a. *Mycobacterium avium* complex (MAC)

   b. Wasting syndrome

   c. Kaposi sarcoma

   d. Candidiasis

11. While caring for a patient with *Pneumocystis pneumonia,* the nurse assesses flat, purplish lesions on the back and trunk. Which condition correlates with this assessment finding?

   a. Molluscum contagiosum

   b. Tuberculosis of the skin

   c. Kaposi sarcoma

   d. Seborrheic dermatitis

12. The nurse receives a phone call at the clinic from the family member of a patient with AIDS. The family member states that the patient started "acting funny" after reporting headache, tiredness, and a stiff neck. Checking the temperature resulted in a fever of 103.2°F. Which response by the nurse is best?

   a. "The patient probably has a case of flu, and you should give Tylenol."

   b. "The patient may have cryptococcal meningitis and will need to be evaluated by the physician."

   c. "This is one of the side effects from antiretroviral therapy and will require changing the medication."

   d. "The patient probably has *Pneumocystis pneumonia* and will need to be evaluated by the physician."

13. A patient is diagnosed with *Pneumocystis pneumonia.* Which medication does the nurse educate the patient about for treatment?

   a. TMP-SMZ

   b. Cephalexin

   c. Azithromycin

   d. Garamycin

14. A patient with AIDS is having a recurrence of 10 to 12 loose stools a day. Which medication may help this patient to control the chronic diarrhea?

   a. Octreotide

   b. Rifaximin

   c. Bismuth subsalicylate

   d. Atropine diphenoxylate

15. The nurse is discussing sex with a patient recently diagnosed with HIV. The patient states, "As long as I have sex with another person who is already infected, I will be okay." Which is the best response by the nurse?

   a. "You should avoid having unprotected sex with a person who is HIV positive because you can increase the severity of the infection in both you and your partner."

   b. "Yes; because you are already infected, it won't make a difference if you have sex with a person who is HIV positive."

   c. "I am not sure why you would want to have sex with another person who is HIV positive. That person may have another sexually transmitted infection."

   d. "If you have sex with another person who is HIV positive, you will develop AIDS sooner."

33

Assessment and Management of Patients with Allergic Disorders

1. Describe the physiologic events involved with allergic reactions and types of hypersensitivity.
2. Use appropriate parameters for assessment of the status of patients with allergic disorders.
3. Identify the pathophysiology, clinical manifestations, and management of patients with allergic disorders.
4. Specify measures to prevent and manage anaphylaxis.
5. Use the nursing process as a framework for care of the patient with allergic rhinitis.

SECTION I: ASSESSING YOUR UNDERSTANDING

Activity A *Fill in the blanks.*

1. Antibodies, the most effective defense mechanisms in the body, react with antigens in three ways: _____, _____, and _____.

2. The classification of immunoglobulin (Ig) that occupies certain receptors on mast cells and produces an inflammatory response is _____.

3. Antibodies formed by lymphocytes and plasma cells in response to an immunogenic stimulus are called _____.

4. Prostaglandins are primary chemical mediators that respond to a stimulus by contracting smooth muscle and increasing capillary permeability. This response causes _____.

5. Type III hypersensitivity reactions involve the binding of antibodies to antigens. List two possible results: _____ and _____.

6. Two examples of a type IV hypersensitivity reaction (occurs 24 to 72 hours after exposure) are _____ and _____.

7. The most common cause of anaphylaxis, accounting for 75% of fatal reactions in the United States, is _____.

8. The initial medication of choice for a severe allergic reaction is _____, administered _____.

9. Patients should be advised that a "rebound" anaphylactic reaction can occur _____ hours after an initial attack, even when epinephrine has been given.

Activity B *Briefly answer the following.*

1. What happens during the physiologic response that causes an allergic reaction?

   _____

   _____

   _____

2. What is the role and function of histamine in response to an allergic threat?

   _____

   _____

   _____

3. What are the four types of hypersensitivity reactions (types I to IV)?

   _____

   _____

   _____

4. What are the three types of skin allergy tests and how are they administered?

   _____

   _____

   _____

5. What is the difference between an *atopic* and *nonatopic* IgE-mediated allergic reaction?

   _____

   _____

   _____

6. What clinical manifestations occur during an anaphylactic reaction?

   _____

   _____

   _____

7. What priority interventions are used in the treatment of an anaphylactic reaction?

   _____

   _____

   _____

8. What are the four types of contact dermatitis and how are they recognized?

   _____

   _____

   _____

Activity C *Match the medication in Column II with the classification in Column I.*

Column I

____ 1. Leukotriene receptor antagonist

____ 2. Leukotriene receptor inhibitor

____ 3. Second-generation H_1 inhibitor

____ 4. First-generation H_1 antihistamines (sedating)

____ 5. Second-generation H_1 antihistamines (nonsedating)

Column II

a. Hydroxyzine

b. Zileuton

c. Montelukast

d. Levocetirizine

e. Cetirizine

SECTION II: APPLYING YOUR KNOWLEDGE

Activity D *Consider the scenarios and answer the questions.*

CASE STUDY: Allergic Rhinitis

Mr. Rock is a 26-year-old contractor who specializes in finished basements and has allergies related to materials used. Because of his job, he is frequently working in environments where there are substances that stimulate an allergic reaction.

1. The nurse is educating him on how he can recognize symptoms that indicate an onset of an allergic reaction. An allergic reaction may be preceded by what symptoms?

   _____

   _____

2. What does the nurse inform Mr. Rock may signal a more severe form of allergic reaction?

   _____

   _____

3. What would the nurse include in the teaching plan regarding his allergies?

   _____

   _____

CASE STUDY: Latex Allergy

Ms. Cauldwell, a student in a nursing program, is beginning her first clinical rotation at the hospital. She and another student are giving a patient a bath, wearing gloves, when Mindy informs the other student that she is itching on both of her hands. When the gloves are removed, Mindy has erythema covering both hands.

1. What type of reaction to the gloves is she experiencing?

   _____

   _____

   _____

2. What can she do to eliminate this type of reaction?

   _____

   _____

3. Ms. Cauldwell asks her instructor if it would help if she used lotion prior to donning gloves. What will the instructor inform her?

   _____

   _____

   _____

4. What types of testing can she receive that will give her a definitive diagnosis of latex allergy?

   _____

   _____

   _____

SECTION III: PRACTICING FOR NCLEX

Activity E *Answer the following questions.*

1. The nurse is preparing to administer a medication that has an affinity for H_1 receptors. Which medication would the nurse administer?
   a. Diphenhydramine
   b. Omeprazole
   c. Cimetidine
   d. Ranitidine

2. An infant is born to a mother who had no prenatal care during her pregnancy. Which type of hypersensitivity reaction does the nurse determine may have occurred?
   a. Bacterial endocarditis
   b. Rh-hemolytic disease
   c. Lupus erythematosus
   d. Rheumatoid arthritis

3. While monitoring the patient's eosinophil level, the nurse suspects a definite allergic disorder when seeing an eosinophil value of which percentage of the total leukocyte count?
   a. 1% to 3%
   b. 3% to 4%
   c. 5% to 10%
   d. 15% to 40%

4. A patient comes to the clinic with pruritus and nasal congestion after eating shrimp for lunch and is suspected to be experiencing an anaphylactic reaction to the shrimp. These symptoms typically occur within how many hours after exposure?
   a. 2 hours
   b. 6 hours
   c. 12 hours
   d. 24 hours

5. A patient is experiencing an allergic reaction after receiving a dose of penicillin. Which signs and symptoms will the nurse look for in the patient's initial assessment?
   a. Dyspnea, bronchospasm, and/or laryngeal edema
   b. Hypotension and tachycardia
   c. The presence and location of pruritus
   d. The severity of cutaneous warmth and flushing

6. The nurse is educating a patient with allergic rhinitis about how the condition is induced. Which factors should the nurse include in the education on this topic?
   a. Airborne pollens or molds
   b. Ingested foods
   c. Parenteral medications
   d. Topical creams or ointments

7. A patient has a sensitivity to ragweed and tells the nurse that it comes at the same time every year. When does the patient typically notice the symptoms?

   a. Early spring

   b. Early fall

   c. Summer

   d. Midwinter

8. A patient asks the nurse if it would be all right to take an over-the-counter antihistamine for the treatment of a rash. Which symptoms will the nurse educate the patient is a major side effect of antihistamines?

   a. Diarrhea

   b. Anorexia

   c. Palpitations

   d. Sedation

9. The nurse is administering a sympathomimetic drug to a patient. Which areas of concern does the nurse have when administering this drug? (Select all that apply.)

   a. Causes bronchodilation.

   b. Constricts integumentary smooth muscle.

   c. Dilates the muscular vasculature.

   d. Causes bronchoconstriction.

   e. Causes laryngospasm.

10. The nurse is administering injected allergens for "hyposensitization," which may produce harmful systemic reactions. Prior to administering these allergens, what medication will the nurse have at the bedside?

    a. Phenergan hydrochloride

    b. Pentazocine

    c. Epinephrine

    d. Meclizine hydrochloride

11. A patient was seen in the clinic for hypertension and received a prescription for a new antihypertensive medication. The patient arrived in the emergency department a few hours after taking the medication with severe angioedema. Which medication prescribed is most likely responsible for the reaction?

    a. Beta-blocker

    b. Angiotensin-converting enzyme (ACE) inhibitor

    c. Angiotensin receptor blocker

    d. Vasodilator

12. A patient has been diagnosed with an allergy to peanuts. Which item is a priority for this patient to carry at all times?

    a. A medical alert bracelet

    b. An H_1 blocker

    c. An EpiPen

    d. An oral airway

13. A patient has had a "stuffy nose" and obtained Afrin nasal spray. Which education should the nurse provide to the patient in order to prevent "rebound congestion"?

    a. Be sure to use the Afrin for at least 10 days to ensure the stuffiness is gone.

    b. Use the medication every 4 hours to prevent congestion from recurring.

    c. Drink plenty of fluids.

    d. Only use the Afrin for 3 to 4 days once every 12 hours.

14. A patient was seen in the clinic 3 days previously for allergic rhinitis and was given a prescription for a corticosteroid nasal spray. The patient calls the clinic and tells the nurse that the nasal spray is not working. Which is the best response by the nurse?

    a. "You need to come back to the clinic to get a different medication since this one is not working for you."

    b. "You may be immune to the effects of this medication and will need something else in its place."

    c. "The full benefit of the medication may take up to 2 weeks to be achieved."

    d. "I am sorry that you are feeling poorly but this is the only medication that will work for your problem."

15. What education should the nurse provide to the patient taking long-term corticosteroids?

    a. The patient should not stop taking the medication abruptly and should be weaned off the medication.

    b. The patient should take the medication only as needed and not take it unnecessarily.

    c. Corticosteroids are relatively safe drugs with very few side effects.

    d. The patient should discontinue using the drug immediately if weight gain is observed.

Assessment and Management of Patients with Inflammatory Rheumatic Disorders

Learning Outcomes

1. Explain the pathophysiology of inflammatory rheumatic diseases and describe the assessment and diagnostic findings seen in patients with these disorders.
2. Use the nursing process as a framework for care of the patient with an inflammatory rheumatic disorder.
3. Devise an education plan for the patient with newly diagnosed inflammatory rheumatic disease.
4. Identify modifications in interventions to accommodate changes in patients' functional ability that may occur with disease progression.

SECTION I: ASSESSING YOUR UNDERSTANDING

Activity A *Fill in the blanks.*

1. The most common symptom of inflammatory rheumatic disease that causes a patient to seek medical attention is _____.

2. In the inflammatory process in rheumatic diseases, a triggering event starts the process by activating _____.

3. Synovial fluid from an inflamed joint is characteristically _____, _____, and _____.

4. The rheumatoid arthritis (RA) reaction produces enzymes that break down _____.

5. In RA, the autoimmune reaction primarily occurs in the _____.

Activity B *Briefly answer the following.*

1. What is the theory of *degradation* as it relates to the pathophysiology of inflammatory rheumatic diseases?

_____

_____

2. What is the difference between *exacerbation* and *remission*?

_____

_____

_____

3. What is the difference between the patho-physiology of inflammatory rheumatic disease and that of degenerative rheumatic disease?

_____

_____

_____

4. Name three goals and corresponding management strategies for the treatment of inflammatory rheumatic diseases.

_____

_____

5. What type of exercises and precautions are used to promote mobility for a patient with an inflammatory rheumatic disease?

_____

_____

_____

6. What is psoriatic arthritis characterized by?

_____

_____

_____

7. When the patient is taking corticosteroids for the treatment of an inflammatory rheumatic disease, which side effects should the nurse educate the patient about?

_____

_____

_____

8. What are the clinical manifestations of gout?

_____

_____

_____

9. What nursing management options exist for fibromyalgia?

_____

_____

_____

Activity C *Match the clinical interpretation/ laboratory significance listed in Column II with its associated test listed in Column I.*

Column I

____ **1.** Uric acid

____ **2.** Complement

____ **3.** Rheumatoid factor

____ **4.** Hematocrit

____ **5.** HLA-B27 antigen

____ **6.** Antinuclear antibody (ANA)

____ **7.** Creatinine

____ **8.** C-reactive protein (CRP)

Column II

a. A decrease can be seen in chronic inflammation.

b. A positive test is associated with systemic lupus erythematosus (SLE), RA, and Raynaud's disease.

c. An increase in this substance is seen with gout.

d. This protein substance is decreased in RA and SLE.

e. This is present in 80% of those who have RA.

f. This is present in 85% of those with ankylosing spondylitis.

g. Frequently positive for RA and SLE.

h. An increase may indicate renal damage, as in scleroderma.

SECTION II: APPLYING YOUR KNOWLEDGE

Activity D *Consider the scenarios and answer the questions.*

CASE STUDY: Diffuse Connective Tissue Disease

Ms. Blount, a 33-year-old mother of two, has joint pain and stiffness, decreased mobility, and increased frequency of fatigue, and is experiencing depression.

1. The nurse is performing an assessment when she comes to the clinic. What symptoms does the nurse identify as characteristic of Rheumatoid Arthritis (RA)?

   _____

   _____

2. Ms. Blount has a series of laboratory studies performed and has a negative RA factor. What is the significance of this result?

   _____

   _____

   _____

3. Ms. Blount has been prescribed methotrexate for initial treatment. When does the nurse inform her that symptom relief will begin?

   _____

   _____

   _____

4. A low-dose corticosteroid regimen is used concurrently with the methotrexate. Ms. Blount wants to know why she should take this medication along with the methotrexate. What explanation will the nurse provide?

   _____

   _____

   _____

CASE STUDY: Systemic Lupus Erythematosus (SLE)

Mrs. Brooke is a 41-year-old mother of two teenagers who has had symptoms of joint tenderness for about 10 years. Lately, she has noticed significant morning stiffness and a slight rash over the bridge of her nose and cheeks. Her health care provider suspects a diagnosis of SLE.

1. When performing an assessment for Mrs. Brooke, what cardiovascular symptoms will the nurse auscultate to determine if present?

   _____

   _____

2. When planning her care, the nurse anticipates providing education regarding the therapeutic medication regimen. What medications does the nurse provide information about?

   _____

   _____

   _____

3. Mrs. Brooke has been placed on corticosteroid therapy. What will the nurse caution her about regarding the risk factors while taking corticosteroids for SLE?

   _____

   _____

   _____

SECTION III: PRACTICING FOR NCLEX

Activity E *Answer the following questions.*

1. A patient is seen in the office for reports of joint pain, swelling, and a low-grade fever. Which laboratory studies reviewed by the nurse indicate a positive diagnosis of RA? (Select all that apply.)

   a. Positive C-reactive protein (CRP)

   b. Positive antinuclear antibody (ANA)

   c. Red blood cell (RBC) count of <4.0 million/mcL

   d. Serum complement level (C3) of >130 mg/dL

   e. Aspartate aminotransferase (AST) and alanine transaminase (ALT) levels of 7 units/L

2. A patient has a serum study that is positive for the rheumatoid factor. Which does the nurse identify is the significance of this test result?

   a. The test results are diagnostic for Sjögren's syndrome.

   b. The test results are diagnostic for systemic lupus erythematosus.

   c. The test results are specific for rheumatoid arthritis.

   d. The test results are suggestive of rheumatoid arthritis.

3. The nurse is caring for a patient who presents with the symptom of blanching of fingers when exposed to cold. Which rheumatic disorder does the nurse prepare to assess the patient for?

   a. Ankylosing spondylitis

   b. Raynaud's phenomenon

   c. Reiter syndrome

   d. Sjögren's syndrome

4. A patient is suspected of having *myositis*. The nurse prepares the patient for which procedure that will confirm the diagnosis?

   a. Bone scan

   b. Computed tomography (CT)

   c. Magnetic resonance imaging (MRI)

   d. Muscle biopsy

5. The nurse is educating a patient about the risks of stroke related to the new prescription for a COX-2 inhibitor and which symptoms should be reported. Which COX-2 inhibitor is the nurse educating the patient about?

   a. Ibuprofen

   b. Celecoxib

   c. Piroxicam

   d. Tolmetin sodium

6. A patient is prescribed a DMARD that is successful in the treatment of rheumatoid arthritis (RA) but has side effects, including retinal eye changes. Which medication does the nurse educate the patient about?

   a. Azathioprine

   b. Diclofenac

   c. Hydroxychloroquine

   d. Aurothioglucose

7. A patient with an acute exacerbation of arthritis is temporarily confined to bed. Which position will the nurse recommend to prevent flexion deformities?

   a. Prone

   b. Semi-Fowler

   c. Side-lying with pillows supporting the shoulders and legs

   d. Supine with pillows under the knees

8. A patient comes to the clinic with an inflamed wrist. How will the nurse splint the joint to immobilize it?

   a. Slight dorsiflexion

   b. Extension

   c. Hyperextension

   d. Internal rotation

9. A patient arrives at the clinic with reports of pain in the left great toe. The nurse assesses a swollen, warm, erythematous left great toe. Which laboratory test will the nurse prepare the patient for to identify the cause?

   a. Uric acid level

   b. Hemoglobin

   c. Potassium level

   d. Erythrocyte sedimentation rate

10. The nurse is educating the patient with gout about ways to prevent reoccurrence of an attack. Which foods will the nurse encourage the patient to avoid?

    a. Baked chicken

    b. Steak

    c. Asparagus

    d. Pineapple

11. The nurse is assessing a patient with a diagnosis of scleroderma. Which clinical manifestations of scleroderma does the nurse assess? (Select all that apply.)

    a. Decreased ventilation owing to lung scarring

    b. Dysphagia owing to hardening of the esophagus

    c. Dyspnea owing to fibrotic cardiac tissue

    d. Productive cough

    e. Butterfly-shaped rash on the face

12. A patient is hospitalized with a severe case of gout. The patient has gross swelling of the large toe and rates pain a 10 out of 10. With a diagnosis of gout, which will the laboratory results reveal?

    a. Glycosuria

    b. Hyperuricemia

    c. Hyperproteinuria

    d. Ketonuria

13. A patient is being placed on a purine-restricted diet. Which food should be suggested by the nurse?

    a. Dairy products

    b. Organ meats

    c. Raw vegetables

    d. Shellfish

14. A patient is taking nonsteroidal anti-inflammatory drugs (NSAIDs) for the treatment of osteoarthritis. Which education should the nurse give the patient about the medication?

    a. Take the medication on an empty stomach in order to increase effectiveness.

    b. Since the medication is able to be obtained over the counter, it has few side effects.

    c. Take the medication with food to avoid stomach upset.

    d. Inform the primary provider if there is ringing in the ears.

15. The nurse is educating a patient that is prescribed adalimumab for the treatment of psoriatic arthritis. Which statement made by the patient indicates that further education is required?

    a. "I will receive a tuberculin skin test prior to beginning this medication."

    b. "I will administer this medication in the muscle of my leg every 2 weeks."

    c. "If I have a fever, I won't administer the medication and will notify my health care provider."

    d. "I should avoid large crowds and protect myself from infections."

Musculoskeletal Function

CHAPTER 35

Assessment of Musculoskeletal Function

Learning Outcomes

1. Describe the basic structure and function of the musculoskeletal system.
2. Discuss the significance of the health history to the assessment of musculoskeletal health.
3. Recognize and evaluate the major manifestations of musculoskeletal dysfunction by applying concepts from the patient's health history and physical assessment findings.
4. Explain clinical indications, patient preparation, and other related nursing implications for common tests and procedures used to assess musculoskeletal function.

SECTION I: ASSESSING YOUR UNDERSTANDING

Activity A   Fill in the blanks.

1. The leading cause of musculoskeletal-related disability in the United States is _____.

2. The approximate percentage of total-body calcium present in the bones is _____.

3. In the human body, there are _____ bones.

4. Approximately _____ mg of calcium daily is essential to maintain adult bone mass.

5. Red bone marrow is located in the shaft of four long and flat bones: the _____, _____, _____, and _____.

6. The major hormonal regulators of calcium homeostasis are _____ and _____.

7. _____ describes the grating, crackling sound heard over irregular joint surfaces like the knee.

Activity B   Briefly answer the following.

1. What are the general functions of the musculoskeletal system?

   _____

   _____

   _____

2. What are the differences in the function of *osteoblasts*, *osteocytes*, and *osteoclasts*?

   _____

   _____

   _____

3. How does vitamin D regulate the balance between bone formation and bone resorption?

   _____

   _____

4. What is the role of the sex hormones testosterone and estrogen on bone remodeling?

_____

_____

_____

5. What is the process of fracture healing, including the three stages of progression?

_____

_____

6. What is the difference between isotonic and isometric contractions?

_____

_____

_____

7. What are the age-related changes of the musculoskeletal system specific to bones, muscles, joints, and ligaments?

_____

_____

8. What is the difference between kyphosis, lordosis, and scoliosis?

_____

_____

Activity C *Match the test used to assess peripheral nerve function sensation in Column II with the nerve being assessed in Column I.*

Column I

____ **1.** Peroneal

____ **2.** Tibial

____ **3.** Radial

____ **4.** Ulnar

____ **5.** Median

Column II

a. Prick the medial and lateral surface of the sole.

b. Prick the distal fat pad of the small finger.

c. Prick the skin midway between the great and second toe.

d. Prick the skin midway between the thumb and second finger.

e. Prick the top or distal surface of the index finger.

SECTION II: APPLYING YOUR KNOWLEDGE

Activity D *Consider the scenario and answer the questions.*

Kevin, age 32, was jogging and tripped over a rock in the path. He fell on his right knee and experienced immediate pain but was able to get up and limp home. The next day, the knee was swollen and painful, and he made an appointment to see his health care provider.

1. The health care provider determines Kevin has an effusion. How was that detected?

_____

_____

2. The health care provider orders a magnetic resonance imaging (MRI) study. What will the nurse educate the patient about prior to having the test?

_____

_____

_____

3. Which procedure will the health care provider perform to remove the fluid from Kevin's knee?

_____

_____

SECTION III: PRACTICING FOR NCLEX

Activity E *Answer the following questions.*

1. A patient has a fracture of the right femur sustained in a motor vehicle crash. Which process of fracture healing does the nurse determine will occur with this patient?

   a. Reactive phase, reparative phase, remodeling phase

   b. Primary phase, secondary phase, third phase

   c. First intention, secondary intention, third intention

   d. Active phase, dormant phase, restructure phase

2. A patient has a fracture treated with open rigid compression plate fixation devices. How will the progress of bone healing be monitored?
   a. Remove the plate and determine if the bone is growing back.
   b. Perform serial x-rays.
   c. Perform an arthroscopy.
   d. The bone will heal on its own without intervention.

3. A patient tells the health care provider about shoulder pain that is present even without any strenuous movement. The health care provider identifies a sac filled with synovial fluid. Which condition will the nurse educate the patient about?
   a. A fracture of the clavicle
   b. Osteoarthritis of the shoulder
   c. Chronic bursitis
   d. Ankylosing spondylitis

4. A patient had a stroke and is unable to move the right upper and lower extremities. During assessment, the nurse picks up the arm and finds it limp and without tone. How will the nurse document this finding?
   a. Rigidity
   b. Flaccidity
   c. Atonic
   d. Tetanic

5. A patient tells the nurse, "I was working out and lifting weights and now that I have stopped, I am flabby and my muscles have gone!" Which is the best response by the nurse?
   a. "While you are lifting weights, endorphins are released, creating increase in muscle mass, but if the muscles are not used, they will atrophy."
   b. "The muscle mass has decreased from the lack of calcium in the cells."
   c. "Your muscles were in a state of hypertrophy from the weight lifting but it will persist only if the exercise is continued."
   d. "Once you stop exercising, the contraction of the muscle does not regain its strength."

6. After a bone density test, an older adult female patient tells the nurse, "I don't understand why I have osteoporosis because I eat well and take my calcium." Which is the best response by the nurse?
   a. "Everyone gets osteoporosis and there is nothing you can do to prevent it."
   b. "Men lose more bone mass than women but women still lose some."
   c. "In order to prevent bone loss, you will have to take hormones."
   d. "The loss is from withdrawal of estrogen and a decrease in activity levels."

7. A patient comes to the clinic and informs the nurse of numbness, tingling, and a burning sensation in the arm from the elbow down to the fingers. Which type of symptom would this be documented as?
   a. Paresthesia
   b. Flaccidity
   c. Atonia
   d. Effusion

8. The nurse is performing an assessment on an older adult patient and observes the patient has an increased forward curvature of the thoracic spine. Which does the nurse identify this common finding as?
   a. Lordosis
   b. Scoliosis
   c. Osteoporosis
   d. Kyphosis

9. The nurse assesses soft subcutaneous nodules along the line of the tendons in a patient's hand and wrist. Which does this finding indicate to the nurse?
   a. The patient has osteoarthritis.
   b. The patient has lupus erythematosus.
   c. The patient has rheumatoid arthritis.
   d. The patient has neurofibromatosis.

10. The nurse is caring for a pregnant patient with pregnancy-induced hypertension. When assessing the reflexes in the ankle, the nurse observes rhythmic contractions of the muscle when dorsiflexing the foot. What would the nurse document this finding as?
   a. Positive Babinski reflex
   b. Clonus
   c. Hypertrophy
   d. Ankle reflex

11. The nurse is performing an assessment for a patient who may have peripheral neurovascular dysfunction. Which signs does the patient present with that indicate circulation is impaired? (Select all that apply.)

    a. Pale, cyanotic, or mottled color

    b. Cool temperature of the extremity

    c. More than 3-second capillary refill

    d. Tenting skin turgor

    e. Limited range of motion

12. A patient is scheduled for a procedure that will allow the primary provider to visualize the knee joint in order to diagnose the patient's pain. Which procedure will the nurse prepare the patient for?

    a. Arthrocentesis

    b. Bone scan

    c. Electromyography

    d. Arthroscopy

13. A patient is having repeated tears of the joint capsule in the shoulder, and the primary provider prescribes an arthrogram. Which intervention will the nurse provide after the procedure is completed? (Select all that apply.)

    a. Apply a compression bandage to the area.

    b. Apply heat to the area for 48 hours.

    c. Administer a mild analgesic.

    d. Inform the patient that a clicking or crackling noise in the joint may persist for a couple of days.

    e. Actively exercise the area immediately after the procedure.

Management of Patients with Musculoskeletal Disorders

Learning Outcomes

1. Describe the pathophysiology, clinical manifestations, and medical and nursing management of low back pain.
2. Discuss common musculoskeletal disorders of the hand, wrist, shoulder, and foot, and nursing management of the patient undergoing surgery to correct these disorders.
3. Identify the pathophysiology, clinical manifestations, and medical, surgical, and nursing management of osteoarthritis.
4. Explain the pathophysiology, clinical manifestations, and medical and nursing management of metabolic bone disorders, including osteoporosis, osteomalacia, and Paget disease.
5. Articulate the pathophysiology, clinical manifestations, and medical and nursing management of musculoskeletal infections, including osteomyelitis and septic arthritis, and of bone tumors.
6. Use the nursing process as a framework for care of the patient undergoing total hip arthroplasty, with select complications of osteoporosis, or with osteomyelitis.

SECTION I: ASSESSING YOUR UNDERSTANDING

Activity A *Fill in the blanks.*

1. The major consequence of osteoporosis is _____.

2. Primary osteoporosis in women usually begins between the ages of _____ and _____.

3. The primary deficit in osteomalacia is _____, which promotes calcium absorption from the gastrointestinal tract.

4. Two medications used to treat Paget disease are _____ and _____.

5. The intervertebral discs that are subject to the greatest mechanical stress and greatest degenerative changes are _____, _____, and _____.

6. The layman's term for onychocryptosis, a common foot condition, is _____.

7. Osteomyelitis with vascular insufficiency, which most commonly affects the feet, is seen most often among patients with _____ and _____.

8. The recommended adequate intake (RAI) level of calcium for all individuals is _____ to _____ mg daily.

9. Bone formation is enhanced by _____, _____, and _____.

10. The most common benign bone tumor is _____.

Activity B *Briefly answer the following.*

1. Identify at least five musculoskeletal problems that can cause acute low back pain.

_____

_____

2. Explain the difference between bursitis and tendonitis.

_____

_____

3. Explain *impingement syndrome* and the measures that are necessary to promote shoulder healing.

_____

_____

_____

4. What technique will assess for Tinel sign?

_____

_____

_____

5. Identify the risk factors (modifiable and nonmodifiable) associated with osteoporosis.

_____

_____

6. Describe the clinical manifestations associated with septic arthritis.

_____

_____

_____

Activity C *Match the diagnostic procedures for low back pain in Column I with their definitions in Column II.*

Column I

____ 1. Bone scan

____ 2. Computed tomography (CT) scan

____ 3. Magnetic resonance imaging (MRI) scan

____ 4. Electromyogram (EMG)

____ 5. Myelogram

____ 6. Ultrasound

Column II

a. Used to evaluate spinal nerve root disorders (radiculopathies)

b. Useful in identifying underlying problems, such as obscure soft tissue lesions adjacent to the vertebral column and problems of vertebral discs

c. May disclose infections, tumors, and bone marrow abnormalities

d. Permits visualization of the nature and location of spinal pathology

e. Permits visualization of segments of the spinal cord that may have herniated or may be compressed (infrequently performed; indicated when MRI scan is contraindicated)

f. Useful in detecting tears in ligaments, muscles, tendons, and soft tissues in the back

SECTION II: APPLYING YOUR KNOWLEDGE

Activity D *Consider the scenario and answer the questions.*

CASE STUDY: Osteoporosis

Ms. Carmichael is a 49-year-old administrative assistant at a community college who has just been diagnosed with osteoporosis. The nurse is planning to educate her about the plan of care and answer questions that she may have.

1. What will the nurse communicate to her about the loss of bone mass?

_____

_____

_____

2. What reasons explain why women develop osteoporosis more frequently than men?

_____

_____

3. The nurse advises Ms. Carmichael that the development of osteoporosis is significantly dependent on what factors?

_____

_____

4. How much calcium should the nurse advise her that she needs daily?

_____

SECTION III: PRACTICING FOR NCLEX

Activity E *Answer the following questions.*

1. A patient comes back to the clinic with continued reports of back pain. Which time frame does the nurse identify as "chronic pain"?
   a. 4 weeks
   b. 3 months
   c. 6 months
   d. 1 year

2. A patient reports experiencing low back pain. Which position will the nurse suggest to relieve this discomfort?
   a. High Fowler to allow for maximum hip flexion
   b. Supine, with the knees slightly flexed and the head of the bed elevated 30 degrees
   c. Prone, with a pillow under the shoulders
   d. Supine, with the bed flat and a firm mattress in place

3. The nurse is educating the patient with low back pain about the proper way to lift objects. Which muscle will the nurse encourage the patient to maximize?
   a. Gastrocnemius
   b. Latissimus dorsi
   c. Quadriceps
   d. Rectus abdominis

4. The nurse educated a patient with low back pain about techniques to relieve the discomfort and prevent further complications. Which statement by the patient demonstrates understanding of the education the nurse provided?
   a. "I will lie prone with my legs slightly elevated."
   b. "I will bend at the waist when I am lifting objects from the floor."
   c. "I will avoid prolonged sitting or walking."
   d. "Instead of turning around to grasp an object, I will twist at the waist."

5. A patient diagnosed with carpal tunnel syndrome (CTS) asks the nurse about numbness in the fingers and pain in the wrist. In responding to the patient, how would the nurse best describe CTS?
   a. "CTS is a neuropathy that is characterized by bursitis and tendonitis."
   b. "CTS is a neuropathy that is characterized by flexion contracture of the fourth and fifth fingers."
   c. "CTS is a neuropathy that is characterized by compression of the median nerve at the wrist."
   d. "CTS is a neuropathy that is characterized by pannus formation in the shoulder."

6. The nurse is assessing the feet of a patient and observes an overgrowth of the horny layer of the epidermis. Which condition will the nurse educate the patient about?

a. Bunion

b. Clawfoot

c. Corn

d. Hammer toe

7. A patient has been diagnosed with osteomalacia. Which common symptoms does the nurse recognize correlate with the diagnosis?

a. Bone fractures and kyphosis

b. Bone pain and tenderness

c. Muscle weakness and spasms

d. Softened and compressed vertebrae

8. A patient stepped on an acorn while walking barefoot in the backyard and developed an infection progressing to osteomyelitis. Which microorganism does the nurse identify is most often the cause of the development of osteomyelitis?

a. *Proteus*

b. *Pseudomonas*

c. *Salmonella*

d. *Staphylococcus aureus*

9. A patient is diagnosed with osteomyelitis of the right leg. Which signs and symptoms does the nurse identify that are associated with this diagnosis? (Select all that apply.)

a. Pain in the right leg

b. Erythema of the right leg

c. Fever

d. Leukopenia

e. Purulent drainage

10. A patient comes to the clinic reporting low back pain radiating down the left leg. After diagnostic studies rule out any pathology, the health care provider prescribes a serotonin–norepinephrine reuptake inhibitor (SNRI). Which medication does the nurse educate the patient about?

a. Amitriptyline

b. Duloxetine

c. Gabapentin

d. Cyclobenzaprine

11. A patient shows the nurse a round, firm nodule on the wrist. The pain is described as aching, with some weakness of the fingers. Which treatment does the nurse assist with? (Select all that apply.)

a. Educate the patient on the use of gabapentin

b. Active range-of-motion exercises

c. Corticosteroid injections

d. Surgical excision

e. Aspiration of the cyst

12. A patient had hand surgery to correct a Dupuytren contracture. Which nursing intervention is a priority postoperatively?

a. Changing the dressing

b. Applying a cock-up splint and immobilization

c. Having the patient exercise the fingers to avoid future contractures

d. Performing hourly neurovascular assessments for the first 24 hours

13. A patient is diagnosed with osteogenic sarcoma. Which laboratory studies will the nurse monitor for the presence of elevation?

a. Magnesium level

b. Potassium level

c. Alkaline phosphatase

d. Troponin levels

14. The nurse is caring for a patient with bone metastasis from a primary breast cancer. The patient reports muscle weakness and nausea and is voiding large amounts frequently. Cardiac arrhythmias are observed on the telemetry monitor. Which does the nurse suspect based on these clinical manifestations?

   a. Hypercalcemia

   b. Hypocalcemia

   c. Hypokalemia

   d. Hyperkalemia

15. The hospice nurse is assigned to care for a patient with metastatic bone cancer who wants to remain at home. Which is the therapeutic goal in the care of this patient?

   a. Prevent the patient from having to go to the hospital for care.

   b. Relieve pain and discomfort while promoting quality of life.

   c. Increase the activity level of the patient to prevent complications related to immobility.

   d. Ensure that the family accepts the patient's imminent death.

Management of Patients with Musculoskeletal Trauma

Learning Outcomes

1. Differentiate between contusions, strains, sprains, dislocations, and subluxations.
2. Identify the clinical manifestations, common treatment modalities, complications, and rehabilitation needs of patients with common types of fractures.
3. Describe the nursing management including the health education needs of the patient with a cast, splint, or brace, or who is in traction.
4. Use the nursing process as a framework for care of the older adult patient with a fracture of the hip.
5. Recognize sports- and occupation-related musculoskeletal disorders and their signs, symptoms, and treatments.
6. Apply the nursing process as a framework for care of the patient with an amputation.

SECTION I: ASSESSING YOUR UNDERSTANDING

Activity A *Fill in the blanks.*

1. A muscle tear that is microscopic and due to overuse is called a _____.

2. The femur fracture that commonly leads to avascular necrosis or nonunion due to an abundant supply of blood vessels in the area is a fracture of the _____.

3. Patients with open fractures risk three major complications: _____, _____, and _____.

4. _____ is the most common fracture of the distal radius.

5. The most common complication of hip fractures in the older adult patient is _____.

6. Common pulmonary complications for the older adult patient following a hip fracture include _____ and _____.

7. Three range-of-motion activities are avoided for a patient with a lower extremity amputation: _____, _____, and _____.

8. The residual limb should never be placed on a pillow to avoid _____.

9. Patients who experience a fracture of the humeral neck are advised that healing will take an average of _____ weeks, with restricted vigorous activity for an additional _____ weeks.

10. The longest immobilization time necessary for fracture union occurs with a fracture of the _____.

Activity B *Briefly answer the following.*

1. A patient with joint dislocation is at risk for the development of avascular necrosis. Which rationale will be provided to this patient?

_____

_____

2. The nurse identifies a grating sensation when moving a patient's extremity. What is this sensation caused by? How would the nurse document this sensation?

_____

_____

_____

3. Name three early and three delayed complications of fractures.

_____

_____

_____

_____

4. A patient is in early shock from a fracture. What five activities are involved in the treatment?

_____

_____

_____

_____

5. Name three early and serious complications associated with immobility and reduced skeletal muscle contractions for a patient with an open fracture.

_____

_____

6. Which immediate nursing and medical management techniques are used for an open fracture?

_____

_____

_____

_____

7. Compare and contrast open and closed reduction as management techniques for fractures.

_____

_____

_____

_____

8. List five factors that can enhance fracture healing and five factors that can inhibit it.

_____

_____

Activity C *Match the type of fracture in Column II with its descriptive terminology listed in Column I.*

PART I

Column I	Column II
____ **1.** A break occurs across the entire section of the bone.	**a.** Avulsion
	b. Comminuted
____ **2.** A fragment of the bone is pulled off by a ligament or tendon.	**c.** Complete
	d. Epiphyseal
____ **3.** Bone is splintered into several fragments.	**e.** Greenstick
____ **4.** One side of a bone is broken and the other side is bent.	
____ **5.** A fracture that occurs through the epiphysis.	

PART II

Column I

Column II

____ **1.** A fracture occurs at an angle across the bone.

____ **2.** Fragments are driven inward.

____ **3.** The fractured bone is compressed by another bone.

____ **4.** The fracture extends through the skin.

____ **5.** A fracture occurring through an area of diseased bone.

a. Compressed

b. Depressed

c. Oblique

d. Open

e. Pathologic

SECTION II: APPLYING YOUR KNOWLEDGE

Activity D *Consider the scenario and answer the questions.*

CASE STUDY: Above-the-Knee Amputation

Mr. William is a 70-year-old patient. He is scheduled to have an above-the-knee amputation of his left leg because of peripheral vascular disease.

1. The nurse is assessing William prior to the surgical procedure. What will the nurse assess to determine the circulatory status of the affected limb?

_____

_____

2. Which factors will be accounted for in determining the level of William's amputation?

_____

_____

_____

3. The nurse will assist Mr. William in exercising the muscles needed for crutch walking. What major muscle is most important to strengthen to improve his rehabilitation potential?

_____

4. Mr. William informs the nurse that he is experiencing sensations that the leg is still present postoperatively. What is the best response by the nurse?

_____

_____

5. Mr. William's amputation is treated with a soft compression dressing. Which nursing action will the nurse perform?

_____

_____

_____

_____

6. The nurse will assess for which complications that can delay prosthetic fittings?

_____

_____

7. The nurse is preparing to apply a bandage to Mr. William's residual limb. Which technique will the nurse use to apply the bandage?

_____

_____

SECTION III: PRACTICING FOR NCLEX

Activity E *Answer the following questions.*

1. A patient fell in a hole in the yard, causing an ankle injury. The ankle is edematous and painful to palpation. How long will the nurse inform the patient that the acute inflammatory stage will last?

a. Less than 24 hours

b. Between 24 and 48 hours

c. About 72 hours

d. At least 1 week

2. The nurse is caring for a patient after arthroscopic surgery for a rotator cuff tear. The nurse informs the patient that full activity can usually resume after what period of time?

a. 3 to 4 weeks

b. 8 weeks

c. 3 to 4 months

d. 6 to 12 months

3. A patient had an above-the-knee amputation of the left leg related to complications from peripheral vascular disease (PVD). The nurse enters the patient's room and observes the dressing and bed covers saturated with blood. Which is the first action by the nurse?

   a. Notify the health care provider.

   b. Apply a tourniquet.

   c. Use skin clips to close the wound.

   d. Reinforce the dressing.

4. A patient sustains an open fracture with extensive soft tissue damage. The nurse identifies this fracture is classified as which grade?

   a. I

   b. II

   c. III

   d. IV

5. A patient sustains an open fracture of the left arm after an accident at the roller-skating rink. Which emergency management plans will be started for this patient? (Select all that apply.)

   a. Cover the area with a clean dressing if the fracture is open.

   b. Immobilize the affected site.

   c. Splint the injured limb.

   d. Have the patient demonstrate mobility of the arm.

   e. Wrap the arm in a compression bandage.

6. The nurse is caring for a patient who sustained an open fracture of the right femur in an automobile crash. Which is the most serious complication this patient will need to be monitored for?

   a. Infection

   b. Muscle atrophy caused by loss of supporting bone structure

   c. Necrosis of adjacent soft tissue caused by blood loss

   d. Nerve damage

7. The nurse is monitoring a patient who sustained an open fracture of the left hip. Which type of shock will the nurse identify may occur with this type of injury?

   a. Cardiogenic

   b. Hypovolemic

   c. Neurogenic

   d. Septicemic

8. A patient sustained an open fracture of the femur 24 hours ago. While assessing the patient, the nurse observes the patient is having difficulty breathing, and oxygen saturation decreases to 88% from a previous 99%. Which complications of the fracture is the patient experiencing?

   a. Spontaneous pneumothorax

   b. Cardiac tamponade

   c. Pneumonia

   d. Fat emboli

9. A patient sustains a fracture of the arm. When will the nurse inform the patient that pendulum exercises will begin?

   a. As soon as tolerated, after a reasonable period of immobilization

   b. In 2 to 3 weeks, when callus ossification prevents easy movements of bony fragments

   c. In about 4 to 5 weeks, after new bone is well established

   d. In 2 to 3 months, after normal activities are resumed

10. A patient falls while skiing and sustains a supracondylar fracture of the humerus. Which serious complication of this injury should the nurse monitor for?

    a. Hemarthrosis

    b. Paresthesia

    c. Malunion

    d. Volkmann ischemic contracture

11. While riding a bicycle on a narrow road, a patient was hit from behind and thrown into a ditch, sustaining a pelvic fracture. Which complications does the nurse monitor for that are common with pelvic fractures?

    a. Paresthesia and ischemia

    b. Hemorrhage and shock

    c. Paralytic ileus and a lacerated urethra

    d. Thrombophlebitis and infection

12. The nurse is caring for a patient with a pelvic fracture. Which nursing assessments for a pelvic fracture will be included? (Select all that apply.)
    a. Checking the urine for hematuria
    b. Palpating peripheral pulses in both lower extremities
    c. Testing the stool for occult blood
    d. Assessing level of consciousness
    e. Assessing pupillary response

13. A patient has suffered a femoral shaft fracture in an industrial injury. Which is an immediate nursing concern for this patient?
    a. Hypovolemic shock
    b. Infection
    c. Knee and hip dislocation
    d. Pain resulting from muscle spasm

14. A nurse is caring for a patient who has had an amputation. Which interventions will the nurse provide to foster a positive self-image? (Select all that apply.)
    a. Encouraging the patient to care for the residual limb
    b. Allowing the expression of grief
    c. Encourage the patient to have family and friends view the residual limb to decrease self-consciousness
    d. Encouraging family and friends to refrain from visiting temporarily because this may increase the patient's embarrassment
    e. Introducing the patient to local amputee support groups

15. A patient was climbing a ladder, slipped on a rung, and fell on the right side of the chest. X-ray studies reveal three rib fractures, and the patient reports pain with inspiration. Which is the priority intervention in the treatment of this patient?
    a. Chest strapping
    b. Mechanical ventilation
    c. Coughing and deep breathing with pillow splinting
    d. Thoracentesis

Digestive and Gastrointestinal Function

Assessment of Digestive and Gastrointestinal Function

Learning Outcomes

1. Describe the structure and function of the organs of the gastrointestinal tract.
2. Explain the mechanical and chemical processes involved in digesting and absorbing nutrients and eliminating waste products.
3. Discriminate between normal and abnormal assessment findings of the gastrointestinal system.
4. Recognize and evaluate the major symptoms of gastrointestinal dysfunction by applying the patient's health history and physical assessment findings.
5. Identify the diagnostic tests used to evaluate gastrointestinal tract function and related nursing implications.

SECTION I: ASSESSING YOUR UNDERSTANDING

Activity A *Fill in the blanks.*

1. Three pancreatic secretions that contain digestive enzymes are _____, _____, and _____.

2. Chyme, partially digested food that is mixed with gastric contents, stimulates segmented contractions, which are _____, and intestinal peristalsis, which is _____.

3. It takes _____ hours after eating for food to pass into the terminal ileum. It takes _____ hours for food to reach and distend the rectum.

4. Structural changes in the esophagus that occur as the result of age-related changes include _____, _____, and _____.

5. Reflux of food into the esophagus from the stomach is prevented by contraction of the _____.

6. The digestion of starches begins in the mouth with the secretion of the enzyme _____.

7. The stomach, which derives its acidity from hydrochloric acid, has a pH of approximately _____.

8. Intrinsic factor is a gastric secretion necessary for the intestinal absorption of vitamin _____, which prevents pernicious anemia.

9. A hormonal regulatory substance that inhibits stomach contraction and gastric secretions is _____.

10. _____, which is secreted by the gallbladder, is responsible for fat emulsification.

11. The stomach has four anatomic regions: the _____, _____, _____, and _____.

12. The major carbohydrate that tissues use for fuel is _____.

Activity B *Briefly answer the following.*

1. What role do the sympathetic and parasympathetic portions of the autonomic nervous system play in GI function?

_____

_____

_____

_____

2. Describe what the outcomes are when there is an obstruction of the GI tract.

_____

_____

_____

3. A flexible sigmoidoscopy permits how much of the lower bowel to be viewed?

_____

4. Prior to performing a guaiac-based fecal occult blood testing (gFOBT), what education will the nurse provide?

_____

_____

_____

_____

5. When is a magnetic resonance imaging (MRI) test contraindicated?

_____

_____

_____

6. What will occur if there is a lack of intrinsic factor secreted by the gastric mucosa?

_____

_____

_____

_____

Activity C *Match the major digestive enzyme in Column II with its associated digestive action listed in Column I.*

Column I

_____ 1. Helps convert protein into amino acids.

_____ 2. Facilitates the production of dextrins and maltose.

_____ 3. Digests protein and helps form polypeptides.

_____ 4. Digests carbohydrates and helps form fructose.

_____ 5. Glucose is a product of this enzyme's action.

_____ 6. Helps form galactose.

Column II

a. Amylase

b. Maltase

c. Sucrase

d. Lactase

e. Pepsin

f. Trypsin

SECTION II: APPLYING YOUR KNOWLEDGE

Activity D *Consider the scenario and answer the questions.*

CASE STUDY: Colonoscopy

Mr. Carl is a 54-year-old patient who comes to the clinic and informs the nurse that he has been having blood in his stools for the past 2 weeks. He states that he has no pain or discomfort and has never had any trouble with his bowel movements. The health care provider schedules him for a colonoscopy.

1. The nurse is giving instructions about preparation of the bowel prior to the procedure. What is the importance of the bowel preparation for a colonoscopy?

_____

_____

2. What information should the nurse provide with regard to the position he will be placed in during the procedure?

_____

_____

_____

3. The nurse informs Mr. Carl that he will be monitored during the entire procedure. What monitoring will occur during the procedure?

_____

_____

4. During the colonoscopy, for what complications should Mr. Carl be continuously monitored?

_____

_____

_____

_____

SECTION III: PRACTICING FOR NCLEX

Activity E *Answer the following questions.*

1. The nurse is performing an initial assessment of a patient reporting increased stomach acid related to stress. Which neuroregulator will have influence over these symptoms?
   a. Gastrin
   b. Cholecystokinin
   c. Norepinephrine
   d. Secretin

2. The nurse is performing an assessment of a patient. During the assessment, the patient informs the nurse of some recent "stomach trouble." Which common symptom does the nurse correlate with GI dysfunction?
   a. Diffuse pain
   b. Dyspepsia
   c. Constipation
   d. Abdominal bloating

3. The nurse is investigating a patient's report of pain in the duodenal area. Where will the nurse perform the assessment?
   a. Epigastric area and consider possible radiation of pain to the right subscapular region
   b. Hypogastrium in the right or left lower quadrant
   c. Left lower quadrant
   d. Periumbilical area, followed by the right lower quadrant

4. A patient reports abdominal pain associated with indigestion. Which is characteristic of this type of pain?
   a. Described as crampy or burning.
   b. Located in the left lower quadrant.
   c. Less severe after an intake of fatty foods.
   d. Relieved by the intake of coarse vegetables, which stimulate peristalsis.

5. The nurse is collecting a stool specimen from a patient. Which characteristic of the stool indicates to the nurse that the patient may have an upper GI bleed?
   a. Clay colored
   b. Greasy and foamy
   c. Tarry and black
   d. Threaded with mucus

6. The nurse is performing an abdominal assessment for a patient in the hospital with reports of abdominal pain. Which part of the assessment will the nurse perform first?
   a. Percussion
   b. Palpation
   c. Auscultation
   d. Inspection

7. The nurse has been requested to position a patient for an examination of the abdomen. Which position will the nurse place the patient in for the examination?
   a. Prone position with pillows positioned to alleviate pressure on the abdomen
   b. Semi-Fowler position with the left leg bent to minimize pressure on the abdomen
   c. Supine position with the knees flexed to relax the abdominal muscles
   d. Reverse Trendelenburg position to facilitate the natural propulsion of intestinal contents

8. The nurse auscultates a patient's abdomen to assess bowel sounds, documenting five to six sounds heard in less than 30 seconds. How will the nurse document the character of the bowel sounds?
   a. Normal
   b. Hypoactive
   c. Hyperactive
   d. Borborygmi

9. The nurse is providing instructions to a patient scheduled for a gastroscopy. Which instructions will the nurse include? (Select all that apply.)

   a. Fast for 8 hours before the examination.

   b. The throat will be sprayed with a local anesthetic.

   c. After gastroscopy, the patient cannot eat or drink until the gag reflex returns (1 to 2 hours).

   d. The health care provider will be able to determine if there is a presence of bowel disease.

   e. There must be bowel cleansing prior to the procedure.

10. A patient is scheduled for a fiberoptic colonoscopy. Which does the nurse inform the patient that fiberoptic colonoscopy is most frequently used to diagnose?

    a. Bowel disease of unknown origin

    b. Cancer screening

    c. Inflammatory bowel disease

    d. Occult bleeding

11. A patient is being prepared for esophageal manometry. The nurse will inform the patient to withhold which medication for 48 hours prior to the procedure?

    a. Amiodarone

    b. Verapamil

    c. Aspirin

    d. Metoprolol

12. The nurse is assisting the health care provider with a gastric acid stimulation test for a patient. Which medication will the nurse prepare to administer subcutaneously to stimulate gastric secretions?

    a. Pentagastrin

    b. Atropine

    c. Glycopyrrolate

    d. Acetylcysteine

13. The nurse is assisting the health care provider with a colonoscopy for a patient with rectal bleeding. For which reason is the nurse asked to administer glucagon during the procedure?

    a. The patient is probably hypoglycemic and requires the glucagon.

    b. To relieve anxiety during the procedure for moderate sedation.

    c. To reduce air accumulation in the colon.

    d. To relax colonic musculature and reduce spasm.

14. A patient is in the outpatient recovery area after having a colonoscopy and informs the nurse of abdominal cramping. Which is the best response by the nurse?

    a. "We may need to go back in and see what is wrong. You shouldn't have discomfort."

    b. "I will call the health care provider and let them know, since there may have been too much air instilled in your colon."

    c. "I will call the health care provider and see if I can give you pain medication. Sometimes the pain can be caused by having a biopsy."

    d. "The cramping is caused by the air insufflated in the colon during the procedure, and it is best to try and expel it."

15. During a colonoscopy with moderate sedation, the patient groans with obvious discomfort and begins bleeding from the rectum. The patient becomes diaphoretic, with an increase in abdominal girth. Which complication of this procedure is the nurse aware may be occurring?

    a. Infection

    b. Bowel perforation

    c. Colonic polyp

    d. Rectal fissure

CHAPTER 39

Management of Patients with Oral and Esophageal Disorders

Learning Outcomes

1. Define the relationship of dental hygiene and dental problems to nutrition and disease.
2. Describe the nursing management of patients with abnormalities of the oral cavity, jaw, and salivary glands including cancer of the oral cavity and disorders of the esophagus.
3. Describe the nursing management of the patient receiving enteral nutrition support.
4. Use the nursing process as a framework for care of the patient undergoing neck dissection, having a gastrostomy or jejunostomy feeding tube placed, or with noncancerous disorders of the esophagus.

SECTION I: ASSESSING YOUR UNDERSTANDING

Activity A *Fill in the blanks.*

1. Digestion normally begins in the _____.

2. Current _____, which increases the likelihood of periodontitis by at least 50%, remains a key modifiable risk factor for periodontitis at all severity levels. (Eke, Wei, Thornton-Evans, et al., 2016).

3. A common lesion of the mouth that is also referred to as a "canker sore" is _____.

4. The incidence of most dental caries is directly related to an increase in the dietary intake of _____.

5. Preventive orthodontics for malocclusion can start as early as age _____.

6. Mumps, a viral infection affecting children, is an inflammation of the _____ gland.

7. _____ is a frequent sequela of oral cancer, particularly when the salivary glands have been exposed to radiation or major surgery.

8. _____ can result after antibiotic use alters normal intestinal flora and promotes the abnormal growth of this potentially dangerous microbe.

Activity B *Briefly answer the following.*

1. What is the process in which tooth decay begins?

2. Which interventions can the nurse encourage patients to take to prevent and control dental caries?

3. Which intervention can be provided to relieve the discomfort of a patient with a tooth abscess in the early stage?

_____

_____

_____

4. Compare and contrast sialadenitis and sialolithiasis.

_____

_____

5. Which potential postoperative complications may be involved with the patient who has had a radical neck dissection?

_____

_____

Activity C *Match the abnormality of the lips, mouth, or gums listed in Column II with its associated symptomatology of the lip, mouth, or gums listed in Column I.*

Column I

_____ 1. Ulcerated and painful, white papules

_____ 2. Reddened area or rash associated with itching

_____ 3. Painful, inflamed, swollen gums

_____ 4. White overgrowth of horny layer of epidermis

_____ 5. Shallow ulcer with a red border and white or yellow center

_____ 6. Hyperkeratotic white patches usually in buccal mucosa

_____ 7. Reddened circum-scribed lesion that ulcerates and becomes encrusted

_____ 8. White patches with rough, hairlike projections usually found on the tongue

Column II

a. Actinic cheilitis

b. Leukoplakia

c. Chancre

d. Canker sore

e. Gingivitis

f. Lichen planus

g. Contact dermatitis

h. Hairy leukoplakia

SECTION II: APPLYING YOUR KNOWLEDGE

Activity D *Consider the scenarios and answer the questions.*

CASE STUDY: Radical Neck Dissection

Mr. Rowly, a 64-year-old patient with a 40-year history of using oral tobacco products, has been diagnosed with a malignancy of the neck and is scheduled for a radical neck dissection. He will be accompanied to the hospital by his wife, who will be assisting with his care after discharge.

1. The nurse is preparing Mr. Rowly for surgery. Which two common morbidities does the nurse identify are associated with a radical neck dissection?

_____

2. Which postoperative complications will the nurse monitor for after Mr. Rowly's surgery?

_____

3. Mr. Rowly is in the postanesthesia care unit (PACU) after surgery. Which position will the nurse maintain the patient in postoperatively?

_____

4. Which finding will be immediately reported to the health care provider indicating airway obstruction?

_____

5. The nurse observes excessive drooling during a postoperative assessment. Which nerve will the nurse assess for damage?

_____

6. What can be done prior to Mr. Rowly's discharge to assist the wife with his care?

_____

_____

CASE STUDY: Mandibular Fracture

William, a 17-year-old student, suffered a mandibular fracture while playing football. He is presently having jaw repositioning surgery under general anesthesia. His parents are in the waiting area.

1. How will the nurse position William in the immediate postoperative period?

_____

2. What should the nurse tell William and his family to explain why nasogastric suctioning is needed?

_____

_____

3. For emergency use, what will the nurse be sure is available at the head of the bed?

_____

4. What initial postoperative diet would be recommended for William?

_____

CASE STUDY: Cancer of the Mouth

Mrs. Eddy, a 64 year old, has been a chain smoker for 20 years. During the past month, she noticed dryness in her mouth and a roughened area that is irritating. She mentioned her symptoms to her dentist, who referred her to a medical internist.

1. On the basis of the patient's health history, the nurse suspects oral cancer. What would the nurse expect the lesion to look like?

_____

2. During the health history, the nurse noted that Mrs. Eddy does not mention a late-occurring symptom of mouth cancer. Which does the nurse identify as a symptom of late mouth cancer?

_____

3. On physical examination, Mrs. Eddy evidences changes associated with cancer of the mouth. What changes would the nurse know are characteristic of cancer of the mouth?

_____

_____

SECTION III: PRACTICING FOR NCLEX

Activity E *Answer the following questions.*

1. The nurse is performing an assessment for a patient who presents to the clinic with a lip lesion. The lesion is erythemic, fissuring, with white hyperkeratosis. Which do these findings indicate?
   a. Actinic cheilitis
   b. Human papillomavirus lesion
   c. Frey syndrome
   d. Sialadenitis

2. A patient is experiencing painful, inflamed, and swollen gums, and when brushing the teeth, the gums bleed. Which common disease of the oral tissue does the nurse educate the patient about?
   a. Candidiasis
   b. Gingivitis
   c. Herpes simplex
   d. Cancer of the oral mucosa

3. The nurse is caring for a patient after drainage of a dentoalveolar or periapical abscess. Which actions will the nurse provide in the postoperative phase? (Select all that apply.)
   a. Soft diet after 24 hours
   b. Fluid restriction for the first 48 hours because the gums are swollen and painful
   c. External heat by pad or compress to hasten the resolution of the inflammatory swelling
   d. Warm saline mouthwashes every 2 hours while awake
   e. Gargle with peroxide and saline every 4 hours

4. A patient reports an inflamed salivary gland below the right ear. Which gland will the nurse assess?
   a. The buccal gland
   b. The parotid gland
   c. The sublingual gland
   d. The submandibular gland

5. An older adult patient who has been living at home alone is diagnosed with parotitis. Which causative bacteria does the nurse identify is the cause of the parotitis?

   a. Methicillin-resistant *Streptococcus aureus* (MRSA)

   b. *Pneumococcus*

   c. *Staphylococcus aureus*

   d. *Streptococcus viridans*

6. A nurse inspects the Stensen duct of the parotid gland to determine inflammation and possible obstruction. Which area in the oral cavity will the nurse assess?

   a. Buccal mucosa next to the upper molars

   b. Dorsum of the tongue

   c. Roof of the mouth next to the incisors

   d. Posterior segment of the tongue near the uvula

7. The nurse is obtaining a history on a patient who comes to the clinic. Which symptom described by the patient is one of the first symptoms associated with esophageal disease?

   a. Dysphagia

   b. Malnutrition

   c. Pain

   d. Regurgitation of food

8. A patient tells the nurse that it feels like food is "sticking" in the lower portion of the esophagus. Which motility disorder correlates with the symptoms the patient describes?

   a. Achalasia

   b. Diffuse spasm

   c. Gastroesophageal reflex disease

   d. Hiatal hernia

9. A patient is brought to the emergency department by a family member, who states that the patient "drank drain cleaner." Which interventions does the nurse provide to treat this patient? (Select all that apply.)

   a. Administer an irritant that will induce vomiting.

   b. Aspirate secretions from the pharynx if respirations are affected.

   c. Neutralize the chemical.

   d. Irrigate the esophagus with large volumes of water.

   e. Administer activated charcoal.

10. The nurse is caring for a patient with a radical neck dissection and observes serosanguineous secretions in the wound suction unit during the first postoperative day. Which amount of drainage in the wound unit will the nurse expect to observe?

    a. Between 40 and 80 mL

    b. Approximately 80 to 120 mL

    c. Between 120 and 160 mL

    d. Greater than 160 mL

11. A patient describes a burning sensation in the esophagus, pain when swallowing, and frequent indigestion. Which does the nurse identify that these clinical manifestations indicate?

    a. This is an indication that the patient has peptic ulcer disease.

    b. This is an indication that the patient may have esophageal cancer.

    c. These symptoms indicate gastroesophageal reflux disease.

    d. The clinical manifestations indicate diverticulitis.

12. A patient has been diagnosed with Zenker's diverticulum. Which treatment does the nurse educate the patient regarding?

    a. A low-residue diet

    b. Chemotherapeutic agents

    c. Radiation therapy

    d. Surgical removal of the diverticulum

13. A patient who has positive human immune deficiency virus (HIV) comes to the clinic reporting white patches with rough hairlike projections on the tongue. The nurse observes the lesions on the lateral border of the tongue. Which abnormality of the mouth does the nurse identify?

    a. Aphthous stomatitis

    b. Nicotine stomatitis

    c. Erythroplakia

    d. Hairy leukoplakia

14. A patient comes to the clinic reporting a sore throat. When assessing the patient, the nurse observes a reddened ulcerated lesion on the lip that the patient states has been there for a couple of weeks but is painless. Which testing will the nurse discuss with the health care provider?

a. HIV

b. Syphilis

c. Gonorrhea

d. Herpes simplex

15. A patient has been taking a 10-day course of antibiotics for pneumonia and now reports white patches that look like milk curds in the mouth. Which treatment will the nurse educate the patient about?

a. Nystatin

b. Cephalexin

c. Fluocinolone acetonide oral base gel

d. Acyclovir

Management of Patients with Gastric and Duodenal Disorders

Learning Outcomes

1. Compare the etiology, pathophysiology, clinical manifestations, and management of acute gastritis, chronic gastritis, and peptic ulcer disease.
2. Use the nursing process as a framework for care of the patient with acute or chronic gastritis, or peptic ulcer.
3. Discuss the etiology, pathophysiology, clinical manifestations, and management of gastric cancer and tumors of the small intestine.
4. Use the nursing process as a framework for care of the patient with gastric cancer or tumors of the small intestine.

SECTION I: ASSESSING YOUR UNDERSTANDING

Activity A *Fill in the blanks.*

1. The most common site for peptic ulcer formation is the _____.

2. People with blood type _____ are more susceptible to the development of peptic ulcers than are those with blood type A, B, or AB.

3. The use of nonsteroidal anti-inflammatory drugs (NSAIDs) such as _____ and _____ is a major risk factor for peptic ulcer disease.

4. The most common complication of peptic ulcer disease that occurs in 10% to 20% of patients is _____.

5. _____ is the preferred diagnostic procedure for peptic ulcers.

6. _____ is the bacillus commonly associated with the formation of gastric, and possibly duodenal ulcers.

7. _____, _____, _____, and _____ are some of the major potential complications of a peptic ulcer.

8. _____ are of value in diagnosing ZES and achlorhydria, hypochlorhydria, or hyperchlorhydria.

Activity B *Briefly answer the following.*

1. Identify the priority action used to treat the ingestion of a corrosive acid or alkali.

_____

_____

_____

2. Explain why patients who have gastritis due to a vitamin deficiency usually have malabsorption of vitamin B_{12}.

_____

_____

3. What two conditions are specifically related to peptic ulcer development?

_____

_____

4. What findings are characteristic of Zollinger-Ellison syndrome?

_____

_____

5. What does the term "stress ulcer" mean?

_____

_____

6. What is the difference between Cushing's and Curling's ulcer in terms of cause and location?

_____

_____

_____

7. Explain the current theory about diet modification for peptic ulcer disease.

_____

_____

_____

_____

8. Describe the clinical manifestations associated with a peptic ulcer perforation.

_____

_____

_____

9. Compare and contrast the clinical manifestations related to gastric ulcers from duodenal ulcers.

_____

_____

Activity C

Pharmacologic Therapy for Peptic Ulcer Disease and Gastritis

Match the specific drug in Column II with the drug type in Column I.

Column I	Column II
_____ **1.** Antibiotics	**a.** Bismuth subsalicylate
_____ **2.** Antidiarrheal	**b.** Clarithromycin
_____ **3.** Histamine-2 receptor antagonist	**c.** Misoprostol
_____ **4.** Proton pump inhibitors	**d.** Famotidine
_____ **5.** Prostaglandin E1 analogue	**e.** Pantoprazole

SECTION II: APPLYING YOUR KNOWLEDGE

Activity D *Consider the scenario and answer the questions.*

CASE STUDY: Gastric Cancer

Mr. Jackson, a 66-year-old African American male, has recently been seen by the health care provider to confirm a diagnosis of gastric cancer. He has a history of tobacco use and was diagnosed 10 years ago with pernicious anemia. He and his family are shocked about the possibility of this diagnosis because he has been asymptomatic prior to recent reports of pain and multiple gastrointestinal symptoms.

1. The nurse is assessing Mr. Jackson and has progressed to palpation of the abdomen. Which indication does the nurse have that metastasis to the liver has occurred?

_____

2. Which type of diagnostic procedures will the nurse educate Mr. Jackson about that will most likely be performed?

_____

_____

3. The surgical team has decided that a Billroth II would be the best approach to treatment. What does the nurse explain to the family that this procedure involves?

_____

_____

4. The nurse explains that combination chemotherapy, more effective than single-agent chemotherapy, frequently follows surgery. What primary agent does the nurse anticipate will be used?

_____

SECTION III: PRACTICING FOR NCLEX

Activity E *Answer the following questions.*

1. A patient has been diagnosed with acute gastritis and asks the nurse what could have caused it. Which is the best response(s) by the nurse? (Select all that apply.)
   a. "It can be caused by ingestion of strong acids."
   b. "You may have ingested some irritating foods."
   c. "Is it possible that you are overusing aspirin."
   d. "It is a hereditary disease."
   e. "It is probably your nerves."

2. The nurse is caring for a patient who has been diagnosed with gastritis. To promote fluid balance when treating gastritis, the nurse educates the patient about the intake of how much fluid per day?
   a. 1.0 L
   b. 1.5 L
   c. 2.0 L
   d. 2.5 L

3. The nurse is preparing to administer medications to a patient with acute gastritis. The patient has a new prescription for a histamine-2 receptor antagonist. Which medication will the nurse administer?
   a. Omeprazole
   b. Famotidine
   c. Lansoprazole
   d. Bismuth salts

4. A patient comes to the clinic, stating, "I think I have an ulcer." Which symptom(s) associated with peptic ulcer pain will the nurse inquire about? (Select all that apply.)
   a. Burning sensation localized in the back or mid-epigastrium
   b. Feeling of emptiness that precedes meals from 1 to 3 hours
   c. Severe gnawing pain that increases in severity as the day progresses
   d. Pain that radiates to the shoulder or jaw
   e. Vomiting without associated nausea

5. The nurse is educating a patient about discharge medications. When will the nurse instruct the patient to take the antacid medication?
   a. With the meal
   b. 30 minutes before the meal
   c. 1 to 3 hours after the meal
   d. Immediately after the meal

6. A patient is scheduled for a Billroth I procedure for ulcer management. Which education will the nurse provide to the patient?
   a. A partial gastrectomy is performed with anastomosis of the stomach segment to the duodenum.
   b. A sectioned portion of the stomach is joined to the jejunum.
   c. The antral portion of the stomach is removed and a vagotomy is performed.
   d. The vagus nerve is cut and gastric drainage is established.

7. The nurse is developing a plan of care for a patient with peptic ulcer disease. Which nursing interventions will be included in the care plan? (Select all that apply.)
   a. Making neurovascular checks every 4 hours
   b. Frequently monitoring hemoglobin and hematocrit levels
   c. Observing stools and vomitus for color, consistency, and volume
   d. Checking the blood pressure and pulse rate every 15 to 20 minutes
   e. Inserting an indwelling catheter for incontinence

8. The nurse is caring for a patient who is suspected to have developed a peptic ulcer hemorrhage. Which action would the nurse perform first?

   a. Place the patient in a recumbent position with the legs elevated.

   b. Prepare a peripheral and central line for intravenous infusion.

   c. Assess vital signs.

   d. Call the health care provider.

9. A patient sustained second- and third-degree burns over 30% of the body surface area approximately 72 hours ago. Which type of ulcer will the nurse monitor for while caring for this patient?

   a. Curling ulcer

   b. Peptic ulcer

   c. Esophageal ulcer

   d. Meckel ulcer

10. A patient is in the hospital for the treatment of peptic ulcer disease. The nurse finds the patient with a boardlike abdomen, vomiting, and reports of a sudden severe pain in the abdomen. Which will the nurse suspect these symptoms indicate?

   a. The treatment for the peptic ulcer is ineffective

   b. A reaction to the medication given for the ulcer

   c. Gastric penetration

   d. Perforation of the peptic ulcer

11. A patient taking metronidazole for the treatment of *Helicobacter pylori* states that the medication is causing nausea. Which suggestion can the nurse provide to the patient to alleviate this problem?

   a. Discontinue the use of the medication.

   b. Tell the patient to ask the health care provider to prescribe another type of antibiotic.

   c. Take the medication with meals to decrease the nausea.

   d. Crush the medication and put it in applesauce.

12. The nurse is educating a patient with peptic ulcer disease about the disease process. Which decreases the secretion of bicarbonate from the pancreas into the duodenum, resulting in increased acidity of the duodenum?

   a. Smoking

   b. Eating spicy foods

   c. Drinking carbonated beverages

   d. Taking antacids

13. The nurse is educating a patient with peptic ulcer about dietary modification. Which will the nurse include when educating this patient?

   a. Avoid extremes of temperature in food and beverages.

   b. Increase the fiber content in the diet.

   c. Decrease the amount of fluid the patient is drinking.

   d. Increase the protein content in the diet.

14. The nurse determines that a patient is at risk for the development of gastric cancer. Which foods will the nurse encourage the patient to avoid? (Select all that apply.)

   a. Fruits

   b. Vegetables

   c. Smoked foods

   d. Pickled foods

   e. Whole grains

15. A patient is having bile reflux after gastric surgery and having the pylorus removed. Which pharmacologic therapy will the nurse educate the patient regarding?

   a. The administration of capecitabine

   b. The administration of omeprazole

   c. The administration of famotidine

   d. The administration of cholestyramine

CHAPTER 41

Management of Patients with Intestinal and Rectal Disorders

Learning Outcomes

1. Describe the pathophysiology, clinical manifestations, and management of patients with constipation, diarrhea, fecal incontinence, and irritable bowel syndrome.
2. Identify celiac disease as a disorder of malabsorption; describe its pathophysiology, clinical manifestations, and management.
3. Discuss the nursing management of the patient with appendicitis, diverticular disease, and intestinal obstruction.
4. Compare Crohn's disease and ulcerative colitis with regard to their pathophysiology; clinical manifestations; diagnostic evaluation; and medical, surgical, and nursing management.
5. Identify the purposes, indications for, types, and administration techniques of parenteral nutrition access devices and formulas.
6. Use the nursing process as a framework for care of the patient with inflammatory bowel disease, or receiving parenteral nutrition, or with colorectal cancer.
7. Explain the nursing management of the patient with an anorectal disorder.

SECTION I: ASSESSING YOUR UNDERSTANDING

Activity A *Fill in the blanks.*

1. _____ may be performed to assess malfunction of the sphincter.

2. _____ is a dilated and atonic colon caused by a fecal mass that obstructs the passage of colon contents.

3. Loss of bicarbonate with diarrhea may lead to _____.

4. The three most common causes of small bowel obstruction are _____, _____, and _____.

5. The majority of large bowel obstructions are caused by _____.

6. A disorder of malabsorption that inactivates pancreatic enzymes is _____ _____.

7. Malabsorption diseases may affect the ability of the digestive system to absorb the major water-soluble _____.

8. A(n) _____ with contrast agent is the diagnostic test of choice to confirm diverticulitis.

9. Common clinical manifestations of Crohn's disease are _____ and _____.

10. The nurse is irrigating a colostomy. The catheter should be advanced into the stoma _____ to _____ inches.

Activity B *Briefly answer the following.*

1. Which four complications are associated with diverticulitis?

   _____

   _____

2. Which common bacteria may be found in a patient who has developed peritonitis?

   _____

   _____

3. Which risk factors for colorectal cancer can the nurse educate the public about?

   _____

   _____

   _____

   _____

   _____

4. Describe the physiologic response that occurs when a patient performs Valsalva maneuver while straining during defecation.

   _____

   _____

   _____

   _____

5. Which are the four classifications for constipation based on their underlying pathophysiologic mechanisms?

   _____

   _____

   _____

   _____

   _____

   _____

6. Which factors are associated with the development of irritable bowel syndrome?

   _____

   _____

   _____

   _____

7. What are the hallmark signs of malabsorption syndrome?

   _____

   _____

   _____

   _____

Activity C

PART 1: Key Terms

Match the term in Column II with its associated definition in Column I.

Column I

___ 1. A tubular fibrous tract that extends from an opening beside the anus into the anal canal

___ 2. Dilated and atonic colon caused by a fecal mass

___ 3. A chemotherapeutic agent used to treat colon cancer

___ 4. A food to avoid for a patient with an ileostomy

___ 5. Straining at stool

___ 6. Another name for regional enteritis

___ 7. A highly reliable blood study used to diagnose appendicitis

___ 8. Painful straining at stool

___ 9. The most common bacteria associated with peritonitis

___ 10. Another term for fecal matter

___ 11. An ileal outlet on the abdomen

___ 12. Intestinal rumbling

___ 13. Another food to avoid for a patient with an ileostomy

___ 14. The most popular over-the-counter medication purchased in the United States

___ 15. Intravenous nutrition used for inflammatory bowel disease

___ 16. The most common complication of colon cancer

Column II

a. Valsalva maneuver

b. Tenesmus

c. Stoma

d. Corn

e. Fistula

f. Peritonitis

g. Crohn's disease

h. TPN

i. 5-FU

j. Effluent

k. CEA

l. Laxatives

m. Megacolon

n. Borborygmus

o. Celery

p. *E. coli*

PART 2: Laxative Classification and Action

Match the type of laxative listed in Column III with its classification in Column II. Then match the classification in Column II with its action listed in Column I.

Column I

___ 1. Magnesium ions alter stool consistency.

___ 2. Surfactant action hydrates stool.

___ 3. Electrolytes induce diarrhea.

___ 4. Polysaccharides and cellulose mix with intestinal contents.

___ 5. Colon is irritated and sensory nerve endings stimulated.

___ 6. Hydrocarbons soften fecal matter.

Column II

___ a. Bulk forming

___ b. Stimulant

___ c. Fecal softener

___ d. Lubricant

___ e. Saline agent

___ f. Osmotic agent

Column III

1. Mineral oil

2. Metamucil

3. Milk of magnesia

4. Dulcolax

5. Colace

6. Colyte

SECTION II: APPLYING YOUR KNOWLEDGE

Activity D *Consider the scenario and answer the questions.*

CASE STUDY: Appendicitis

Rory, age 18, is admitted to the hospital with a possible diagnosis of appendicitis. She reports pain in the right lower quadrant of the abdomen, nausea, and a fever of 101°F prior to her hospital admission.

1. Since Rory has been symptomatic for 24 hours, which assessment data correlates with a diagnosis of appendicitis?

   _____

   _____

   _____

   _____

2. Before the nurse sends Rory to have any diagnostic x-rays, which procedure will be performed?

   _____

   _____

3. Two hours after admission, the nurse observes Rory lying motionless and supine in the bed and she tells the nurse that she feels worse. What does this finding indicate to the nurse?

   _____

   _____

SECTION III: PRACTICING FOR NCLEX

Activity E *Answer the following questions.*

1. The nurse is assessing a patient with appendicitis. The nurse is attempting to elicit a Rovsing sign. Where will the nurse palpate for this indicator of acute appendicitis?
   a. Right lower quadrant
   b. Left lower quadrant
   c. Right upper quadrant
   d. Left upper quadrant

2. A patient is not having daily bowel movements and has begun regular laxative use. Which education will the nurse provide regarding laxative use?
   a. When taking the laxatives, plenty of fluids should be taken as well.
   b. The laxatives should be taken no more than three times a week or laxative addiction will result.
   c. Laxatives should not be routinely taken due to destruction of nerve endings in the colon.
   d. Laxatives should never be the first treatment of constipation; natural methods should be employed first.

3. A patient is admitted to the hospital after not having had a bowel movement in several days. The nurse observes the patient is having small liquid stools, a distended abdomen with cramping. Which complication will the nurse monitor the patient for?
   a. Appendicitis
   b. Rectal fissures
   c. Bowel perforation
   d. Diverticulitis

4. The nurse is performing an abdominal assessment for a patient with diarrhea and auscultates a loud rumbling sound in the left lower quadrant. How will the nurse document this sound on the nurse's notes?
   a. Loud bowel sounds
   b. Borborygmus
   c. Tenesmus
   d. Peristalsis

5. The nurse is caring for an older adult patient experiencing fecal incontinence. When planning the care of this patient, which will the nurse designate as a priority goal?
   a. Maintaining skin integrity
   b. Beginning a bowel program to establish continence
   c. Instituting a diet high in fiber and increase fluid intake
   d. Determining the need for surgical intervention to correct the problem

6. A patient with irritable bowel syndrome has been having more frequent symptoms lately and is not sure what lifestyle changes may have occurred. Which suggestion can the nurse provide to identify a trigger for the symptoms?

   a. Document how much fluid is being taken to determine if the patient is overhydrating.

   b. Discontinue the use of any medication presently being taken to determine if medication is a trigger.

   c. Begin an exercise regimen and biofeedback to determine if external stress is a trigger.

   d. Keep a 1- to 2-week symptom and food diary to identify food triggers.

7. The nurse is caring for a patient who has malabsorption syndrome with an undetermined cause. Which procedure will the nurse assist with that is the best diagnostic test for this illness?

   a. Ultrasound

   b. Endoscopy with mucosal biopsy

   c. Stool specimen for ova and parasites

   d. Pancreatic function tests

8. A patient arrives in the emergency department reporting right lower abdominal pain that began 4 hours ago and is getting worse. The nurse assesses rebound tenderness at McBurney point. Which does this assessment data indicate to the nurse?

   a. Crohn's disease

   b. Ulcerative colitis

   c. Appendicitis

   d. Diverticulitis

9. The nurse is caring for a patient who has had an appendectomy. Which is the best position for the nurse to maintain the patient in after the surgery?

   a. Prone

   b. Sims left lateral

   c. High Fowler

   d. Supine with head of bed elevated 15 degrees

10. A patient is suspected to have diverticulosis without symptoms of diverticulitis. Which diagnostic test does the nurse anticipate educating the patient about prior to scheduling?

    a. Colonoscopy

    b. Barium enema

    c. Flexible sigmoidoscopy

    d. CT scan

11. The nurse is admitting a patient with a diagnosis of diverticulitis and assesses that the patient has a boardlike abdomen, no bowel sounds, and reports severe abdominal pain. Which is the nurse's first action?

    a. Start an IV with lactated Ringer solution.

    b. Notify the health care provider.

    c. Administer a retention enema.

    d. Administer an opioid analgesic.

12. The nurse is assigned to care for a patient 2 days after an appendectomy due to a ruptured appendix with resultant peritonitis. The nurse has just assisted the patient with ambulation to the bedside commode when the patient points to the surgical site and informs the nurse that "something gave way." Which complication does the nurse suspect may have occurred?

    a. A drain may have become dislodged.

    b. Wound dehiscence has occurred.

    c. Infection has developed.

    d. The surgical wound has begun to bleed.

13. A patient is having a diagnostic workup for reports of frequent diarrhea, right lower abdominal pain, and weight loss. The nurse is reviewing the results of the barium study and notes the presence of "string sign." Which is the significance of this in relation to the patient's condition?

    a. Crohn's disease

    b. Ulcerative colitis

    c. Irritable bowel syndrome

    d. Diverticulitis

14. A patient is being seen in the clinic reporting painful hemorrhoids. The nurse assesses the patient and observes the hemorrhoids are prolapsed but able to be placed back in the rectum manually. The nurse documents the hemorrhoids as which degree?

a. First degree

b. Second degree

c. Third degree

d. Fourth degree

15. The nurse is irrigating a colostomy when the patient says, "You will have to stop, I am cramping so badly." Which is the priority action by the nurse?

a. Inform the patient that it will only last a minute and continue with the procedure.

b. Clamp the tubing and give the patient a rest period.

c. Stop the irrigation and remove the tube.

d. Replace the fluid with cooler water since it is probably too warm.

Metabolic and Endocrine Function

Assessment and Management of Patients with Obesity

Learning Outcomes

1. Describe the causes, risks, and pathophysiology associated with obesity.
2. Discriminate between normal and abnormal assessment findings identified in the patient with obesity.
3. Identify strategies aimed at preventing and treating obesity, including lifestyle modification, pharmacologic therapy, and nonsurgical interventions.
4. Explain nursing management considerations for the patient with obesity using nonsurgical interventions.
5. Compare and contrast surgical modalities indicated to treat patients with obesity in terms of preoperative, postoperative, and long-term management and complications.
6. Use the nursing process as a framework for care of the patient who undergoes bariatric surgery.

SECTION I: ASSESSING YOUR UNDERSTANDING

Activity A Fill in the blanks.

1. _____ is an abnormal or excessive fat accumulation that may impair health.

2. It is estimated that _____% of American adults have obesity.

3. The causes of obesity include _____, _____, _____, and _____ factors.

4. Increase in fat stores, or adipose tissue, results in increases in the hormone _____, which is secreted by fat cells.

5. Patient _____ and _____ is measured to determine body mass index (BMI).

6. Women with waist circumference more than _____ inches and men with waist circumference more than _____ inches have greater risks for obesity-related morbidity than those with smaller waistlines.

7. Treatment of obesity includes _____ aimed at weight loss and then weight maintenance.

Activity B Briefly answer the following.

1. Explain the "thrifty gene" hypothesis.

_____

_____

2. What types of food are considered to be obesogenic?

_____

_____

3. Which multicomponent behavioral intervention should be discussed with a patient that has a BMI in excess of 30 kg/m²?

_____

_____

4. Which type of physical activity should be recommended for all adults?

_____

_____

5. Describe techniques for promoting adequate sleeping patterns.

_____

_____

6. What are the indications for a patient being prescribed antiobesity medications?

_____

_____

Activity C *Match the medication for treating obesity in Column I with the associated classification in Column II.*

Column I

____ 1. Phentermine

____ 2. Lorcaserin

____ 3. Liraglutide

____ 4. Orlistat

____ 5. Naltrexone/ bupropion

Column II

a. GLP-1 receptor agonist

b. Sympathomimetic amines

c. Dual agents

d. Selective serotonergic 5-HT2C receptor agonist

e. Gastrointestinal lipase inhibitor

SECTION II: APPLYING YOUR KNOWLEDGE

Activity D *Consider the scenario and answer the questions.*

CASE STUDY: Obesity

Ms. Carly is a 32-year-old teacher who reports being overweight all of her life. She presently weighs 350 lb with a BMI of 66.1 and reports that her primary health care provider informed her that she is prediabetic. She arrives at the bariatric outpatient center requesting surgery to decrease her weight and states that she has researched having the Roux-en-Y gastric bypass surgery.

1. Which contraindication should be assessed for when discussing gastric bypass?

_____

_____

2. Which prescreening testing is performed prior to gastric bypass surgery?

_____

_____

3. When discussing complications related to the Roux-en-Y bypass, what will the nurse be sure that the patient understands?

_____

_____

SECTION III: PRACTICING FOR NCLEX

Activity E *Answer the following questions.*

1. The nurse is assessing a patient with android obesity. Which risk factors will the nurse consider during the assessment of this patient? (Select all that apply.)

   a. Previous diagnosis of hyperthyroidism

   b. A diagnosis of hypertension

   c. A history of coronary artery disease

   d. A diagnosis of type 2 diabetes

   e. A history of multiple sclerosis

2. The nurse is providing education for a patient with obesity about caloric reduction. Which calorie deficit should the nurse recommend daily from the baseline?

  a. 100 to 250 calories

  b. 250 to 400 calories

  c. 500 to 1000 calories

  d. 1000 to 1500 calories

3. The nurse is educating a patient with obesity about weight loss with healthy dietary habits. Which statement made by the patient indicates that further education is required?

  a. "I need to adopt a diet heavy with plant-based food items."

  b. "The DASH diet will help me lose weight and maintain the weight loss."

  c. "In addition to dietary adjustments, I should exercise daily."

  d. "The only way I will be successful is if I purchase a commercial diet plan."

4. A patient is prescribed antiobesity medications to assist with a 75-lb weight loss goal. Which statement made by the patient indicates further education is needed?

  a. "Since I will be taking this medication, I won't have to change my dietary habits."

  b. "The weight loss medication may have unfavorable side effects."

  c. "Once I stop taking the medication, I may gain some or all of the weight back."

  d. "I will exercise daily and be sure to drink plenty of fluids."

5. The nurse is preparing a patient for a bariatric surgical procedure that will result in diminishing gastric contraction, limit ghrelin secretion, and decrease pancreatic enzyme secretion. Which procedure is the nurse preparing the patient for?

  a. Intragastric balloon therapy

  b. Vagal blocking therapy

  c. Sleeve gastrectomy

  d. Roux-en-Y gastric bypass

6. A patient that will undergo bariatric surgery asks the nurse when they will be allowed to eat after surgery. Which is the best response by the nurse?

  a. "You will most likely be able to have clear liquids within 24 to 48 hours."

  b. "You will not feel like eating anything for about 1 week."

  c. "You will be able to have some clear liquids when you return from surgery."

  d. "You will be started on a bland diet within 24 hours."

7. After bariatric surgery, the nurse is positioning the patient in the bed. Which position best promotes comfort and emptying of the stomach?

  a. Left lateral Sims position

  b. High-Fowler position

  c. Prone position

  d. Low-Fowler position

8. An older adult patient with morbid obesity had Roux-en-Y gastric bypass surgery. On postoperative day 2, the patient reports abdominal pain, and the nurse assesses a temperature of 102°F, heart rate of 126, and an elevated white blood cell count. Based on the assessment data, which does the nurse suspect is occurring with this patient?

  a. The patient is experiencing dumping syndrome.

  b. An anastomotic leak has occurred from the bypass surgery.

  c. The patient is dehydrated from lack of fluids.

  d. The patient likely has a small bowel obstruction.

9. The nurse is caring for a patient after Roux-en-Y bypass surgery for the treatment of morbid obesity. In order to prevent pernicious anemia, which prescribed medication will the nurse educate the patient about?

   a. Taking over-the-counter multivitamins daily

   b. Taking iron preparations orally once a month

   c. The administration of vitamin B_{12} injections monthly

   d. Taking oral thiamine tablets daily

10. A patient who recently had bariatric surgery states, "I feel ashamed at the way I look because of the sagging skin everywhere. I may have looked better heavier." Which is the best response by the nurse?

    a. "You should have been informed that this could occur after weight loss."

    b. "It is better than being overweight and so unhealthy."

    c. "This isn't anything that can be fixed, so you will just have to adjust to the sagging skin."

    d. "These feelings are understandable and not unusual. Let me give you support group information."

CHAPTER 43

Assessment and Management of Patients with Hepatic Disorders

Learning Outcomes

1. Identify the metabolic functions of the liver, the pathophysiologic alterations and clinical manifestations that occur with hepatic disorders, and the significance of liver function test findings.
2. Explain and demonstrate the proper techniques to perform a health history and physical assessment and discriminate between normal and abnormal findings identified in the patients with alterations of the liver.
3. Relate jaundice, portal hypertension, ascites, varices, nutritional deficiencies, and hepatic encephalopathy and coma to pathophysiologic alterations of the liver.
4. Describe the medical, surgical, and nursing management of patients with esophageal varices.
5. Compare the various types of hepatitis and their causes, prevention, clinical manifestations, management, prognosis, and home health care needs.
6. Use the nursing process as a framework for care of the patient with cirrhosis of the liver.
7. Specify nonsurgical management, surgical management, and nursing care of patients with cancer of the liver and of patients undergoing liver transplantation.

SECTION I: ASSESSING YOUR UNDERSTANDING

Activity A *Fill in the blanks.*

1. Liver function tests are not abnormal until _____% of the liver is revealed to be damaged.

2. The two major complications of a liver biopsy are _____ and _____.

3. HBV is transmitted primarily through _____.

4. The most common reason for liver transplantation is exposure to _____.

5. Hepatocellular carcinoma is caused by _____, _____, _____, and _____.

6. The leading cause of death after liver transplantation is _____.

7. The majority of blood supply to the liver, which is rich in nutrients from the gastrointestinal tract, comes from the _____.

8. The liver synthesizes prothrombin only if there is enough _____.

9. The substance necessary for the manufacture of bile salts by hepatocytes is _____.

10. Hepatic lobectomy for cancer can be successful when the primary site is localized. Because of the regenerative capacity of the liver, a surgeon can remove up to _____% of liver tissue.

11. _____, caused by contaminated needles shared by drug users, is also the most common reason for liver transplantation.

12. _____ is the most common single cause of death in patients with cirrhosis.

Activity B *Briefly answer the following.*

1. What age-related changes are significant in the hepatobiliary system?

   _____

   _____

2. What role does the liver play in glucose metabolism?

   _____

   _____

3. Compare and contrast hemolytic, hepatocellular, and obstructive jaundice in regard to etiology.

   _____

   _____

   _____

   _____

4. Identify the main function of bile salts.

   _____

5. What are the indications for postexposure vaccination with hepatitis B immunoglobulin?

   _____

   _____

6. Which chemicals most commonly are implicated in toxic hepatitis?

   _____

7. Cirrhosis results in shunting of portal system blood into collateral blood vessels in the gastrointestinal tract. Which are the most common sites of engorged collateral blood vessels?

   _____

   _____

8. Name three signs of advanced liver disease.

   _____

Activity C *Match the vitamin listed in Column II with the signs of deficiency due to severe chronic liver disease listed in Column I.*

Column I

____ 1. Hypoprothrombinemia

____ 2. Beriberi and polyneuritis

____ 3. Hemorrhagic lesions of scurvy

____ 4. Night blindness

____ 5. Macrocytic anemia

____ 6. Skin and neurologic changes

____ 7. Mucous membrane lesions

Column II

a. Vitamin A

b. Vitamin C

c. Vitamin K

d. Folic acid

e. Thiamine

f. Riboflavin

g. Pyridoxine

SECTION II: APPLYING YOUR KNOWLEDGE

Activity D *Consider the scenarios and answer the questions.*

CASE STUDY: Liver Biopsy

Mrs. Veronica Myers, age 46, is scheduled for a liver biopsy to determine if she has cirrhosis of the liver. The nurse assigned to care for Mrs. Myers is to accompany her to the treatment room.

1. Which preparation is required by the nurse prior to beginning the procedure?

   _____

   _____

2. The nurse is positioning Mrs. Myers for the biopsy. Which position will the nurse place her in to ensure adequate access to the biopsy site?

   _____

3. What will the nurse instruct Mrs. Myers to do immediately before needle insertion?

   _____

   _____

4. Which position will the nurse assist Mrs. Myers to maintain immediately after the biopsy is performed?

_____

_____

CASE STUDY: Paracentesis

Ms. Wendy Gamble, age 62, is scheduled for a paracentesis due to ascites formation subsequent to cirrhosis of the liver.

1. Before the procedure, the nurse obtains several drainage bottles. What is the maximum amount of fluid to be aspirated during the procedure?

_____

2. Which position of comfort will the nurse assist the patient to maintain during the paracentesis?

_____

_____

3. The nurse is monitoring Ms. Gamble for signs of vascular collapse. Which signs and symptoms will indicate to the nurse that this is occurring?

_____

_____

CASE STUDY: Alcoholic or Nutritional Cirrhosis

Mr. Nathan Farmer, a 50-year-old physically disabled veteran, has lived alone for 30 years. He has maintained his independence despite chronic back pain resulting from a war injury. He has a long history of depression and limited food intake. He drinks 6 to 10 bottles of beer daily. He was recently admitted to a veterans' hospital with a diagnosis of alcoholic or nutritional cirrhosis. He is asymptomatic for ascites.

1. Which early clinical manifestation indicative of alcoholic or nutritional cirrhosis does the nurse assess?

_____

2. Nathan is 5 feet 8 inches tall and weighs 154 lb. The health care provider recommends 50 cal/kg for weight gain. What will Nathan's daily caloric intake be?

_____

_____

3. The health care provider recommends a sodium-restricted diet. What will the suggested sodium intake to be?

_____

CASE STUDY: Liver Transplantation

Ms. Denise Davis, a 54-year-old mother of three, is scheduled for a liver transplantation subsequent to an extensive hepatic malignancy with multifocal tumors greater than 8 cm in diameter.

1. Which postoperative complication that is common after liver transplant will the nurse monitor Ms. Davis for?

_____

2. Ms. Davis is prescribed cyclosporine to prevent rejection of the transplanted liver. Which potential side effects of the medication may Ms. Davis experience?

_____

3. Which interventions will the nurse provide for Ms. Davis prior to the liver transplant to assist her psychologically to prepare for the procedure?

_____

_____

_____

SECTION III: PRACTICING FOR NCLEX

Activity E *Answer the following questions.*

1. The nurse is educating a patient with cirrhosis about the importance of maintaining a low-sodium diet. Which statement made by the patient indicates that the education is effective?

    a. "Peanut butter will be a good option for me since it will also add protein."

    b. "Fresh fruit like the pear I ate for lunch will be a low-sodium option."

    c. "It's alright if I just have a couple of hot dogs with ketchup at dinner."

    d. "Canned soup is a light meal that will be low in calories and healthy."

2. The nurse is caring for a patient with ascites as a result of hepatic dysfunction. Which intervention will the nurse provide to determine if the ascites is increasing? (Select all that apply.)

   a. Measure urine output every 8 hours.

   b. Assess and document vital signs every 4 hours.

   c. Measure abdominal girth daily.

   d. Perform daily weights.

   e. Monitor number of bowel movements per day.

3. The nurse is concerned about potassium loss when a diuretic is prescribed for a patient with ascites and edema. Which diuretic may be prescribed that spares potassium and prevents hypokalemia?

   a. Furosemide

   b. Spironolactone

   c. Acetazolamide

   d. Bumetanide

4. The nurse is caring for a patient with ascites due to cirrhosis of the liver. Which position does the nurse determine will activate the renin–angiotensin–aldosterone and sympathetic nervous system and decrease responsiveness to diuretic therapy?

   a. Prone

   b. Supine

   c. Left-lateral Sims'

   d. Upright

5. A patient is scheduled for a diagnostic paracentesis, but when coagulation studies are reviewed, the nurse observes results outside of normal parameters. How will the nurse proceed with preparation for the paracentesis?

   a. An ultrasound-guided paracentesis will be performed.

   b. The procedure will be canceled until the laboratory results are within normal parameters.

   c. The paracentesis will be performed at the bedside.

   d. The nurse will administer packed red blood cells (RBCs) prior to the paracentesis.

6. The nurse is caring for a patient with ascites. Which intervention will the nurse perform to correct the decrease in effective arterial blood volume that will lead to sodium retention?

   a. Administer diuretic therapy.

   b. Assist with a therapeutic paracentesis.

   c. Infuse platelets.

   d. Infuse albumin.

7. The nurse provides care to a patient with gross ascites who is maintaining a position of comfort in the high semi-Fowler position. Which is the nurse's priority assessment of this patient?

   a. Respiratory assessment related to increased thoracic pressure

   b. Urinary output related to increased sodium retention

   c. Peripheral vascular assessment related to immobility

   d. Skin assessment related to increase in bile salts

8. A patient with suspected esophageal varices is scheduled for an upper endoscopy with moderate sedation. After the procedure is performed, how long will the nurse withhold food and fluids?

   a. For 2 hours after the last dose of medication is given

   b. Until the gag reflex returns

   c. Until the patient expresses thirst

   d. For 6 hours after the procedure

9. A patient who had a recent myocardial infarction was brought to the emergency department with bleeding esophageal varices and is presently receiving fluid resuscitation. Which first-line pharmacologic therapy will the nurse prepare to administer to control the bleeding from the varices?

   a. Vasopressin

   b. Epinephrine

   c. Octreotide

   d. Glucagon

10. A patient with bleeding esophageal varices has had pharmacologic therapy with octreotide and endoscopic therapy with esophageal varices banding but continues to bleed. Which procedure will the nurse prepare for that will lower portal pressure?

    a. Transjugular intrahepatic portosystemic shunting (TIPS)

    b. Administration of vasopressin

    c. Sclerotherapy

    d. Balloon tamponade

11. The nurse is educating a patient being treated for hepatic encephalopathy about dietary restrictions to prevent ammonia accumulation. Which statement made by the patient indicates that the patient understands the education?

    a. "I will decrease the amount of fats in my diet."

    b. "I need to eat foods that are high in potassium."

    c. "I need to decrease the amount of protein in my diet."

    d. "It is necessary to increase the amount of magnesium in my diet."

12. The nurse is caring for a patient with cirrhosis of the liver and observes that the patient is having hand-flapping tremors. How will the nurse document this finding?

    a. Constructional apraxia

    b. Fetor hepaticus

    c. Ataxia

    d. Asterixis

13. The nurse is administering lactulose to decrease the ammonia level in a patient who has hepatic encephalopathy. Which will the nurse carefully monitor for that may indicate a medication overdose?

    a. Watery diarrhea

    b. Vomiting

    c. Ringing in the ears

    d. The presence of asterixis

14. A patient with severe chronic liver dysfunction comes to the clinic with bleeding of the gums and blood in the stool. Which vitamin deficiency does the nurse identify the patient may be experiencing?

    a. Riboflavin deficiency

    b. Folic acid deficiency

    c. Vitamin A deficiency

    d. Vitamin K deficiency

15. A patient must begin receiving the hepatitis B series of injections. The patient asks when the next two injections should be administered. Which is the best response by the nurse?

    a. "You must have the second one in 2 weeks and the third in 1 month."

    b. "You must have the second one in 1 month and the third in 6 months."

    c. "You must have the second one in 6 months and the third in 1 year."

    d. "You must have the second one in 1 year and the third the following year."

CHAPTER 44

Management of Patients with Biliary Disorders

Learning Outcomes

1. Identify the structure and function of the biliary tract and pancreas.
2. Describe the pathophysiology, clinical manifestations, and medical management of cholelithiasis.
3. Differentiate between acute and chronic pancreatitis.
4. Apply the nursing process as a framework for care of the patient with cholelithiasis, undergoing laparoscopic or open cholecystectomy, or with acute pancreatitis.
5. Explain the nutritional and metabolic effects of surgical treatment of tumors of the pancreas.

SECTION I: ASSESSING YOUR UNDERSTANDING

Activity A *Fill in the blanks.*

1. The capacity of the gallbladder for bile storage is _____ to _____ mL.

2. The endocrine secretions of the pancreas are _____, _____, and _____.

3. Digestive enzymes are secreted by the pancreas: _____ aids in the digestion of carbohydrates, _____ aids in protein digestion, and _____ aids in the digestion of fats.

4. _____ is the cause of more than 90% of cases of acute cholecystitis.

5. The most serious complication after a laparoscopic cholecystectomy is _____ _____.

6. A major cause of morbidity and mortality in patients with acute pancreatitis is _____.

7. Bile is stored in the _____.

8. The major stimulus for increased bicarbonate secretion from the pancreas is _____ _____.

9. Statistics show that there is a greater incidence of gallbladder disease for women who are _____, _____, and _____.

Activity B *Briefly answer the following.*

1. Describe what occurs when a gallstone obstructs the cystic duct.

   _____

   _____

2. Why does jaundice occur in patients with gallbladder disease?

   _____

   _____

3. A patient is scheduled for an outpatient laparoscopic cholecystectomy. Because the patient will only be at the hospital for less than a day, intensive education is necessary. Which information will the nurse include in the education?

_____

_____

_____

4. Percutaneous cholecystostomy has been used in the treatment and diagnosis of acute cholecystitis in patients who are poor risks for any surgical procedure or for general anesthesia. Which type of patients fit these conditions?

_____

_____

5. What are some of the clinical signs for predicting the severity of pancreatitis and associated mortality?

_____

_____

Activity C *Match the diagnostic study in Column I with the description/purpose of the study in Column II.*

Column I

____ **1.** Cholecystogram, cholangiogram

____ **2.** Celiac axis arteriography

____ **3.** Laparoscopy

____ **4.** Endoscopic retrograde cholangiopancreatography

____ **5.** Endoscopic ultrasound (EUS)

Column II

a. Identifies small tumors and facilitates fine-needle aspiration biopsy.

b. Visualizes the gallbladder and bile duct.

c. Visualizes the liver and pancreas.

d. Visualizes the biliary structure.

e. Visualizes the pancreas via endoscopy.

SECTION II: APPLYING YOUR KNOWLEDGE

Activity D *Consider the scenario and answer the questions.*

CASE STUDY: Cholecystectomy: Preoperative Situation

Mrs. Lockhart, a 33-year-old mother of four with obesity, is diagnosed as having acute gallbladder inflammation. She is 5 feet 4 inches tall and weighs 198 lb. The surgeon decides to delay surgical intervention until the acute symptoms subside.

1. What does the nurse anticipate that the initial course of treatment will likely consist of?

_____

2. As foods are added to the diet, which type of foods will the nurse educate her to avoid?

_____

_____

3. Mrs. Lockhart is being medicated with chenodeoxycholic acid. Which education will the nurse provide to her about the decreased effectiveness of the drug when taken in conjunction with certain items?

_____

_____

CASE STUDY: Cholecystectomy: Postoperative Situation

Because Mrs. Lockhart's symptoms continue to recur, she is scheduled for gallbladder surgery.

1. She is scheduled for a laparoscopic cholecystectomy under general anesthesia. The surgeon determines that the common bile duct may be obstructed by a gallstone. What will be performed prior to the surgery?

_____

_____

2. What will the nurse assess for postoperatively in order to prevent complications?

_____

_____

3. Mrs. Lockhart will be educated that dietary fat restriction is usually lifted after the biliary ducts dilate to accommodate bile once held by the gallbladder. How long will the nurse inform her that this will take?

_____

SECTION III: PRACTICING FOR NCLEX

Activity E *Answer the following questions.*

1. A patient is diagnosed with gallstones in the bile ducts. Which laboratory result will the nurse review that is indicative of this disorder?
   a. Serum ammonia concentration of 90 mg/dL
   b. Serum albumin concentration of 4.0 g/dL
   c. Serum bilirubin level greater than 1.0 mg/dL
   d. Serum globulin concentration of 2.0 g/dL

2. A patient is admitted to the hospital with a possible common bile duct obstruction. Which symptoms assessed by the nurse are indicators of this problem? (Select all that apply.)
   a. Amber-colored urine
   b. Clay-colored feces
   c. Pruritus
   d. Jaundice
   e. Pain in the left upper abdominal quadrant

3. A patient is admitted to the hospital with possible cholelithiasis. Which test will the nurse prepare the patient for to confirm diagnosis?
   a. X-ray
   b. Oral cholecystography
   c. Cholecystography
   d. Ultrasonography

4. A patient is receiving pharmacologic therapy with ursodeoxycholic acid or chenodeoxycholic acid for treatment of small gallstones. The patient asks the nurse how long the therapy will take to dissolve the stones. Which is the best answer by the nurse?
   a. 1 to 2 months
   b. 3 to 5 months
   c. 6 to 8 months
   d. 6 to 12 months

5. A patient is diagnosed with mild acute pancreatitis. Which condition is characteristic of this disorder?
   a. Edema and inflammation
   b. Pleural effusion
   c. Sepsis
   d. Disseminated intravascular coagulopathy

6. The nurse is admitting a patient to the intensive care unit with a diagnosis of acute pancreatitis. When performing a health history, which statement made by the patient is likely the reason that the patient came to the acute care facility?
   a. "I was having severe pain in the abdomen."
   b. "I have had a temperature of 99.5°F for several days."
   c. "My skin started looking a little yellow."
   d. "I started losing some of my short-term memory."

7. The nurse will assess for an important early indicator of acute pancreatitis. Which prolonged and elevated level would the nurse identify as an early indicator?
   a. Serum calcium
   b. Serum lipase
   c. Serum bilirubin
   d. Serum amylase

8. When caring for the patient with acute pancreatitis, pain relief measures are essential. Which nursing actions will be provided? (Select all that apply.)
   a. Encourage bed rest to decrease the metabolic rate.
   b. Assist the patient into the prone position.
   c. Withhold oral feedings to limit the release of secretin.
   d. Administer parenteral opioid analgesics as prescribed.
   e. Administer prophylactic antibiotics.

9. A patient is suspected to have pancreatic carcinoma and is having diagnostic testing to determine insulin deficiency. Which will the nurse identify is an indicator for insulin deficiency in this patient? (Select all that apply.)

   a. An abnormal glucose tolerance

   b. Glucosuria

   c. Hyperglycemia

   d. Elevated lipase level

   e. Hypoglycemia

10. A nurse will monitor blood glucose levels for a patient diagnosed with hyperinsulinism. Which blood value does the nurse identify as inadequate to sustain normal brain function?

    a. 30 mg/dL

    b. 50 mg/dL

    c. 70 mg/dL

    d. 90 mg/dL

11. The nurse is caring for a patient with acute pancreatitis. The patient has a prescription for an anticholinergic medication. Which education will the nurse provide about the reason the patient is taking the medication?

    a. To decrease metabolism

    b. To depress the central nervous system and increase the pain threshold

    c. To reduce gastric and pancreatic secretions

    d. To relieve nausea and vomiting

12. The patient admitted with acute pancreatitis has passed the acute stage and is now able to tolerate solid foods. Which type of diet will increase caloric intake without stimulating pancreatic enzymes beyond the ability of the pancreas to respond?

    a. Low-sodium, high-potassium, low-fat diet

    b. High-carbohydrate, high-protein, low-fat diet

    c. Low-carbohydrate, high-potassium diet

    d. High-carbohydrate, low-protein, low-fat diet

13. The nurse is caring for a patient with acute pancreatitis. Which action can be provided in order to prevent atelectasis and prevent pooling of respiratory secretions?

    a. Frequent change of positions

    b. Placing the patient in the prone position

    c. Perform chest physiotherapy

    d. Suction the patient every 4 hours

14. A patient with acute pancreatitis puts the call bell on to tell the nurse about an increase in pain. The nurse observes the patient guarding; the abdomen is boardlike and no bowel sounds are detected. Which is the major concern for this patient?

    a. The patient requires more pain medication.

    b. The patient is developing a paralytic ileus.

    c. The patient has developed peritonitis.

    d. The patient has developed kidney disease.

15. The nurse is caring for a patient with chronic pancreatitis. When observing the stool of the patient, which indication does the nurse have that fat absorption is impaired?

    a. The stools are streaked with blood.

    b. The stools are frothy and foul smelling.

    c. The stools are pale and pencil thin.

    d. The stools are watery.

16. A patient undergoes a laparoscopic cholecystectomy for the treatment of cholelithiasis and is discharged several hours later. The patient calls the nurse and reports pain in the right shoulder. Which is the best response by the nurse?

    a. "You need to have someone bring you back to the hospital immediately since this is a complication of the procedure."

    b. "This is due to the gas used to insufflate the abdomen and you can use a heating pad for 15 to 20 minutes every hour."

    c. "The health care provider will need to insert a drain since there may be an accumulation of fluid in the abdominal cavity."

    d. "Sometimes during a laparoscopic cholecystectomy, the liver is lacerated and causes bleeding, but it will stop on its own."

Assessment and Management of Patients with Endocrine Disorders

1. Describe the functions of each of the endocrine glands and their hormones.
2. Differentiate diagnostic studies and clinical manifestations for endocrine disorders.
3. Demonstrate knowledge of management strategies for endocrine disorders.
4. Explain nursing interventions in the care of patients with endocrine disorders.
5. Use the nursing process as a framework for care of the patient with an endocrine disorder.

SECTION I: ASSESSING YOUR UNDERSTANDING

Activity A *Fill in the blanks.*

1. The term used to describe the regulation of hormone concentration in the bloodstream is _____.

2. The _____ is the major structure that balances the rapid action of the nervous system with slower hormonal action.

3. The two major hormones secreted by the posterior lobe of the pituitary gland are _____, which controls _____, and _____, which facilitates _____.

4. Oversecretion of adrenocorticotropic hormone (ACTH), or the growth hormone, results in _____ or _____.

5. A deficiency of ADH or vasopressin can result in the disorder known as _____, which is characterized by_____ _____ and _____.

6. The thyroid gland produces three hormones: _____, _____, and _____.

7. The most common cause of hypothyroidism is _____.

8. Primary hyperthyroidism occurs two to four times more often in _____ than in ____.

9. The most common type of hyperthyroidism is _____.

10. The two most common medications used to treat hyperthyroidism are _____ and _____.

11. Tetany is evidenced when these signs are positive: _____ or _____.

12. The three types of steroid hormones produced by the adrenal cortex are _____, _____, and _____.

13. One of the most important and frequently occurring complications of hyperparathyroidism is _____.

14. _____ is the most common cause of thyrotoxicosis in the older adult patient.

Activity B *Briefly answer the following.*

1. Name the hormones that the anterior pituitary gland is responsible for secreting.

_____

_____

2. List four ways that hormones are classified.

_____

_____

3. What are the objectives in the management of hypothyroidism?

_____

_____

_____

4. Describe how radioactive iodine would be administered to a patient with cancer of the thyroid gland.

_____

_____

_____

Activity C *Match the hormonal function listed in Column II with its corresponding hormone listed in Column I.*

Column I

____ 1. Glucagon

____ 2. Aldosterone

____ 3. Oxytocin

____ 4. Somatotropin

____ 5. Vasopressin

____ 6. Calcitonin

____ 7. Prolactin

____ 8. Melatonin

____ 9. Parathormone

____ 10. Insulin

Column II

a. Controls excretion of water by the kidneys.

b. Lowers blood sugar.

c. Inhibits bone resorption.

d. Influences metabolism that is essential for normal growth.

e. Supports sexual maturation.

f. Promotes the secretion of milk.

g. Stimulates the reabsorption of sodium and the elimination of potassium.

h. Promotes glycogenolysis.

i. Increases the force of uterine contractions during parturition.

j. Regulates serum calcium.

SECTION II: APPLYING YOUR KNOWLEDGE

Activity D *Consider the scenarios and answer the questions.*

CASE STUDY: Primary Hypothyroidism

Mrs. Conrad, age 28, has been hospitalized for 2 days for symptoms leading to the diagnosis of primary hypothyroidism.

1. What tests does the nurse know will assist with the confirmation of diagnosis of primary hypothyroidism for Mrs. Conrad?

_____

_____

2. Which clinical manifestations that are consistent with Mrs. Conrad's diagnosis should be monitored?

_____

_____

_____

3. Which comfort measures will the nurse include in Mrs. Conrad's care?

_____

_____

4. Mrs. Conrad is prescribed levothyroxine 0.125 mg orally daily. What education will the nurse provide?

_____

_____

_____

_____

CASE STUDY: Hyperparathyroidism

Ms. Boone, age 65, reports continued emotional irritability. Her family describes her as always being "on edge" and acting "neurotic." After several months of exacerbated symptoms, she underwent a complete physical examination with laboratory studies and was diagnosed with hyperparathyroidism.

1. Ms. Boone is having difficulty closing her eyes and has to use artificial tears because her eyes are so dry. Which condition does the nurse observe that has caused this problem?

_____

2. Ms. Boone also reports "feeling like my heart is beating out of my chest." Which education will the nurse provide related to this symptom?

_____

3. Ms. Boone is started on methimazole for treatment of the hyperthyroidism. What education will the nurse provide about the medication?

_____

_____

CASE STUDY: Subtotal Thyroidectomy

Mr. Darrell, age 37, has just returned to the clinical area from the postanesthesia care unit (PACU) after undergoing a subtotal thyroidectomy.

1. Postoperatively, he is assisted from the stretcher to the bed. Which position of comfort should the nurse help to maintain?

_____

2. The nurse will assess for the common manifestation of recurrent laryngeal nerve damage. Which assessment finding is an indicator for this type of nerve damage?

_____

3. What will the nurse have available to administer if tetany occurs?

_____

SECTION III: PRACTICING FOR NCLEX

Activity E *Answer the following questions.*

1. A patient is receiving levothyroxine for prolonged hypothyroidism. Which will the nurse inform the patient to monitor for closely?

    a. Angina

    b. Depression

    c. Mental confusion

    d. Hypoglycemia

2. A patient comes to the clinic reporting severe thirst and drinking up to 10 L of cold water daily. The nurse observes that the patient's urine looks like water. Which diagnostic test does the nurse identify the health care provider will prescribe for diagnosis?

    a. Complete blood count (CBC)

    b. Fluid deprivation test

    c. Urine specific gravity

    d. Thyroid-stimulating hormone (TSH) test

3. A patient is exhibiting signs of hyperthyroidism. Which clinical manifestations reported by the patient correlate with this diagnosis? (Select all that apply.)

    a. A pulse rate slower than 90 bpm

    b. An elevated systolic blood pressure

    c. Muscular fatigability

    d. Weight loss

    e. Intolerance to cold

4. The nurse is caring for a patient with hyperthyroidism who suddenly develops symptoms related to thyroid storm. Which symptoms does the nurse identify are indicative of this emergency?

   a. Heart rate of 62

   b. Blood pressure 90/58 mm Hg

   c. Oxygen saturation of 96%

   d. Temperature of 102°F

5. A patient is experiencing a thyroid storm. Which medication will the nurse administer to reverse the effects of the excess thyroid hormone? (Select all that apply.)

   a. Acetaminophen

   b. Iodine

   c. Propylthiouracil

   d. Synthetic levothyroxine

   e. Dexamethasone

6. The nurse assesses a patient with an obvious goiter. Which type of deficiency does the nurse identify as the most likely cause of the goiter?

   a. Thyrotropin

   b. Iodine

   c. Thyroxine

   d. Calcitonin

7. The nurse is assisting a patient with hyperthyroidism to choose breakfast items. Which breakfast items are the best choice for the nurse to recommend?

   a. Cereal with milk and bananas

   b. Fried eggs and bacon

   c. Orange juice and toast

   d. Pork sausage and cranberry juice

8. A patient is suspected of having a pheochromocytoma and is having diagnostic tests performed in the hospital. Which symptoms does the nurse identify as most significant for a patient with this disorder?

   a. Blood pressure varying between 120/86 and 240/130 mm Hg

   b. Heart rate of 56 to 64 bpm

   c. Shivering

   d. Reports of nausea

9. A patient is diagnosed with overactivity of the adrenal medulla. Which epinephrine value does the nurse identify as a positive diagnostic indicator for overactivity of the adrenal medulla?

   a. 50 pg/mL

   b. 100 pg/mL

   c. 100 to 300 pg/mL

   d. 450 pg/mL

10. The nurse is caring for a patient with hyperparathyroidism and observes a calcium level of 16.2 mg/dL. Which action(s) does the nurse prepare to provide to reduce the calcium level? (Select all that apply.)

    a. Administration of calcitonin

    b. Administration of calcium carbonate

    c. Intravenous isotonic saline solution in large quantities

    d. Monitoring the patient for fluid overload

    e. Administration of a bronchodilator

11. A patient is prescribed desmopressin for the treatment of diabetes insipidus. Which therapeutic response does the nurse determine the patient will experience?

    a. A decrease in blood pressure

    b. A decrease in blood glucose levels

    c. A decrease in urine output

    d. A decrease in appetite

12. The nurse auscultates a bruit over the thyroid glands. Which is the significance of this finding?

    a. The patient may have hypothyroidism.

    b. The patient may have thyroiditis.

    c. The patient may have hyperthyroidism.

    d. The patient may have Cushing's disease.

13. A patient with a history of hypothyroidism is admitted to the intensive care unit unconscious and with a temperature of 95.2°F. A family member informs the nurse that the patient has not taken thyroid medication in over 2 months. Which do these findings indicate to the nurse?

    a. Thyroid storm

    b. Myxedema coma

    c. Diabetes insipidus

    d. Syndrome of inappropriate antidiuretic hormone (SIADH)

14. The nurse on the telemetry floor is caring for a patient with long-standing hypothyroidism who has been taking synthetic thyroid hormone replacement sporadically. Which is a priority that the nurse will monitor for in this patient?

    a. Symptoms of acute coronary syndrome

    b. Dietary intake of foods with saturated fats

    c. Symptoms of pneumonia

    d. Heat intolerance

15. A patient taking corticosteroids for exacerbation of Crohn's disease comes to the clinic and informs the nurse of the desire to stop taking them because of the increase in acne and moon face. Which education will the nurse provide regarding these symptoms?

    a. The symptoms are permanent side effects of the corticosteroid therapy.

    b. The moon face and acne will resolve when the medication is tapered off.

    c. Those symptoms are not related to the corticosteroid therapy.

    d. The dose of the medication must be too high and should be lowered.

16. A patient has been taking tricyclic antidepressants for many years for the treatment of depression. The patient has developed SIADH and has been admitted to the acute care facility. Which will the nurse carefully monitor when caring for this patient? (Select all that apply.)

    a. Strict intake and output

    b. Neurologic function

    c. Urine and blood chemistry

    d. Liver function tests

    e. Signs of dehydration

46

Management of Patients with Diabetes

1. Differentiate between the types of diabetes, associated etiologic factors, and pathophysiologic alterations.
2. Identify the diagnostic and clinical significance of blood glucose test results.
3. Describe the relationships among diet and dietary modifications, exercise, and medication (i.e., insulin or oral antidiabetic agents) for people with diabetes.
4. Use the nursing process as a framework for care of the patient who has hyperglycemia with diabetic ketoacidosis or hyperglycemic hyperosmolar syndrome.
5. Describe management strategies for a person with diabetes to use during "sick days."
6. Outline the major complications of diabetes and the self-care behaviors that are important in their prevention.

SECTION I: ASSESSING YOUR UNDERSTANDING

Activity A *Fill in the blanks.*

1. It is estimated that more than _____ million people in the United States have diabetes, although almost one third of these cases are undiagnosed.

2. In the United States, diabetes is the leading cause of _____, _____, and _____.

3. The major classifications of diabetes are: _____, _____, _____, and diabetes associated with other conditions or syndromes.

4. Because insulin normally inhibits _____ and _____, these processes occur in an unrestrained fashion in people with insulin deficiency and contribute further to hyperglycemia.

5. When excess glucose is excreted in the urine, it is accompanied by excessive loss of fluids and electrolytes, which is called _____.

6. Insulin resistance refers to a _____ tissue sensitivity to insulin.

7. Uncontrolled type 2 diabetes may lead to an acute problem—_____ _____.

8. Gestational diabetes occurs in as many as
   _____% of pregnant women and increases
   their risk for hypertensive disorders during
   pregnancy.

9. Goals for blood glucose levels during pregnancy are _____ or less before meals
   and _____ or less 2 hours after meals.

10. Classic clinical manifestations of diabetes
    include the "three Ps": _____,
    _____, and _____.

11. A finding of _____
    is the basic criterion for the diagnosis of
    diabetes.

12. Type 2 diabetes is the _____
    leading cause of death and affects approxi-
    mately _____% of older adults.

13. A woman at average risk for the develop-
    ment of hyperglycemia during pregnancy
    should be tested at _____ weeks of
    gestation.

14. _____ is the most common risk
    of insulin pump therapy.

15. _____, _____, and
    _____ are the three
    metabolic derangements that occur in dia-
    betic ketoacidosis.

Activity B *Briefly answer the following.*

1. Why does the economic cost of diabetes continue to increase?

   _____

   _____

2. Why does hyperglycemia develop during
   pregnancy?

   _____

   _____

3. Identify two main problems related to insulin
   in type 2 diabetes.

   _____

   _____

4. When educating a patient with diabetes about
   increasing fiber intake, which risks will be discussed?

   _____

   _____

   _____

5. Describe how insulin regulation is altered in
   the diabetic state.

   _____

   _____

   _____

   _____

6. List the clinical manifestations characteristic
   of hyperglycemic hyperosmolar syndrome.

   _____

   _____

7. Describe the action of sulfonylureas for
   patients who have type 2 diabetes.

   _____

   _____

Activity C *Match the physiologic change listed in Column II with its associated term listed in Column I.*

Column I

_____ 1. Gluconeogenesis

_____ 2. Glucosuria

_____ 3. Glycogenolysis

_____ 4. Nephropathy

_____ 5. Retinopathy

Column II

a. Filtered glucose
   that the kidney
   cannot absorb
   spills over into
   urine.

b. Glycogen breaks
   down in the
   liver through
   the action of
   glucagon.

c. New glucose is
   produced from
   amino acids.

d. Microvascular
   changes develop
   in the eyes.

e. Small vessel
   disease affects
   the kidneys.

SECTION II: APPLYING YOUR KNOWLEDGE

Activity D *Consider the scenarios and answer the questions.*

CASE STUDY: Type 1 Diabetes

Albert Weiss, a 35-year-old patient with insulin dependent diabetes, is admitted to the hospital with a diagnosis of pneumonia. He has been febrile since admission. His daily insulin requirement is 24 units of neutral protamine Hagedorn (NPH).

1. Each morning, Mr. Weiss is given NPH insulin at 7:30 AM. Meals are served at 8:30 AM, 12:30 PM, and 6:30 PM. Between which hours does the nurse expect that the NPH insulin will reach its maximum effect (peak)?

_____

2. A bedtime snack is provided for Mr. Weiss. This is based on the knowledge that intermediate-acting insulins are effective for what duration of time?

_____

3. Mr. Weiss refuses his bedtime snack. Which is a priority for the nurse to assess due to his refusal of a snack?

_____

_____

CASE STUDY: Hypoglycemia

Betty Anderson, an 18-year-old patient with diabetes mellitus type 1, is unconscious when admitted to the hospital. Her daily dose of insulin has been 32 units of NPH each morning. Her mother informs the nurse that Betty and her boyfriend just broke up prior to both going away to college and she hasn't been eating well since the breakup.

1. Which factors likely contributed to the development of Betty's hypoglycemia?

_____

2. Betty is given 1 mg of glucagon hydrochloride, subcutaneously, in the emergency department. Which latent symptoms will the nurse monitor for related to the action of the glucagon?

_____

_____

3. After Betty is medically stabilized, she is admitted to the clinical area for observation and education about diabetes type 1. Which warning symptoms should the nurse educate Betty about associated with hypoglycemia?

_____

_____

4. What information can the nurse provide to Betty to help prevent future events of hypoglycemia?

_____

_____

_____

CASE STUDY: Diabetic Ketoacidosis

Danae Blanks, age 62, is admitted to the clinical area with a diagnosis of diabetic ketoacidosis. Ms. Blanks lives alone and is frequently nonadherent with her dietary and medication regimen. She has had several admissions prior to this one. On admission, she is drowsy yet responsive.

1. Which priority actions will the nurse take in caring for Ms. Blanks?

_____

_____

_____

2. Which rehydrating intravenous solution will the nurse infuse as prescribed?

_____

3. Which laboratory result will the nurse find that may be associated with Ms. Blanks' condition?

_____

4. The health care provider prescribes an insulin drip to be started at 5 units/hr. When hanging the drip, what should the nurse do prior to connecting the drip to the patient?

_____

_____

_____

5. As blood glucose levels approach normal, which electrolyte imbalance will the nurse assess for?

_____

SECTION III: PRACTICING FOR NCLEX

Activity E *Answer the following questions.*

1. A patient is diagnosed with type 1 diabetes. Which clinical characteristics does the nurse determine will likely be associated with this patient? (Select all that apply.)

   a. Ketosis prone

   b. Little endogenous insulin

   c. Obesity at diagnoses

   d. Younger than 30 years of age

   e. Older than 65 years of age

2. When the nurse is caring for a patient with type 1 diabetes, which clinical manifestation would be a priority to closely monitor?

   a. Hypoglycemia

   b. Hyponatremia

   c. Ketonuria

   d. Polyphagia

3. A female patient with diabetes who weighs 130 lb has an ideal body weight of 116 lb. For weight reduction of 2 lb/wk, approximately what will her daily caloric intake be?

   a. 1000 calories

   b. 1200 calories

   c. 1500 calories

   d. 1800 calories

4. The nurse is preparing to administer intermediate-acting insulin to a patient with diabetes. Which insulin will the nurse administer?

   a. NPH

   b. Iletin II

   c. Humalog

   d. Glargine

5. An older adult patient with diabetes type 2 comes to the emergency department with second-degree burns to the bottom of both feet and states, "I didn't feel too hot but my feet must have been too close to the heater." Which does the nurse understand is most likely the reason for the decrease in temperature sensation?

   a. A faulty heater

   b. Autonomic neuropathy

   c. Peripheral neuropathy

   d. Sudomotor neuropathy

6. The nurse is caring for a patient with an abnormally low blood glucose concentration. Which glucose level will the nurse observe when assessing laboratory results?

   a. Lower than 50 to 60 mg/dL

   b. Between 60 and 80 mg/dL

   c. Between 75 and 90 mg/dL

   d. 95 mg/dL

7. A patient with diabetic ketoacidosis has had a large volume of fluid infused for rehydration. Which potential complication from rehydration will the nurse monitor for?

   a. Hypokalemia

   b. Hyperkalemia

   c. Hyperglycemia

   d. Hyponatremia

8. The nurse is assessing a patient with nonproliferative (background) retinopathy. When examining the retina, what will the nurse expect to assess? (Select all that apply.)

   a. Leakage of fluid or serum (exudates)

   b. Microaneurysms

   c. Focal capillary single closure

   d. Detachment

   e. Blurred optic discs

9. A nurse is caring for a patient with diabetes who has a diagnosis of nephropathy. What will the nurse expect the urinalysis report to indicate?

   a. Albumin

   b. Bacteria

   c. Red blood cells

   d. White blood cells

10. The nurse is preparing to administer insulin to a patient with type 1 diabetes in the morning prior to a surgical procedure. Which percentage of the usual morning dose of insulin will the nurse administer preoperatively?

    a. 10% to 20%

    b. 25% to 40%

    c. 50% to 60%

    d. 85% to 90%

11. An older adult patient is in the hospital with urosepsis. The patient begins to experience an altered level of consciousness, profound dehydration, and hypotension. Which condition does the nurse suspect the patient is experiencing?

    a. Systemic inflammatory response syndrome

    b. Hyperglycemic hyperosmolar syndrome

    c. Multiple-organ dysfunction syndrome

    d. Diabetic ketoacidosis

12. The nurse is preparing to administer IV fluids for a patient with ketoacidosis who has a history of hypertension and congestive heart failure. Which prescription for fluids will the nurse infuse for this patient?

    a. D_5W

    b. 0.9% normal saline

    c. 0.45% normal saline

    d. D_5 normal saline

13. A patient has been newly diagnosed with type 2 diabetes, and the nurse is assisting with the development of a meal plan. Which step will be taken into consideration prior to making the meal plan?

    a. Make sure that the patient is aware that quantity of foods will be limited.

    b. Ensure that the patient understands that some favorite foods may not be allowed on the meal plan.

    c. Determine whether the patient is on insulin or taking oral antidiabetic medication.

    d. Review the patient's diet history to identify eating habits, and lifestyle and cultural eating patterns.

14. The nurse is educating a patient with diabetes about the importance of increasing dietary fiber. Which will the nurse explain is the reason for the increase? (Select all that apply.)

    a. May improve blood glucose levels

    b. Decrease the need for exogenous insulin

    c. Help reduce cholesterol levels

    d. May reduce postprandial glucose levels

    e. Increase potassium levels

15. The nurse is educating a patient about the benefits of fruit versus fruit juice in the diabetic diet. The patient states, "What difference does it make if you drink the juice or eat the fruit? It is all the same." Which is the best response by the nurse?

    a. "Eating the fruit is more satisfying than drinking the juice. You will get full faster."

    b. "Eating the fruit will give you more vitamins and minerals than the juice will."

    c. "The fruit has less sugar than the juice."

    d. "Eating the fruit instead of drinking juice decreases the glycemic index by slowing absorption."

16. The nurse is administering an insulin drip to a patient in ketoacidosis. Which insulin does the nurse administer that can be used intravenously?

    a. NPH

    b. Regular

    c. Lispro

    d. Lantus

Kidney and Urinary Tract Function

Assessment of Kidney and Urinary Function

SECTION I: ASSESSING YOUR UNDERSTANDING

Activity A *Fill in the blanks.*

1. The functional unit of each kidney is the _____, located in the _____ of the kidney.

2. Normal adult bladder capacity is _____ mL of urine.

3. The urine osmolality level that indicates an early sign of kidney disease is _____.

4. The regulation of the amount of sodium excreted depends on the hormone _____.

5. When a person is dehydrated, the urine osmolality is _____.

6. Water is reabsorbed, rather than excreted, under the control of the _____ _____.

7. The normal serum pH is _____; urine pH is ____.

8. The major waste product of protein metabolism is _____, with approximately _____ g produced and excreted daily.

9. The test that most accurately reflects glomerular filtration and renal excretory function is the _____ test.

Activity B *Briefly answer the following.*

1. When will a patient need to receive renal replacement therapy?

_____

_____

2. Name the three areas of the ureters that have a propensity for obstruction by renal calculi.

_____

_____

3. Where are amino acids and glucose usually filtered?

_____

_____

4. Where is the antidiuretic hormone (ADH), or vasopressin, secreted?

_____

_____

5. What does the regulation of sodium volume excreted depend on?

_____

_____

Activity C *Match the description of pain in Column II with the pain location in Column I.*

Column I

_____ **1.** Kidney

_____ **2.** Bladder

_____ **3.** Ureteral

_____ **4.** Prostatic

_____ **5.** Urethral

Column II

a. Severe, sharp, stabbing, colicky

b. Dull, constant ache

c. Vague discomfort

d. Dull continuous pain, intense when voiding

e. Pain variable, most severe during and immediately after voiding.

SECTION II: APPLYING YOUR KNOWLEDGE

Activity D *Consider the scenario and answer the questions.*

Mrs. Carol, age 55, is having a kidney biopsy to determine the cause of her frequent episodes of hematuria. Mrs. Carol has had several other diagnostic tests performed with inconclusive results and is experiencing blood in her urine.

1. Before the biopsy is carried out, which laboratory studies will be conducted for Mrs. Carol in order to identify any risk of postbiopsy bleeding?

_____

_____

2. Which position will the nurse assist Mrs. Carol in maintaining during the procedure?

_____

_____

3. Which intervention does the nurse provide to clear any blood from the urine after the procedure?

_____

_____

SECTION III: PRACTICING FOR NCLEX

Activity E *Answer the following questions.*

1. The nurse is reviewing the laboratory values for a patient and observes an increase in blood osmolality. Which is the significance of this increase?

a. ADH stimulation

b. An increase in urine volume

c. Diuresis

d. Less reabsorption of water

2. A patient is being seen in the clinic for possible kidney disease. Which major sensitive indicator of kidney disease does the nurse prepare the patient for?

a. Blood urea nitrogen level

b. Creatinine clearance level

c. Serum potassium level

d. Uric acid level

3. The nurse is caring for a patient with end-stage kidney disease in the hospital and smells a fetid odor from the patient's breath. Which major manifestation of uremia will be present?

a. A decreased serum phosphorus level

b. Hyperparathyroidism

c. Hypocalcemia with bone changes

d. Increased secretion of parathormone

4. The nurse assesses a patient upon admission to the hospital. Which significant nursing assessment data is relevant to renal function? (Select all that apply.)

a. Any voiding disorders

b. The patient's occupation

c. The presence of hypertension or diabetes

d. The patient's financial status

e. The ability of the patient to manage activities of daily living

5. The nurse is assigned to care for a patient in the oliguric phase of kidney failure. When does the nurse document that oliguria is present?

   a. When the urine output is less than 30 mL/h

   b. When the urine output is about 100 mL/h

   c. When the urine output is between 300 and 500 mL/h

   d. When the urine output is between 500 and 1000 mL/h

6. A 24-hour urine collection is scheduled to begin at 8:00 AM. When should the nurse initiate the procedure?

   a. After discarding the 8:00 AM specimen

   b. At 8:00 AM, with or without a specimen

   c. 6 hours after the urine is discarded

   d. With the first specimen voided after 8:00 AM

7. The nurse is educating a patient about preparation for an IV urography. Which will the nurse include in the preparation instructions?

   a. A liquid restriction for 8 to 10 hours before the test is required

   b. The patient may have liquids before the test

   c. The patient will have enemas until the urine is clear

   d. The patient is restricted from eating or drinking from midnight until after the test

8. A patient had a renal angiography and is being brought back to the hospital room. Which nursing actions will the nurse perform after the procedure to detect complications? (Select all that apply.)

   a. Assess peripheral pulses.

   b. Compare color and temperature between the involved and uninvolved extremities.

   c. Examine the puncture site for swelling and hematoma formation.

   d. Apply warm compresses to the insertion site to decrease swelling.

   e. Increase the amount of IV fluids to prevent clot formation.

9. A patient is having an MAG3 renogram and is informed that radioactive material will be injected to determine kidney function. Which will the nurse instruct the patient to do during the procedure?

   a. Lie still on the table for approximately 35 minutes.

   b. Drink contrast material at various intervals during the procedure.

   c. Turn from side to side to get a variety of views during the procedure.

   d. Take deep breaths and hold them at various times throughout the procedure.

10. A patient is scheduled for a test with contrast to determine kidney function. Which statement made by the patient should the nurse inform the health care provider about prior to testing?

    a. "I don't like needles."

    b. "I am allergic to shrimp."

    c. "I take medication to help me sleep at night."

    d. "I have had a test similar to this one in the past."

CHAPTER 48

Management of Patients with Kidney Disorders

Learning Outcomes

1. Describe the key factors associated with the development of kidney disorders.
2. Explain the pathophysiology, clinical manifestations, medical management, and nursing management for patients with kidney disorders.
3. Differentiate between causes and understand the nursing management of patients with chronic kidney disease and acute kidney injury.
4. Compare and contrast the renal replacement therapies, including hemodialysis, peritoneal dialysis, continuous renal replacement therapies, and kidney transplantation.
5. Identify the nursing management of the hospitalized patient who is undergoing dialysis.
6. Develop a postoperative plan of nursing care for the patient undergoing kidney surgery and transplantation.

SECTION I: ASSESSING YOUR UNDERSTANDING

Activity A *Fill in the blanks.*

1. _____ and _____ cause approximately 70% of the cases of chronic kidney disease.

2. The two forms of nephrosclerosis are _____ and _____.

3. Two blood levels that are significantly increased in acute kidney injury (AKI) are _____ and _____.

4. _____, likely due to the use of glucose containing dialysate, is common in patients on long-term PD.

5. The most common and serious complication of continuous ambulatory peritoneal dialysis (CAPD) is _____.

6. Two complications of renal surgery that are believed to be caused by reflex paralysis of intestinal peristalsis and manipulation of the colon or duodenum during surgery are _____ and _____.

7. The most accurate indicator of fluid loss or gain in an acutely ill patient is _____.

8. The major manifestation of nephrotic syndrome is _____.

9. The most common type of renal carcinoma arises from the renal epithelium and accounts for more than ____% of all kidney tumors.

10. The four phases of AKI are _____, _____, _____, and _____.

11. _____ is the type of kidney disease characterized by increased glomerular permeability and manifested by massive proteinuria.

Activity B *Briefly answer the following.*

1. Which clinical manifestations may be present to indicate that a patient with chronic glomerulonephritis is likely developing heart failure?

_____

_____

_____

2. What assessment findings are significant for the patient who has nephrotic syndrome?

_____

_____

_____

3. Compare and contrast the difference between autosomal dominant and autosomal recessive polycystic kidney disease.

_____

_____

_____

_____

4. How can the nurse assist the patient with all of the testing required to detect a possible renal tumor?

_____

_____

_____

5. What factors influence mortality rate in patients with AKI?

_____

_____

Activity C *Match the symptom listed in Column II with its associated fluid or electrolyte imbalance listed in Column I.*

Column I

_____ 1. Calcium deficit

_____ 2. Calcium excess

_____ 3. Fluid volume deficit

_____ 4. Fluid volume excess

_____ 5. Magnesium deficit

_____ 6. Potassium deficit

_____ 7. Potassium excess

_____ 8. Protein deficit

_____ 9. Sodium deficit

_____ 10. Sodium excess

Column II

a. Carpopedal spasm and tetany

b. Muscle hypotonicity and flank pain

c. Oliguria and weight loss

d. Positive Chvostek sign

e. Crackles and dyspnea

f. Chronic weight loss and fatigability

g. Fingerprinting on the sternum

h. Irritability and intestinal colic

i. Rough, dry tongue and thirst

j. Soft, flabby muscles and weakness

SECTION II: APPLYING YOUR KNOWLEDGE

Activity D *Consider the scenarios and answer the questions.*

CASE STUDY: Continuous Ambulatory Peritoneal Dialysis (CAPD)

Mr. Edwards is a 29-year-old patient with diabetes and end-stage kidney disease (ESKD). He had a kidney transplant that was rejected and chose CAPD as a way of managing his ESKD. The nurse has been educating Mr. Edwards about the use of CAPD and will have a home health nurse come in to the home and ensure that he will be able to manage the regimen.

1. Why does the nurse believe that Mr. Edwards chose to manage his ESKD with CAPD?

_____

_____

2. Using CAPD, how often would he need to dialyze himself?

_____

3. Mr. Edwards is aware that toxic wastes are exchanged during the equilibration or dwell time. How long is he instructed to allow the fluid to dwell?

_____

4. The nurse is educating Mr. Edwards about the dietary modifications that are necessary to decrease the amount of accumulated waste products. What will the nurse include in the education?

_____

CASE STUDY: Acute Kidney Injury

Mr. Frank, a 42-year-old patient, is hospitalized with a diagnosis of AKI resulting from the administration of gentamicin sulfate for a _Pseudomonas aeruginosa_ infection. He is acutely ill upon admission and experiencing an altered level of consciousness.

1. The nurse is concerned that Mr. Frank is experiencing reduced kidney blood flow. Which clinical manifestations will the nurse assess for?

_____

2. During the oliguric phase of AKI, what will Mr. Frank's protein intake for his 156-lb body weight be?

_____

3. When he has passed the diuretic phase, which diet will the nurse recommend for him?

_____

4. After the oliguric phase, Mr. Frank will experience a period of recovery. How long does the nurse expect the recovery period to last?

_____

SECTION III: PRACTICING FOR NCLEX

Activity E _Answer the following questions._

1. The nurse notes that a patient who is retaining fluid had a 1-kg weight gain. Documentation will indicate that this is equivalent to about how many milliliters?
- **a.** 250 mL
- **b.** 500 mL
- **c.** 750 mL
- **d.** 1000 mL

2. A patient admitted with electrolyte imbalance has carpopedal spasm, ECG changes, and a positive Chvostek sign. Which deficit does the nurse evaluate the patient for?
- **a.** A calcium deficit
- **b.** A magnesium deficit
- **c.** A phosphorus deficit
- **d.** A sodium deficit

3. The nurse is reviewing a patient's laboratory results. Which findings does the nurse assess that are consistent with acute glomerulonephritis? (Select all that apply.)
- **a.** Red blood cells in the urine
- **b.** Polyuria
- **c.** Proteinuria
- **d.** White cell casts in the urine
- **e.** Hemoglobin of 12.8 g/dL

4. The nurse is caring for a patient in the oliguric phase of AKI. Which does the nurse determine the daily urine output will be?
- **a.** 1.5 L
- **b.** 1.0 L
- **c.** Less than 400 mL
- **d.** Less than 50 mL

5. The nurse is educating a patient who is required to restrict potassium intake. Which foods will the nurse suggest the patient eliminate that are rich in potassium?
- **a.** Butter
- **b.** Citrus fruits
- **c.** Cooked white rice
- **d.** Salad oils

6. A patient has AKI with a negative nitrogen balance. How much weight does the nurse expect the patient to lose?
- **a.** 0.5 kg/day
- **b.** 1.0 kg/day
- **c.** 1.5 kg/day
- **d.** 2.0 kg/day

7. A patient has stage 3 chronic kidney failure. Which will the nurse expect the patient's glomerular filtration rate (GFR) to be?
- **a.** A GFR of 90 mL/min/1.73 m^2
- **b.** A GFR of 30 to 59 mL/min/1.73 m^2
- **c.** A GFR of 120 mL/min/1.73 m^2
- **d.** A GFR of 85 mL/min/1.73 m^2

8. A patient with chronic kidney failure experiences decreased levels of erythropoietin. Which serious complication related to those levels will the nurse assess for when caring for this patient?
   a. Anemia
   b. Acidosis
   c. Hyperkalemia
   d. Pericarditis

9. At the end of five peritoneal exchanges, a patient's fluid loss was 500 mL. How much is this loss equal to?
   a. 0.5 lb
   b. 1.0 lb
   c. 1.5 lb
   d. 2 lb

10. The nurse is caring for a patient after kidney surgery. Which major danger will the nurse closely monitor for?
    a. Abdominal distention owing to reflex cessation of intestinal peristalsis
    b. Hypovolemic shock caused by hemorrhage
    c. Paralytic ileus caused by manipulation of the colon during surgery
    d. Pneumonia caused by shallow breathing because of severe incisional pain

11. A patient undergoing a CT scan with contrast has a baseline creatinine level of 3 mg/dL. Which is the most effective intervention to reduce the risk of developing radiocontrast-induced nephropathy (CIN)?
    a. Performing the test without contrast
    b. Administering gentamicin sulfate prophylactically
    c. Hydrating with saline intravenously before the test
    d. Administering sodium bicarbonate after the procedure

12. The nurse is reviewing the potassium level of a patient with kidney disease. The results of the test are 6.5 mEq/L, and the nurse observes peaked T waves on the ECG. Which priority action will the nurse perform as prescribed to reduce the potassium level?
    a. Administration of an insulin drip
    b. Administration of a loop diuretic
    c. Administration of sodium bicarbonate
    d. Administration of sodium polystyrene sulfonate

13. The nurse is administering calcium acetate to a patient with ESKD. When is the best time for the nurse to administer this medication?
    a. With food
    b. 2 hours before meals
    c. 2 hours after meals
    d. At bedtime with 8 oz of fluid

14. A patient with ESKD is scheduled to have an arteriovenous fistula created. The nurse explains that the patient will have a temporary dialysis catheter because the fistula has to "mature." The nurse will explain that the patient will have to wait how long before using the fistula?
    a. 1 to 2 weeks
    b. 2 to 3 weeks
    c. 1 month
    d. 2 to 3 months

15. A patient is placed on hemodialysis for the first time. The patient reports a headache with nausea and begins to vomit, and the nurse observes a decreased level of consciousness. Which does the nurse identify has occurred with the patient?
    a. The dialysis was performed too rapidly.
    b. The patient is having an allergic reaction to the dialysate.
    c. The patient is experiencing a cerebral fluid shift.
    d. Too much fluid was pulled off during dialysis.

CHAPTER 49

Management of Patients with Urinary Disorders

Learning Outcomes

1. Explain the factors contributing to upper and lower urinary tract infections.
2. Use the nursing process as a framework for care of the patient with a lower urinary tract infection.
3. Differentiate between the various adult dysfunctional voiding patterns and develop an education plan for a patient who has urinary incontinence.
4. Identify potential causes of an obstruction of the urinary tract along with the medical, surgical, and nursing management of the patient with this condition.
5. Describe the pathophysiology, clinical manifestations, medical management, and nursing management for patients with genitourinary trauma and urinary tract cancers.
6. Use the nursing process as a framework for care of the patient with renal calculi and for care of the patient undergoing urinary diversion surgery.

SECTION I: ASSESSING YOUR UNDERSTANDING

Activity A *Fill in the blanks.*

1. The three natural defenses to bacterial invasion of the urinary tract are _____ (protein), _____ (immunoglobulin), and _____, which interfere with the adherence of *Escherichia coli.*

2. Three organisms most frequently found in UTIs are _____, _____, and _____.

3. Fifty percent of all hospital-acquired infections are UTIs, and in the majority of cases these are _____.

4. The most common site of a lower UTI is the _____.

5. The type of incontinence that results from a sudden increase in intra-abdominal pressure is _____.

6. Fluid management as a method of behavioral therapy for incontinence requires a daily liquid intake of _____ mL.

7. The major complication of neurogenic bladder is _____.

8. The major cause of death for patients with neurologic impairment of the bladder is _____.

9. A woman is taught to catheterize herself by inserting the catheter _____ inches into the urethra.

10. A major clinical manifestation of renal stones is _____.

269

Activity B *Briefly answer the following.*

1. What are the six categories of risk factors for UTIs?

_____

_____

2. Which factors commonly contribute to UTIs in older adult patients?

_____

_____

_____

3. Which common risk factors are responsible for urinary incontinence?

_____

_____

_____

_____

4. What are the various causes of transient incontinence?

_____

_____

_____

5. Explain the general principles/guidelines that the nurse will adhere to in order to prevent infection in a patient with an indwelling urinary catheter.

_____

_____

6. What are eight risk factors for bladder cancer?

_____

_____

_____

_____

Activity C *Match the type of medication in Column II with the specific medication used to treat UTIs and pyelonephritis in Column I.*

Column I

____ 1. Nitrofurantoin

____ 2. Cephalexin

____ 3. Ciprofloxacin

____ 4. Ampicillin

____ 5. Co-trimoxazole

____ 6. Phenazopyridine

Column II

a. Trimethoprim–sulfamethoxazole

b. Urinary analgesic agent

c. Penicillin antibiotic

d. Anti-infective, urinary tract

e. Fluoroquinolone antibiotic

f. Bactericidal antibiotic

SECTION II: APPLYING YOUR KNOWLEDGE

Activity D *Consider the scenario and answer the questions.*

CASE STUDY: Acute Pyelonephritis

Ms. Jones, age 24, arrives in the emergency department reporting chills, low back pain, pain with urination, nausea, and vomiting. The symptoms began approximately 8 hours ago and she has been taking acetaminophen for a fever of 102°F. The patient is exhibiting the clinical manifestations of acute pyelonephritis.

1. The nurse is aware that a test must be performed to isolate the causative organism in order that the appropriate antibiotic be given. Which type of specimen will the nurse collect?

_____

2. The nurse is performing an assessment of the patient and identifies which findings correlate with the diagnosis of acute pyelonephritis?

_____

_____

3. The patient is suspected to have an obstruction in the urinary tract. Which type of testing will be performed in order to locate and confirm the obstruction?

_____

SECTION III: PRACTICING FOR NCLEX

Activity E *Answer the following questions.*

1. A patient comes to the clinic suspecting a possible UTI. Which symptoms of a UTI does the nurse identify from the assessment data gathered?
   a. Rebound tenderness at McBurney point
   b. An output of 200 mL with each voiding
   c. Cloudy urine
   d. Urine with a specific gravity of 1.005 to 1.022

2. A patient has been diagnosed with a urinary tract infection (UTI) and is prescribed an antibiotic. Which first-line fluoroquinolone antibacterial agent for UTIs does the nurse administer as prescribed that is highly effective for treatment?
   a. Trimethoprim–sulfamethoxazole
   b. Ciprofloxacin
   c. Nitrofurantoin
   d. Phenazopyridine

3. A patient with a urinary tract infection (UTI) is having burning and pain when urinating. Which urinary analgesic does the nurse administer as prescribed for relief of these symptoms?
   a. Sulfamethoxazole/trimethoprim
   b. Levofloxacin
   c. Phenazopyridine
   d. Amoxicillin

4. The nurse is educating a patient with urolithiasis about preventative measures to avoid another occurrence. Which intervention does the nurse educate the patient to perform?
   a. Increase fluid intake so that the patient can excrete 2500 to 4000 mL every day, which will help prevent additional stone formation.
   b. Participate in strenuous exercises so that the tone of smooth muscle in the urinary tract can be strengthened to help propel calculi.
   c. Add calcium supplements to the diet to replace losses to renal calculi.
   d. Limit voiding to every 6 to 8 hours so that increased volume can increase hydrostatic pressure, which will help push stones along the urinary system.

5. The nurse is providing an education program for the nursing assistants in a long-term care facility in order to decrease the number of urinary tract infections (UTIs) in the female population. Which interventions will the nurse discuss in the program? (Select all that apply.)
   a. For those patients who are incontinent, insert indwelling catheters.
   b. Perform hand hygiene prior to patient care.
   c. Assist the patients with frequent toileting.
   d. Provide careful perineal care.
   e. Encourage patients to wear briefs.

6. The nurse is caring for a patient with dementia in the long-term care facility when the patient has a change in cognitive function. Which condition does the nurse identify is likely occurring with the patient?
   a. A UTI
   b. A stroke
   c. An aneurysm
   d. Fecal impaction

7. The nurse is educating a female patient with a urinary tract infection (UTI) regarding the pharmacologic regimen for treatment. Which education is important for the nurse to provide to the patient?
   a. Take the antibiotic as well as an antifungal for the yeast infection she will probably have.
   b. Take the antibiotic for 3 days as prescribed.
   c. Understand that if the infection reoccurs, the dose will be higher next time.
   d. Be sure to take the medication with grapefruit juice.

8. A patient informs the nurse that every time she sneezes or coughs, she urinates in her pants. Which type of incontinence does the nurse identify the patient is experiencing?
   a. Urge incontinence
   b. Functional incontinence
   c. Stress incontinence
   d. Iatrogenic incontinence

9. A patient taking an alpha-adrenergic medication for the treatment of hypertension is having a problem with incontinence. Which education does the nurse provide to the patient?

   a. The medication has caused permanent damage to the bladder sphincter and will require surgical correction.

   b. Relaxation of the supporting ligaments has occurred and the patient will need to perform pelvic floor exercises to strengthen them.

   c. The patient will require a medication regimen to decrease the overactivity of the bladder.

   d. When the medication is discontinued or changed, the incontinence will resolve.

10. The patient has been diagnosed with urge incontinence. Which classification of medication does the nurse educate the patient about to help alleviate the symptoms?

    a. Antispasmodic agents

    b. Urinary antispasmodic agents

    c. Antibiotics

    d. Anticholinergic agents

11. A patient has a suprapubic catheter inserted postoperatively. Which are the advantages of the suprapubic catheter versus a urethral catheter? (Select all that apply.)

    a. The suprapubic catheter can be kept in longer than a urethral catheter.

    b. The patient can void sooner than with a urethral catheter.

    c. The suprapubic catheter allows for more mobility.

    d. The patient is not at risk for a UTI with a suprapubic catheter.

    e. The suprapubic catheter permits measurement of residual urine without urethral instrumentation.

12. The nurse is educating a patient who will be performing self-catheterization at home. Which information provided by the nurse will help reduce the incidence of infection?

    a. Clean the catheter with antibacterial soap, thoroughly rinse, and dry before reinsertion.

    b. Sterilize the catheter by boiling it in water for 20 minutes.

    c. Insert the catheter for urine drainage three times per day.

    d. A new catheter must be used each time catheterization is required.

13. The nurse is caring for a patient with severe pain related to ureteral colic. Which medication will the nurse administer as prescribed that will inhibit the synthesis of prostaglandin E, reducing swelling and facilitating passage of the stone?

    a. Morphine sulfate

    b. Aspirin

    c. Ketorolac

    d. Meperidine

14. A patient who has been treated with uric acid for stones is being discharged from the hospital. Which type of diet does the nurse discuss with the patient?

    a. Low-calcium diet

    b. High-protein diet

    c. Low-phosphorus diet

    d. Low-purine diet

15. A patient has had surgery to create an ileal conduit for urinary diversion. Which is a priority intervention by the nurse in the postoperative phase of care?

    a. Turn the patient every 2 hours around the clock.

    b. Administer pain medication every 2 hours.

    c. Monitor urine output hourly and report output greater than 30 mL/h.

    d. Clean the stoma with soap and water after the patient voids.

Reproductive Function

CHAPTER 50

Assessment and Management of Patients with Female Physiologic Processes

Learning Outcomes

1. Describe the structures and functions of the female reproductive system as well as approaches to assessment of female physiologic processes.
2. Identify the diagnostic examinations and tests used to determine alterations in female reproductive function, and describe the nurse's role before, during, and after these examinations and procedures.
3. Compare and contrast the different methods of contraception and the causes of infertility; describe implications for nursing care and education for the patient who wishes to practice contraception or to conceive.
4. Use the nursing process as a framework for care of the patient with an ectopic pregnancy.
5. Develop an education plan for women who are approaching or have completed menopause.

SECTION I: ASSESSING YOUR UNDERSTANDING

Activity A *Fill in the blanks.*

1. Puberty usually begins from ages _____ to _____ but may occur as early as age _____.

2. The pituitary gland releases two essential hormones: _____ hormone causes the ovaries to secrete estrogen and _____ hormone stimulates the production of progesterone.

3. Menopause usually begins at age _____ to _____ years with a median age of _____ years. Perimenopause can begin as early as age _____ years.

4. The menstrual cycle is dependent on hormone production. The hormone responsible for stimulating progesterone is _____.

5. Intimate partner violence involves four main types of violence: _____, _____, _____, and _____ (Centers for Disease Control and Prevention [CDC], 2019a).

6. Youth who identify as LGBTQ are at higher risk of _____ and _____ (Wingo et al., 2018).

7. The most accurate outpatient procedure for evaluating a woman for endometrial cancer is _____.

8. _____ is probably the most significant form of menstrual dysfunction because it may signal cancer, benign tumors of the uterus, or other gynecologic problems.

9. Many women currently use oral contraceptive preparations of synthetic _____ and _____.

10. The _____ is an effective contraceptive device that consists of a round, flexible spring (50 to 90 mm wide) covered with a domelike latex rubber cup.

Activity B *Briefly answer the following.*

1. A woman comes to the clinic frequently with reports of chronic pelvic pain. What does the nurse identify can be associated with this issue?

_____

_____

2. Why is Pap smear follow-up important if a woman has atypical cells from the first test?

_____

3. Describe the education that will be provided to a patient who has had a surgical cone biopsy.

_____

_____

_____

4. Why would a hysteroscopy be indicated for a patient experiencing abnormal uterine bleeding?

_____

_____

5. What is the premenstrual syndrome?

_____

_____

6. Describe four possible options for the treatment of an ectopic pregnancy.

_____

_____

7. List six possible causes of ectopic implantation.

_____

_____

_____

Activity C *Match the term in Column II with its corresponding definition in Column I.*

Column I	Column II
____ 1. Painful sexual intercourse	**a.** Adnexa
	b. Amenorrhea
____ 2. Bladder protruding into the vagina	**c.** Chandelier sign
____ 3. Beginning of menstruation	**d.** Cystocele
	e. Dysmenorrhea
____ 4. Description of ovaries and fallopian tubes	**f.** Dyspareunia
	g. Endometriosis
____ 5. Painful menstruation	**h.** Menarche
____ 6. Implantation of endometrial tissue in other areas of the pelvis	
____ 7. Pain on movement of the cervix	
____ 8. Absence of menstrual flow	

SECTION II: APPLYING YOUR KNOWLEDGE

Activity D *Consider the scenario and answer the questions.*

Ms. Clary, a 50-year-old patient, informs the nurse that she is experiencing some of the symptoms of menopause. She has not had a menstrual period in 8 months and states that she is having hot flashes.

1. What does the nurse explain to Ms. Clary is the cause of the hot flashes?

_____

_____

2. Ms. Clary asks the nurse about the benefits of hormone therapy. Compare and contrast the advantages and disadvantages of hormone therapy.

_____

_____

_____

_____

3. What other methods can the nurse inform her are available to treat the hot flashes?

_____

_____

_____

_____

SECTION III: PRACTICING FOR NCLEX

Activity E *Answer the following questions.*

1. A patient informs the nurse about experiencing vaginal bleeding for the past several days. She is postmenopausal and has not had a menstrual period for the past 4 years. Which will the nurse educate the woman to do?

   a. See the gynecologist or health care provider as soon as possible.

   b. Discuss the bleeding episode with the health care provider at the next appointment.

   c. Disregard this bleeding episode, because it is probably normal.

   d. Use a birth control method, because she may be fertile with her next ovulation.

2. During an internal vaginal examination, the health care provider notes a frothy and malodorous discharge. Which bacterium is suspected to cause this disorder?

   a. *Candida*

   b. *Eschar*

   c. *Trichomonas*

   d. *Escherichia coli*

3. A postmenopausal patient is experiencing dyspareunia. Which will the nurse recommend to diminish the discomfort?

   a. Ibuprofen

   b. Petroleum jelly

   c. Water-based lubricant

   d. Aspirin

4. The nurse is discussing nutritional needs for a postmenopausal patient. Which dietary increase will the nurse recommend to the patient?

   a. Calcium

   b. Iron

   c. Salt

   d. Vitamin K

5. The nurse is educating a patient with premenstrual syndrome (PMS) about changing dietary practices. Which will the nurse recommend the patient increase intake of?

   a. Magnesium

   b. Vitamin D

   c. Iron

   d. Zinc

6. An adolescent patient reports "terrible pain" during menstruation. Which will the nurse document this subjective data as?

   a. Dysmenorrhea

   b. Amenorrhea

   c. Menorrhagia

   d. Metrorrhagia

7. The nurse is discussing contraception with a patient interested in transdermal contraceptives. Which will the nurse inform the patient is the most common side effect of transdermal contraceptives?

   a. Breast cancer

   b. Withdrawal bleeding

   c. Thrombophlebitis

   d. Application site allergic reactions

8. A patient is scheduled for a gynecologic examination and Pap smear but informs the nurse that she just began her menstrual cycle. Which is the best response by the nurse?

   a. "This will have no bearing on your test today."

   b. "We will proceed with the examination and reschedule your Pap smear for next week."

   c. "We will reschedule your examination when you have finished menstruating."

   d. "We will do the test and take into consideration that you are menstruating."

9. A patient informs the nurse that she believes she has premenstrual syndrome (PMS) and is having physical symptoms as well as moodiness. Which physical symptoms does the nurse identify are consistent with PMS? (Select all that apply.)

   a. Fluid retention

   b. Low back pain

   c. Fever

   d. Headache

   e. Hypotension

10. A patient asks the nurse if there are any available nonsurgical options to terminate a pregnancy if she is only 2 weeks pregnant. Which information will the nurse provide to the patient about a medication that blocks progesterone?

    a. Mifepristone is used only in early pregnancy to terminate a pregnancy nonsurgically.

    b. Methotrexate is used only in early pregnancy to terminate a pregnancy nonsurgically.

    c. Clomiphene is used only in early pregnancy to terminate a pregnancy nonsurgically.

    d. Birth control pills can be used to terminate the pregnancy.

11. The nurse is preparing a patient for a gynecologic examination when the patient states, "I hope the examination doesn't hurt as much as intercourse with my husband does." Which will the nurse document this finding as?

    a. Dysmenorrhea

    b. Dyspareunia

    c. Dysuria

    d. Dysthymia

12. The nurse is providing information at the local YMCA about screenings for breast and cervical cancer. The nurse will inform young women that they should begin their screenings at what time?

    a. Annual breast and pelvic examinations are important for all women 21 years of age or older and for those who are sexually active, regardless of age.

    b. Annual breast and pelvic examinations should begin at age 14.

    c. Annual breast and pelvic examinations should begin when a woman becomes sexually active.

    d. Annual breast and pelvic examinations should be performed when a woman begins taking birth control.

13. The nurse is assisting a patient in preparing for a pelvic examination. Which position will the nurse place the patient in for the examination?

    a. Left lateral

    b. Prone

    c. Jackknife

    d. Lithotomy

14. When the nurse places the patient in the stirrups for a pelvic examination she observes a bulge caused by rectal cavity protrusion. How will the nurse document this finding?

    a. Cystocele

    b. Rectocele

    c. Uterine prolapse

    d. Hemorrhoids

Management of Patients with Female Reproductive Disorders

1. Compare the various types of vaginal infections and the signs, symptoms, and treatments of each.
2. Discuss the signs and symptoms, management, and nursing care of patients with inflammatory processes, structural disorders, and benign and malignant conditions of the female reproductive tract.
3. Use the nursing process as a framework for care of the patient with a vulvovaginal infection or with genital herpes, or who is undergoing a hysterectomy.
4. Describe the nursing management of the patient undergoing radiation therapy for cancer of the female reproductive tract.

SECTION I: ASSESSING YOUR UNDERSTANDING

Activity A *Fill in the blanks.*

1. The vagina is protected against infection by its normally low pH (3.5 to 4.5), which is maintained in part by the actions of _____, the dominant bacteria in a healthy vaginal ecosystem.

2. The epithelium of the vagina is highly responsive to _____.

3. Bacterial vaginosis is characterized by a _____ odor.

4. Bacterial vaginosis is not usually considered a serious condition, although it can be associated with _____, _____, and _____.

5. Human papillomavirus (HPV) can be found in lesions of the _____, _____, _____, _____, _____, and _____.

6. There are more than _____ types of HPV.

7. The most common strains of HPV, 6 and 11, usually cause _____ on the vulva.

8. Women with HPV should have annual Pap smears because of the potential of HPV to cause _____.

9. The most effective treatment for trichomoniasis is _____ or _____.

10. A woman with vulvovaginal symptoms should be instructed not to _____, because it will remove the discharge needed to make the diagnosis.

11. The treatment of polycystic ovarian syndrome consists of _____ including _____ and _____.

Activity B *Briefly answer the following.*

1. Which patient-teaching points may decrease the 10 common risk factors for vulvovaginal infections?

_____

_____

2. Explain why a decrease in estrogen can lead to vaginal infections.

_____

_____

_____

3. List the treatment options available for the patient who has vulvovaginitis.

_____

_____

_____

4. Explain the extent of organ involvement with pelvic inflammatory disease (PID).

_____

_____

_____

5. Vulvovaginal candidiasis can occur at any time, although certain populations may be infected more than others. Which people are at an increased risk for this condition?

_____

_____

_____

Activity C *Match the word in Column II with its associated definition in Column I.*

Column I

____ 1. Intense burning and inflammation of the vulva

____ 2. A preferred treatment for candidiasis

____ 3. The recommended treatment for trichomoniasis

____ 4. The drug of choice for herpes genitalis

____ 5. A potential complication of toxic shock syndrome

____ 6. The downward displacement of the bladder toward the vaginal orifice

____ 7. Test used for diagnosis of cervical cancer

____ 8. Term used to describe the surgical procedure in which the uterus, cervix, and ovaries are removed

____ 9. A term used to describe vaginal bleeding

____ 10. Another name for benign tumors of the uterus

____ 11. In utero exposure to this drug increases the incidence of vaginal cancer

____ 12. A risk factor for uterine cancer

____ 13. Exercises that strengthen the pelvic muscles

____ 14. An opening between two hollow organs

____ 15. Displacement of the uterus into the vaginal canal

____ 16. Cysts that arise from parts of the ovum

Column II

a. Fibroids

b. Fistula

c. Cystocele

d. Mycostatin

e. Acyclovir

f. Vulvodynia

g. Dermoid

h. Septic shock

i. Menorrhagia

j. Diethylstilbestrol (DES)

k. Kegel

l. Prolapse

m. Hormone replacement therapy (HRT)

n. Pap smear

o. Total hysterectomy

p. Metronidazole

SECTION II: APPLYING YOUR KNOWLEDGE

Activity D *Consider the scenarios and answer the questions.*

CASE STUDY: Bacterial Vaginosis

Mary Barner, a 19-year-old college student, has recently noticed increased vaginal discharge that is gray to yellowish-white in color and comes into the clinic for treatment.

1. The nurse will educate Mary Barner on reduction of risk factors that cause bacterial vaginosis. Which risk factors does the nurse include when educating?

_____

_____

_____

2. What is a diagnostic sign of bacterial vaginosis?

_____

3. Metronidazole is prescribed to be taken twice a day for 1 week. While taking this medication, what should Mary Barner be instructed to do?

_____

_____

CASE STUDY: Pelvic Inflammatory Disease

Donna Worley is a 26-year-old graduate student who has been sexually active with multiple partners for 5 years. Last year she experienced several incidences of cervicitis. She now comes to the clinic reporting severe lower abdominal discomfort and is walking with a shuffling gait.

1. What negative outcomes are possible for Donna to have if she is not treated immediately?

_____

_____

2. What type of treatment does the nurse anticipate instructing Donna about?

_____

_____

3. What organisms should Donna be tested for prior to treatment?

_____

SECTION III: PRACTICING FOR NCLEX

Activity E *Answer the following questions.*

1. A patient has been diagnosed with a vaginal infection and received a prescription for metronidazole. The nurse informs the client that this infection is caused by which organism?
   a. *Candida albicans*
   b. *Escherichia coli*
   c. *Streptococcus*
   d. *Trichomonas vaginalis*

2. A patient is diagnosed with Bartholinitis. Which organism does the nurse identify the patient is most likely infected with?
   a. *Candida albicans*
   b. *Chlamydia*
   c. *Gardnerella vaginalis*
   d. *Trichomonas vaginalis*

3. A patient is infected with a vulvovaginal infection. Which interventions for the relief of pain and discomfort can the nurse educate the patient about? (Select all that apply.)
   a. Warm perineal irrigations
   b. Sitz baths
   c. Cornstarch for chafed inner thighs
   d. Cold compresses to the vagina
   e. A vaginal douche

4. A patient has had a pessary inserted for long-term treatment of a prolapsed uterus. As part of the teaching plan, which will the nurse advise the patient to do?
   a. See her gynecologist to remove and clean the pessary at regular intervals.
   b. Keep the insertion site clean and dry.
   c. Avoid penile-vaginal intercourse.
   d. Avoid climbing stairs as much as possible.

5. A patient diagnosed with endometriosis asks for an explanation of the disease. Which will the nurse explain to the patient?

   a. She has developed an infection in the lining of her uterus.

   b. Tissue from the lining of the uterus has implanted in areas outside the uterus.

   c. The lining of the uterus is thicker than usual, causing heavy bleeding and cramping.

   d. The lining of the uterus is too thin because endometrial tissue has implanted outside the uterus.

6. A patient is taking oral danazol, 800 mg/day, for 9 months for the treatment of endometriosis. How does the nurse describe this medication to the patient?

   a. "It is a gonadotropin that decreases ovarian and pituitary stimulations."

   b. "It is an antigonadotropin that increases pituitary stimulation and decreases ovarian stimulation."

   c. "It is a gonadotropin that decreases pituitary stimulation and increases ovarian stimulation."

   d. "It is an antigonadotropin that decreases pituitary and ovarian stimulations."

7. The nurse in the gynecology clinic is interviewing a patient who informs the nurse that her mother and aunt had carcinoma of the cervix. Which two chief symptoms of early carcinoma will the patient be questioned about?

   a. Leukoplakia and metrorrhagia

   b. Dyspareunia and foul-smelling vaginal discharge

   c. "Strawberry" spots and menorrhagia

   d. Leukorrhea and irregular vaginal bleeding or spotting

8. The nurse is reviewing a patient's lab work and notes a stage II Pap smear result. Which will this indicate for the patient?

   a. Cancer in situ

   b. Vaginal invasion

   c. Pelvic wall invasion

   d. Bladder extension

9. A perimenopausal woman informs the nurse that she is having irregular vaginal bleeding. Which will the nurse encourage the patient to do?

   a. Stop taking her hormonal therapy.

   b. See her gynecologist as soon as possible.

   c. Disregard this phenomenon because it is common during this life stage.

   d. Mention it to the health care provider during her next annual examination.

10. A patient has been diagnosed with a vulvar malignancy. Which primary treatment for vulvar malignancy will the nurse prepare the patient for?

    a. Chemotherapy creams

    b. Laser vaporization

    c. Radiation

    d. Wide excision

11. The nurse is caring for a patient postoperatively who had a simple vulvectomy. Which nursing actions will be provided to this patient? (Select all that apply.)

    a. Cleanse the wound daily.

    b. Offer a low-residue diet.

    c. Position the patient with pillows.

    d. Sit in a warm tub of water.

    e. Apply an antibiotic ointment.

12. A patient has a diagnosis of stage III ovarian cancer and wants to know what organs are involved. Which information will be provided to the patient?

    a. The cancer involves only the ovaries.

    b. The cancer involves the ovaries with pelvic extension.

    c. The cancer involves metastases outside the pelvis.

    d. The cancer involves distant metastases.

13. A patient reports to the nurse that she has a sense of pelvic pressure and urinary problems such as incontinence, frequency, and urgency. The problem has gotten much worse since the birth of her third child. Which does the nurse suspect the patient is experiencing?

    a. A cystocele

    b. A rectocele

    c. An enterocele

    d. A urinary tract infection

14. A woman who has been trying to conceive is diagnosed with fibroid tumors of the uterus and is scheduled to have a procedure using a laser through a hysteroscope passed through the cervix. Which type of procedure will the nurse prepare the patient for?

   a. A hysteroscopic resection of myomas

   b. Laparoscopic myomectomy

   c. Laparoscopic myolysis

   d. Laparoscopic cryomyolysis

15. The nurse is encouraging a patient to have a cervical examination and Pap smear. It has been many years since the patient's last examination, and she was diagnosed with HPV 6 years ago. The patient states, "I am not having any trouble down there, so it is best to leave things alone." Which is the best response by the nurse?

   a. "Early cervical cancer rarely produces any symptoms."

   b. "If you are not having any problems, then there is no reason to have one."

   c. "You could have another type of sexually transmitted infection."

   d. "If your insurance is paying for it, you should have an examination."

Assessment and Management of Patients with Breast Disorders

Learning Outcomes

1. Describe the anatomy and physiology of the breast as well as identify the assessment and diagnostic studies used to diagnose breast disorders.
2. Compare and contrast the pathophysiology of benign and malignant breast disorders.
3. Summarize evidence-based guidelines for the early detection of breast cancer and develop a plan for educating patients and consumer groups about breast self-awareness.
4. Use the nursing process as a framework for care of the patient undergoing surgery for the treatment of breast cancer.
5. Recognize the physical, psychosocial, and rehabilitative needs of the patient who has had breast surgery for the treatment of breast cancer.

SECTION I: ASSESSING YOUR UNDERSTANDING

Activity A *Fill in the blanks.*

1. The breasts are located between the _____ and _____ ribs over the pectoralis muscle from the sternum to the midaxillary line.

2. Fascial bands, called _____, support the breast on the chest wall.

3. A thorough breast examination, including instruction in breast self-examination (BSE), takes at least _____ minutes.

4. _____ is the firm enlargement of glandular tissue beneath and immediately surrounding the areola of the male.

5. Mastitis, an inflammation or infection of breast tissue, occurs most commonly in _____ women.

Activity B *Briefly answer the following.*

1. What are the major risk factors for a woman to develop breast cancer?

_____

_____

2. Which role does the nurse have when educating a patient in breast self-examination (BSE)?

_____

_____

_____

_____

3. When do variations in breast tissue occur?

_____

4. What are at least six causes of nipple discharge in a nonlactating woman?

_____

_____

_____

_____

5. Research suggests that there are racial disparities in cancer mortality. What are these disparities driven by?

_____

_____

Activity C *Match the term in Column II with its corresponding definition in Column I.*

Column I

____ 1. Overdeveloped breast tissue usually seen in boys

____ 2. Breast augmentation

____ 3. Mammography after injection of dye

____ 4. Breast cancer in the ductal system

____ 5. Breast pain, usually hormonal in nature

____ 6. Infection of breast tissue

____ 7. Partial breast radiation

Column II

a. Galactography

b. Mastalgia

c. Paget disease

d. Mastitis

e. Gynecomastia

f. Brachytherapy

g. Mammoplasty

SECTION II: APPLYING YOUR KNOWLEDGE

Activity D *Consider the scenario and answer the questions.*

CASE STUDY: Total Mastectomy (Simple Mastectomy)

Louise Carter, age 53, has biopsy results indicating a malignancy in her breast. She is scheduled for a simple mastectomy.

1. On examination, Louise's tumor is found in the anatomic area where tumors usually develop. Where does the nurse determine that the tumor will be palpated?

_____

2. Postoperatively, what type of sensations other than discomfort might Ms. Carter feel?

_____

_____

_____

3. The nurse informs Ms. Carter that it is time to change her dressing for the first time. Which preparation will the nurse provide for her before and during this time?

_____

_____

_____

_____

SECTION III: PRACTICING FOR NCLEX

Activity E *Answer the following questions.*

1. The nurse is educating a patient about the best time to perform BSE. When does the nurse inform her is the best time after menses to perform BSE?

   a. 3 to 4 days

   b. 5 to 7 days

   c. 8 to 9 days

   d. After the 10th day

2. The nurse is assessing the breast of a female patient and observes a prominent venous pattern on the left breast. Which does the nurse identify this is indicative of?

   a. Increased blood supply required by a tumor

   b. Infection

   c. Ulceration of the nipple

   d. Thrombus formation

3. The nurse is assessing an older adult female who has not seen her health care provider in 2 years. The nurse is assisting the patient into a gown and observes edema and pitting of the skin on the right breast. Which is the significance of this finding?
   a. Inflammation due to mastitis while the patient is breast-feeding
   b. This finding is not uncommon and is significant only when of recent origin
   c. A neoplasm blocking lymphatic drainage, a classic sign of advanced breast cancer
   d. Likely related to benign cysts of the breast in the nipple area

4. The nurse is educating a group of women at a local event about breast cancer. Which does the nurse understand is the current practice that will be focused on rather than BSE?
   a. Breast self-awareness
   b. Mammography every year
   c. Hormone replacement
   d. Ultrasound with mammography

5. The nurse is discussing mammography with a female patient at the clinic. The patient asks at which age she should begin getting yearly mammograms. Which response will the nurse provide to the patient?
   a. 35
   b. 40
   c. 50
   d. 55

6. A patient is having a fine-needle biopsy (FNB) of a mass in the left breast for diagnosis. When the needle is inserted and the mass is no longer palpable, which has most likely occurred?
   a. The mass has been absorbed into the tissues of the breast.
   b. The mass may be cystic and was ruptured when the needle was inserted.
   c. The mass may not have been located correctly.
   d. The mass is not palpable because it is an inflammatory lesion.

7. A patient is having a biopsy that will remove the entire mass, plus a margin of surrounding tissue. Which type of biopsy will be documented on the operative permit?
   a. Excisional biopsy
   b. Incisional biopsy
   c. Core biopsy
   d. Ultrasound-guided core biopsy

8. The nurse is providing preoperative instruction for a patient who will be having an excisional breast biopsy. The patient asks the nurse what type of bra should be used after the procedure. Which will the nurse discuss with the patient?
   a. Avoid the use of a bra for 24 hours after the procedure.
   b. Wear a bra as long as it is an underwire bra.
   c. Wear a supportive bra after the procedure.
   d. Do not wear a bra until the sutures are removed.

9. A female patient comes to the clinic reporting a greenish-colored discharge from the nipple, and the breast feels warm to touch. Which does the nurse suspect these symptoms may indicate?
   a. Infection
   b. Cancer
   c. A ruptured cyst
   d. Blocked lymph duct

10. The nurse is assisting a patient with breast-feeding. The patient said that with her last baby, there was problem with her nipples becoming irritated. Which information will the nurse suggest to the patient? (Select all that apply.)
    a. Daily washing with water
    b. Massage with breast milk or lanolin
    c. Exposure to air
    d. Hot compresses
    e. Aspirin

11. A patient is considering use of chemoprevention because she is at high risk for developing breast cancer. Which will the nurse do to assist the patient with her decision?

   a. Inform the patient that medication should not be used prophylactically due to the many side effects.

   b. Inform the patient that she should take every measure available to her to prevent this disease.

   c. Provide the patient with information regarding the benefits, risks, and possible side effects.

   d. Provide the patient with information about bilateral mastectomy for the prevention of this disease.

12. A patient is told that she has a common form of breast cancer where the tumor arises from the duct system and invades the surrounding tissues, often forming a solid irregular mass. Which type of cancer does the nurse discuss with the patient?

   a. Infiltrating ductal carcinoma

   b. Infiltrating lobular carcinoma

   c. Medullary carcinoma

   d. Mucinous carcinoma

13. A patient had a sentinel node biopsy and states, "Something is very wrong with me." The patient explains that she had a bowel movement and urinated and both are blue in color. Which explanations should the nurse provide to the patient?

   a. The cancer may be invasive and holding on to some of the dye that is used.

   b. The patient must be having a reaction to the dye that was used.

   c. The dye that was used during the biopsy is safe and being excreted.

   d. The health care provider will have to discuss this with her.

14. A patient has had a total mastectomy 12 hours ago and the nurse is assessing the surgical wound. The nurse observes ecchymosis, swelling, and tightness around the wound, and the patient states that it is painful. Which does the nurse suspect has occurred?

   a. The patient has developed an infection.

   b. The patient has developed a hematoma.

   c. The patient has developed lymphedema.

   d. The patient has developed a cyst.

15. A patient is scheduled to receive radiation therapy for 6 weeks after her lumpectomy. The patient states that she is worried about the side effects of the radiation. Which information will the nurse discuss about the side effects of the radiation?

   a. "The radiation can make you very nauseated, but something will be given for nausea."

   b. "The radiation can cause you to lose your hair, but you can wear a wig or scarves."

   c. "The radiation can cause musculoskeletal fatigue and you may not be able to continue to work while receiving the radiation."

   d. "The radiation can cause some skin breakdown toward the end of treatment in the axillary folds."

CHAPTER 53

Assessment and Management of Patients with Male Reproductive Disorders

Learning Outcomes

1. Describe structures and function of the male reproductive system.
2. Discuss nursing assessment of the male reproductive system, identifying diagnostic tests used and their related nursing implications.
3. Explain the causes and management of male sexual dysfunction.
4. Compare the types of prostatectomy with regard to advantages and disadvantages.
5. Use the nursing process as a framework for care of the patient with male reproductive disorders and conditions, including prostate, testicular, and penis disorders.

SECTION I: ASSESSING YOUR UNDERSTANDING

Activity A *Fill in the blanks.*

1. Two specific tests used to diagnose prostate cancer are _____ and _____.

2. The most common isolated organism that causes prostatitis is _____.

3. The most commonly used medication for estrogen therapy in the treatment of prostate cancer is _____; other hormonal therapies such as _____, _____, _____, _____, and _____ suppress testicular androgen.

4. Five major potential complications after prostatectomy are _____, _____, _____, _____, and _____.

5. Two tumor markers that may be elevated in testicular cancer are _____ and _____.

6. The testes have a dual function: _____ and secretion of the male sex hormone _____, which induces and preserves the male sex characteristics.

7. _____ and _____ often decrease in as many as two thirds of men older than 70 years of age.

8. Men older than 50 years of age are at increased risk for genitourinary tract cancers including those of the _____, _____, _____, and _____.

9. The cells within the prostate gland produce a protein called the _____ _____, which can be measured in the blood.

10. _____ occurs when semen travels toward the bladder instead of exiting through the penis, resulting in infertility.

11. _____, a complication of prostatectomy, occurs in 80% to 95% of patients.

12. _____ are the oral medications that are considered first-line therapy in the treatment of erectile dysfunction.

Activity B *Briefly answer the following.*

1. List four symptoms associated with prostatitis.

   _____

   _____

2. Identify seven symptoms that a patient with benign prostatic hyperplasia might display.

   _____

   _____

   _____

   _____

3. Which factors will be considered when a patient is choosing a penile implant?

   _____

   _____

   _____

   _____

Activity C *Match each disorder of the male reproductive system listed in Column II with its description listed in Column I.*

Column I

___ 1. Collection of fluid in the testes

___ 2. An obstructive complex characterized by increased urinary frequency

___ 3. Constricted foreskin of the penis

___ 4. Failure of the testes to descend into the scrotum

___ 5. Inflammation of the testes

___ 6. Abnormal dilation of the veins in the scrotum

___ 7. Inflammation of the prostate gland

___ 8. Infection of the epididymis

Column II

a. Cryptorchidism
b. Epididymitis
c. Hydrocele
d. Orchitis
e. Phimosis
f. Prostatism
g. Prostatitis
h. Varicocele

SECTION II: APPLYING YOUR KNOWLEDGE

Activity D *Consider the scenario and answer the questions.*

CASE STUDY: Prostatectomy

Tom Jones, age 65, is scheduled for a robotic-assisted laparoscopic radical prostatectomy after undergoing medical management of his prostate cancer for 1 year. His wife will be accompanying him to the hospital and staying during his surgical procedure.

1. Mr. Jones asks the nurse if he will be able to have sex again. What is the best response by the nurse?

   _____

   _____

   _____

   _____

2. The day after Mr. Jones has his surgery, he reports a feeling of fullness in the lower abdomen and feeling as though he needs to void. He says he sees blood around his penis where the catheter is. What concern is related to these symptoms?

_____

_____

3. Which interventions can the nurse provide to alleviate Mr. Jones' discomfort from this problem?

_____

_____

_____

SECTION III: PRACTICING FOR NCLEX

Activity E *Answer the following questions.*

1. A patient comes to the clinic reporting an inability to sustain an erection and is prescribed a PDE-5 inhibitor, sildenafil. Which medication will the nurse caution the patient about taking with this medication?
   a. Isosorbide
   b. Lisinopril
   c. Diphenhydramine
   d. Levothyroxine

2. A patient is having a digital rectal examination (DRE) in the health care provider's office, and the nurse is to assist in the examination. Which education will the nurse provide to decrease the discomfort from the examination?
   a. Take a deep breath and hold it when the health care provider inserts a gloved finger into the rectum.
   b. Take a deep breath and exhale when the health care provider inserts a gloved finger into the rectum.
   c. When bending over the examining table, point the feet outward to decrease the discomfort.
   d. Inform the patient that the examination is not uncomfortable and will be over in a short period of time.

3. The nurse is demonstrating the technique for performing a testicular self-examination (TSE) to a group of men for a company health fair. One of the men asks the nurse at what age a man should begin performing TSE. Which is the best response by the nurse?
   a. "It should begin in adolescence."
   b. "It should begin in men over age 50."
   c. "It should be performed in high-risk males over age 30."
   d. "It should begin at age 40."

4. A patient comes to the emergency department and tells the nurse, "I took a pill to help me perform sexually and then passed out." The nurse is assessing the patient and finds a nitroglycerin patch on his back. Which is the first intervention the nurse must perform?
   a. Take the patient's blood pressure.
   b. Ask the patient to obtain a urine specimen.
   c. Start an IV.
   d. Administer atropine 0.5 mg.

5. A patient has demonstrated interest in obtaining a penile implant. Which will the patient consider prior to making this decision? (Select all that apply.)
   a. Activities of daily living (ADLs)
   b. Social activities
   c. Expectations of the patient and partner
   d. Financial status
   e. Occupation

6. A patient is planning to use a negative-pressure (vacuum) device to maintain and sustain an erection. Which will the nurse caution the patient about with the use of this device?
   a. "Do not use the device while taking nitrates."
   b. "Do not leave the constricting band in place for longer than 1 hour to avoid penile injury."
   c. "Watch for erosion of the prosthesis through the skin."
   d. "Watch for the development of infection."

7. When developing an educational program for a group of adolescents about sexually transmitted infections (STIs), which will the nurse inform the group about the single greatest risk factor for contracting an STI?

   a. Type of contraception used

   b. Number of times the person has contact with a partner

   c. Number of sexual partners

   d. Where the patient lives

8. A patient is being treated for prostatitis and the nurse is providing education about the treatment. Which will the nurse include in the education of this patient?

   a. Force fluid to prevent urine from backing up and distending the bladder.

   b. Take several cool baths during the day to alleviate discomfort.

   c. Be sure to take the 3-day course of anti-fungal medication.

   d. Avoid foods and liquids with diuretic action or that increase prostatic secretions.

9. A patient informs the nurse that his father died of prostate cancer, and he wants to know ways in which to reduce risk factors for developing it. Which education will the nurse give to the patient to decrease modifiable risk factors?

   a. Limit red meat and dairy products high in fat.

   b. Quit smoking.

   c. Avoid wearing tight pants and underwear.

   d. Monitor blood pressure.

10. A patient is suspected to have prostate cancer related to observed clinical symptoms. Which definitive test can the nurse assist with to confirm a diagnosis of prostate cancer?

    a. DRE

    b. PSA

    c. Prostate biopsy

    d. Cystoscopy

11. A patient is having brachytherapy for the treatment of prostate cancer and asks the nurse if he can have sex after radiation therapy is completed. Which is the best response by the nurse?

    a. "You most likely will not be able to have sexual intercourse after radiation therapy."

    b. "You must be sure to use a condom for 2 weeks after implantation and then it will no longer be necessary."

    c. "There are no restrictions to sex during radiation."

    d. "You must use a condom for at least 6 months after beginning radiation therapy."

12. A patient with an indwelling catheter after a radical prostatectomy is having bladder spasms. Which medication prescribed by the primary provider can the nurse administer to help alleviate the discomfort?

    a. Cephalexin

    b. Phenazopyridine

    c. Oxybutynin

    d. Tadalafil

13. The nurse is educating a patient about performing testicular self-examination (TSE). Which will the nurse inform the patient is the best time to perform the examination?

    a. In the morning when arising

    b. After exercise

    c. After a warm bath or shower

    d. At bedtime

14. A patient experiences hypotension, lethargy, and muscle spasms while receiving bladder irrigations after a transurethral resection of the prostate (TURP). Which is the first action the nurse should take?

    a. Discontinue the irrigations.

    b. Increase the rate of the IV fluids.

    c. Administer a unit of packed red blood cells.

    d. Prepare the patient for an ECG.

15. The nurse is providing education to a patient about decreasing the risk of penile cancer. Which will the nurse tell the patient is the best way to decrease the risk of developing penile cancer?

    a. Avoid sex with multiple partners.

    b. Use good genital hygiene.

    c. Use a condom when having sex.

    d. Perform self-examinations.

CHAPTER 54

Assessment and Management of Patients Who Are LGBTQ

Learning Outcomes

1. Describe the importance of providing inclusive health care environments for people who are lesbian, gay, bisexual, transgender, and queer.
2. Use inclusive terminology when communicating and conducting an assessment with a person who is lesbian, gay, bisexual, transgender, and queer.
3. Explain and demonstrate the proper techniques to perform a health history and physical assessment and discriminate between normal and abnormal findings identified in the patient who is lesbian, gay, bisexual, transgender, and queer.
4. Describe the various medical procedures and hormone treatments available for the person who is undergoing gender reassignment.
5. Compare and contrast surgical procedures available to people seeking gender reassignment in terms of indications and preoperative and postoperative complications.
6. Use the nursing process as a framework for care of the patient who undergoes gender reassignment surgery.

SECTION I: ASSESSING YOUR UNDERSTANDING

Activity A *Fill in the blanks.*

1. _____ is the way people experience and express themselves sexually.

2. _____ is an umbrella term that refers to romantic, emotional, or sexual attraction to people of the opposite gender, the same gender, or to more than one gender.

3. Women have _____ chromosomes, a uterus and ovaries, and the primary sex hormone is _____; men have _____ chromosomes, a penis and testicles, and the primary sex hormone is _____.

4. The biggest challenge to estimating the LGBTQ population in the United States is the lack of _____.

5. In understanding older adults who are LGBTQ, it is important to recognize their _____, _____, and _____ experiences.

6. To achieve the secondary sex characteristics of the opposite gender, _____ are needed.

Activity B *Briefly answer the following.*

1. Which effects of sex hormones are not able to be reversed?

   _____

2. Name some of the common androgen-reducing medications that may be used to decrease testosterone levels.

   _____

   _____

   _____

   _____

3. Why would progesterone not be used in the feminization process?

   _____

   _____

   _____

4. For a transgender man (female-to-male), which changes will occur with the administration of testosterone?

   _____

   _____

   _____

5. Discuss the two primary medical treatments of hair removal for long-term results.

   _____

   _____

   _____

6. What are the goals for the patient undergoing male-to-female genital reassignment surgery?

   _____

   _____

   _____

Activity C *Match the term in Column I with its associated description in Column II.*

Column I

_____ 1. Bisexual

_____ 2. Cisgender

_____ 3. Intersex

_____ 4. Queer

_____ 5. Questioning

_____ 6. Transgender

Column II

a. people who identify with the gender that matches the sex assigned to them at birth

b. people who are romantically, emotionally, or sexually attracted to numerous genders (male, female, transgender, intersex, etc.) or people who identify as nonheterosexual but do not want to use labels such as gay, lesbian, or bisexual

c. umbrella term used to describe the full range of people whose gender identity does not match with the sex assigned to them at birth

d. people who are romantically, emotionally, or sexually attracted to both male and female genders

e. a person who is born with biologic traits that do not fit into those that traditionally characterize either male or female

f. a person who is unsure or is still exploring their sexual orientation or is concerned about applying a social label to themselves

SECTION II: APPLYING YOUR KNOWLEDGE

Activity D *Consider the scenario and answer the questions.*

CASE STUDY: Care of the Transgender Female Undergoing Orchiectomy and Vaginoplasty

Kit Fallon is a 36-year-old transgender female who has made the decision to undergo vaginoplasty. She underwent breast augmentation and chondrolaryngoplasty approximately 6 months ago and had no difficulty in the intraoperative or postoperative phase of the surgery.

1. What is the goal of gender reassignment surgery?

_____

_____

2. What are the two major goals of postoperative care for this patient?

_____

_____

3. What immediate postoperative education about the need for a vaginal dilator will the nurse provide to the patient?

_____

_____

4. What discharge instructions will it be important for the nurse to discuss with the patient to maintain patency and reduce the risk for infection?

_____

_____

SECTION III: PRACTICING FOR NCLEX

Activity E *Answer the following questions.*

1. The nurse is admitting a patient who identifies with the LGBTQ community. Which actions by the nurse will foster a therapeutic nurse–patient relationship? (Select all that apply.)
   a. Inform the patient that they have to identify as male or female on the forms being filled out.
   b. Inform the patient that they will be asked about gender/sexual identity so that they may be provided personalized care.
   c. When asking assessment questions, inform the patient that the questions are asked of every patient admitted.
   d. Indicate to the patient that if they are uncomfortable answering the questions asked, the patient may choose not to answer the questions.
   e. When asking questions that identify the patient's personal preference of pronouns, explain what this means.

2. A patient with gender dysphoria is discussing with the nurse their wish to progress to gender reassignment surgery. Which statements by the patient indicates that the process toward gender reassignment is realistic?
   a. "I can make an appointment with a surgeon to schedule my surgery as soon as possible."
   b. "I am going to ask the health care provider to begin my hormonal therapy."
   c. "I will see the mental health provider for an appointment to begin the process."
   d. "I just am afraid that if I start the process, I will change my mind."

3. A patient who is a transgender woman is preparing to take sex hormones. Which previous effects of the androgens cannot be reversed by the hormones? (Select all that apply.)
   a. Breast tissue
   b. Size and shape of the hands
   c. Shape of the jaw
   d. Shape of the pelvic structures
   e. Facial hair

4. A patient who is a transgender male is taking testosterone to produce desired changes. Which statements by the patient indicates that the testosterone is having the desired effect?

   a. "I have noticed that my face is much oilier, and I have hair growth on my chest."

   b. "My breast size is increasing, and I have a heavier menstrual period."

   c. "Someone told me that my voice has gotten higher than it usually is."

   d. "I have an increase in body fat, and my muscle mass is decreasing."

5. A patient who is a transgender female is prescribed cyproterone acetate. Which statements by the patient indicates to the nurse that the patient has developed an adverse effect from the medication?

   a. "I am having shortness of breath, and my chest hurts."

   b. "I checked my blood pressure, and it is 90/50 mm Hg."

   c. "I am having difficulty passing my urine, and it is very cloudy."

   d. "I have been seeing and hearing things that aren't really there."

6. A patient is preparing to have laser hair removal treatments. In which situations will the nurse inform the patient to avoid these treatments?

   a. The patient is planning a trip to the beach and will have sun exposure.

   b. The patient has had an allergic reaction to latex products and foods.

   c. The patient has previously used depilatory creams for facial hair removal.

   d. The patient is taking isotretinoin for the treatment of acne.

7. A patient who is a transgender male is taking testosterone and is seeking treatment for acne. The health care provider prescribes minocycline. What education will the nurse include when discussing these medications? (Select all that apply.)

   a. "Be sure to take the medications together at the same time each day."

   b. "As soon as the acne clears up, you can stop taking both of the medications."

   c. "Frequent monitoring of liver function will be required."

   d. "If planning on reassignment surgery, wound healing may be delayed."

   e. "All other medications will be discontinued while you are taking the drug."

8. A patient underwent a phalloplasty 1 week ago. Which procedure will the nurse assist with so that the patient may begin voiding?

   a. Removal of an indwelling urethral catheter

   b. Clamping of the suprapubic catheter and removal of a transurethral catheter

   c. Applying suprapubic pressure to express the urine from the bladder

   d. Needle aspiration of the urine from the bladder

9. The nurse is preparing a patient for phalloplasty surgery and assessing whether the patient has met all of the criteria for surgery. Which statements by the patient will be immediately reported to the surgeon because it may cause a delay or cancellation of the procedure?

   a. "I quit smoking about 6 months ago and now only use e-cigarettes."

   b. "I took my bowel preparation yesterday."

   c. "I stopped taking my hormone treatment 3 weeks ago."

   d. "I am able to attend all of my follow-up visits after surgery."

10. A patient underwent phalloplasty surgery yesterday; the nurse assesses that the skin of the reconstructed shaft is dark blue, and the patient reports severe pain in the area. Which is the priority action by the nurse?

    a. Apply an ice pack to the area.

    b. Administer ibuprofen 600 mg po.

    c. Notify the health care provider.

    d. Assist the patient to a side-lying position.

Integumentary Function

CHAPTER 55

Assessment of Integumentary Function

Learning Outcomes

1. Describe the structures and functions of the skin, hair, and nails.
2. Discriminate between normal and abnormal assessment findings of the skin, hair, and nails.
3. Recognize and evaluate the major alterations in skin, hair, and nails by applying the patient's health history and physical assessment findings.
4. Compare and contrast the patterns and typical distributions of primary and secondary skin lesions.
5. Distinguish common skin manifestations associated with systemic disease.
6. Identify the common diagnostic tests used in evaluating skin disorders and related nursing implications.

SECTION I: ASSESSING YOUR UNDERSTANDING

Activity A *Fill in the blanks.*

1. There are three layers of the skin: _____, _____, and _____.

2. The epidermis is composed of three types of cells: _____, _____, and _____.

3. The epidermis is almost completely replaced every _____.

4. The subcutaneous tissue, which is primarily composed of _____ tissue, has a major role in _____ regulation.

5. The term used to describe hair loss is _____.

6. _____ and _____ are two types of skin glands.

7. Skin needs to be exposed to sunlight to manufacture vitamin _____.

8. Jaundice can first be observed by examining the _____ and _____.

9. The nurse should know that clubbing of the nails is usually an indicator of _____.

10. _____, _____, and _____ are the major physical processes involved in loss of heat from the body to the environment.

Activity B *Briefly answer the following.*

1. Describe how the production of melanin is controlled.

   _____

   _____

   _____

   _____

2. Describe what function the hair of the skin serves.

_____

_____

_____

_____

3. What is the function of the receptor endings of nerves in the skin?

_____

_____

_____

_____

4. When assessing the skin of an older adult, which major age-related changes are seen in the skin?

_____

_____

_____

_____

Activity C *Match the description in Column II with the associated key term in Column I.*

Column I

____ **1.** Dermatosis

____ **2.** Erythema

____ **3.** Hirsutism

____ **4.** Hyperpigmentation

____ **5.** Hypopigmentation

____ **6.** Keratin

____ **7.** Melanin

____ **8.** Petechiae

____ **9.** Telangiectasia

____ **10.** Vitiligo

Column II

a. Pinpoint red spots that appear on the skin as a result of blood leakage into the skin

b. A localized or widespread condition characterized by destruction of the melanocytes in circumscribed areas of the skin, resulting in white patches

c. The substance responsible for coloration of the skin

d. Decrease in the melanin of the skin, resulting in a loss of pigmentation

e. Red marks on the skin caused by distention of the superficial blood vessels

f. An insoluble, fibrous protein that forms the outer layer of skin

g. Increase in the melanin of the skin, resulting in an increase in pigmentation

h. Any abnormal skin condition

i. Redness of the skin caused by congestion of the capillaries

j. The condition of having excessive hair growth

SECTION II: APPLYING YOUR KNOWLEDGE

Activity D *Consider the scenario and answer the questions.*

Mrs. Paul, age 72, is being seen in the clinic for a regular checkup. She asks the nurse to check several small lesions on her back and arms. Mrs. Paul has diabetes that is well controlled with diet.

1. The nurse is assessing the various lesions on Mrs. Paul's back and arms. What will the nurse document related to the assessment findings?

   _____

   _____

2. The nurse observes dull, red bumps smaller than a pencil eraser on Mrs. Paul's arms. They are bilateral and occur in linear clusters. How will the nurse document these lesions?

   _____

3. Why would it be important for the nurse to assess the legs and feet for skin changes?

   _____

   _____

   _____

   _____

SECTION III: PRACTICING FOR NCLEX

Activity E *Answer the following questions.*

1. The nurse is caring for an adult patient with a body temperature within normal range. Which is the approximate insensible water loss per day in this patient?
   a. 250 mL/day
   b. 600 mL/day
   c. 800 mL/day
   d. 1000 mL/day

2. The nurse is applying a cold towel to a patient's neck to reduce body heat. How will the nurse determine that the heat is reduced?
   a. Conduction
   b. Convection
   c. Evaporation
   d. Radiation

3. The nurse is assessing the fingernails of a patient at the clinic. The nurse observes pitting on the surface of the nail. Which disorder is this finding indicative of?
   a. Psoriasis
   b. Vitiligo
   c. Diabetes
   d. Melanoma

4. The nurse is caring for a patient with dark skin who is having gastrointestinal bleeding. How will the nurse determine from skin color change that shock may be present?
   a. The skin is ashen gray and dull
   b. The skin is dusky blue
   c. The skin is reddish pink
   d. The skin is whitish pink

5. The nurse assesses a dark-skinned patient who has cherry-red nail beds, lips, and oral mucosa. Which disorder does the nurse identify correlates with this assessment finding?
   a. Anemia
   b. Carbon monoxide poisoning
   c. Polycythemia
   d. Shock

6. The nurse is assessing a patient with a primary skin lesion called a macule. Which does the nurse identify is a clinical example of this lesion?
   a. Hives
   b. Impetigo
   c. Port-wine stains
   d. Psoriasis

7. The nurse assesses a patient and observes a herpes simplex/zoster skin lesion. How will the nurse document this lesion?

   a. Macule

   b. Papule

   c. Vesicle

   d. Wheal

8. The nurse is assessing a patient with risk factors related to human immune deficiency virus (HIV). Which assessment finding does the nurse identify as a manifestation of the disease?

   a. Telangiectasia

   b. Ecchymosis

   c. Fluid-filled vesicles

   d. Purplish cutaneous lesions

9. A patient is visiting the health care provider to determine what type of allergy is causing a rash. Which type of testing will be appropriate in order to determine the cause of this finding?

   a. Skin biopsy

   b. Skin scrapings

   c. Tzanck smear

   d. Patch test

10. The nurse is assisting with the collection of a Tzanck smear. Which is the suspected diagnosis of the patient?

    a. Fungal infection

    b. Herpes zoster

    c. Psoriasis

    d. Seborrheic dermatosis

11. A patient has a serum bilirubin concentration of 3 mg/100 mL. Which will the nurse observe when performing a skin assessment on this patient?

    a. Jaundice

    b. Pallor

    c. Bronzed appearance

    d. Cherry-red face

12. A patient comes to the clinic and asks the nurse why the skin of the forehead, palms, and soles has a yellow-orange tint. There is no yellowing of the sclera or mucous membranes. Which question would be most appropriate to ask the patient to identify a potential cause of the skin discoloration?

    a. "Have you been ingesting large quantities of alcohol?"

    b. "Have you been diagnosed with Addison disease?"

    c. "Have you been in the sun a lot?"

    d. "Have you been eating a large amount of carotene-rich foods?"

13. A patient has contact dermatitis on the hand, and the nurse observes an area that is thickened and rough between the thumb and forefinger. How will the nurse document this finding?

    a. Atrophy

    b. Lichenification

    c. Keloid

    d. Scales

14. The nurse assesses a patient with silvery-white, thick scales on the scalp, elbows, and hand of a patient that bleed when picked off. Which skin disorder correlates with this assessment finding?

    a. Vitiligo

    b. Psoriasis

    c. Melanoma

    d. Petechiae

15. The nurse observes an African American patient with a large hypertrophied area of scar tissue on the left ear lobe. Which does the nurse document this finding as?

    a. Atrophy

    b. Scar

    c. Lichenification

    d. Keloid

CHAPTER 56

Management of Patients with Dermatologic Disorders

Learning Outcomes

1. Describe the medical and nursing management of the patient with a wound, pruritus, dermatologic secretory disorder, infections of the skin, parasitic skin diseases, or noninfectious inflammatory dermatoses.
2. Use the nursing process as a framework for care of the patient with a pressure injury, or with a blistering disorder including toxic epidermal necrolysis and Stevens–Johnson syndrome.
3. Discuss the medical and nursing management of the patient with skin tumors (benign, malignant, and metastatic).
4. Identify the medical and nursing management of the patient undergoing plastic and cosmetic procedures.

SECTION I: ASSESSING YOUR UNDERSTANDING

Activity A *Fill in the blanks.*

1. The most common skin condition in adolescents and young adults between the ages of 12 and 35 years is _____.

2. There are three types of wound dressings: _____, _____, and _____.

3. Autolytic _____ is a process that uses the body's own digestive enzymes to break down necrotic tissue.

4. Corticosteroids are widely used in treating dermatologic conditions to provide _____, _____, and _____ effects.

5. The main secretory function of the skin is performed by the _____, which help regulate body temperature.

6. Scabies is an infestation of the skin by the itch mite _____.

7. Bullous impetigo, a deep-seated infection characterized by large, fluid-filled blisters, is caused by the bacteria _____.

8. Pemphigus vulgaris is a(n) _____ disease in which the immunoglobulin G (IgG) antibody is directed against a specific cell surface antigen in epidermal cells.

9. _____ is an important principle of psoriasis treatment.

10. There are three types of therapy indicated for the treatment of psoriasis: _____, _____, and _____.

11. _____ is the leading cause of death in people with blistering diseases.

Activity B *Briefly answer the following.*

1. List four major objectives of therapy for patients with dermatologic problems.

_____

_____

_____

2. Describe why moisture-retentive dressings are efficient at removing exudate.

_____

_____

_____

3. How do cytokines work?

_____

_____

4. The nurse is applying foam dressing to an exudative sacral decubitus ulcer. After application of the foam dressing, what is important for the nurse to do?

_____

_____

5. What are the potential complications of Stevens–Johnson syndrome (SJS) and toxic epidermal necrolysis (TEN)?

_____

_____

6. List five risk factors related to the development of melanoma.

_____

_____

_____

_____

Activity C *Match the term in Column I with the definition in Column II.*

Column I

_____ 1. Comedone

_____ 2. Cheilitis

_____ 3. Carbuncle

_____ 4. Furuncle

_____ 5. Tinea

_____ 6. Pyodermas

_____ 7. Liniments

_____ 8. Xerosis

_____ 9. Santyl

_____ 10. Gel

_____ 11. Fluocinonide

_____ 12. Famvir

_____ 13. Scabies

_____ 14. Permethrin

_____ 15. Toxic epidermal necrolysis (TEN)

Column II

a. A potentially fatal skin disorder

b. An enzymatic débriding agent

c. A prescription scabicide

d. Localized skin infection involving only one hair follicle

e. Primary lesion of acne

f. Dry crackling skin at corners of mouth

g. Localized skin infection involving hair follicles

h. A semisolid emulsion that becomes liquid when applied to the skin or scalp

i. Most common fungal infection of skin or scalp

j. Bacterial skin infections

k. Overly dry skin

l. Lotions with added oil to soften skin

m. A topical corticosteroid with medium to high potency

n. An antiviral agent used to treat herpes zoster

o. An infestation caused by the itch mite

SECTION II: APPLYING YOUR KNOWLEDGE

Activity D *Consider the scenarios and answer the questions.*

CASE STUDY: Acne Vulgaris

Brian Vargo is a 15-year-old boy who has been experiencing facial eruptions of acne for about a year. The numerous lesions are inflamed and present on the face and neck. He has tried many over-the-counter medications and nothing seems to help. His father had a history of severe acne when he was a teenager.

1. What type of dietary advice can the nurse provide to Brian that may assist in preventing the "flare-ups" related to acne?

_____

_____

_____

_____

2. The health care provider prescribes an oral antibiotic for Brian to take for 1 month and then wants to see him at that time to determine effectiveness. Which type of antibiotic is generally prescribed for treatment?

_____

3. Which nursing interventions will assist Brian in coping with his acne?

_____

_____

_____

_____

CASE STUDY: Malignant Melanoma

Steve Cantorelli is a 26-year-old professional baseball player for a Florida farm team. He spends many hours in the sun practicing between 9:00 AM and 4:00 PM. His V-neck uniform leaves little protection for his chest. Steve had a mole on his chest for 5 years, and one day last October he noticed that the margins of the mole were elevated and palpable and the color had become darker. Since his father had melanoma when he was 32 years old, Steve decided to see the health care provider.

1. On examination, a circular lesion with irregular outer edges and a pinkish hue in the center is observed on Steve's chest. Which type of lesion is consistent with this finding?

_____

2. Which procedure will the nurse prepare the patient for to obtain confirmation of the diagnosis?

_____

3. The nurse measures the lesion and documents that it is greater than 14 mm in thickness and growing vertically. Which prognosis does the nurse expect the health care provider to discuss with the patient after the biopsy results are returned?

_____

_____

SECTION III: PRACTICING FOR NCLEX

Activity E *Answer the following questions.*

1. The nurse is changing the dressing of a chronic wound. There is no sign of infection or heavy drainage. How long will the nurse leave the wound covered?
   a. 6 to 12 hours
   b. 12 to 24 hours
   c. 24 to 36 hours
   d. 48 to 72 hours

2. A patient has a moisture-retentive dressing for the treatment of a sacral decubitus ulcer. How long will the nurse leave the dressing in place before replacing it?

a. 4 to 6 hours

b. 8 hours

c. 12 to 24 hours

d. 24 to 36 hours

3. A patient is advised to apply a suspension-type lotion to a dermatosis site. The nurse will advise the patient to apply the lotion how often to be most effective?

a. Every hour

b. Every 3 hours

c. Every 12 hours

d. Every day at the same time

4. Which will the nurse assess for to determine if a patient using corticosteroids for a dermatologic condition is having local side effects? (Select all that apply.)

a. Skin atrophy

b. Striae

c. Telangiectasia

d. Comedones

e. Ecchymosis

5. The nurse is instructing a patient on how to apply a corticosteroid cream to lesions on the arm. Which intervention will the nurse instruct the patient to do to increase the absorption of the medication?

a. Apply an occlusive dressing over the site after application.

b. Make sure that the skin is slightly dehydrated so that the medication can absorb through the skin cracks.

c. Apply a thick layer of cream over the lesions so that if some rubs off, there is more to absorb.

d. Apply the medication every 2 hours.

6. The nurse will assess all possible causes of pruritus for a patient reporting generalized pruritus. Which does the nurse understand can be other causes for this condition?

a. End-stage kidney disease

b. Hypothyroidism

c. Pneumonia

d. Myasthenia gravis

7. A patient is being evaluated for nodular cystic acne. Which systemic pharmacologic agent may be prescribed for the treatment of this disorder?

a. Isotretinoin

b. Benzoyl peroxide

c. Tretinoin

d. Salicylic acid

8. A patient reports severe itching that intensifies at night. The nurse assesses the skin using a magnifying glass and penlight to look for the "itch mite." Which skin condition does the nurse assess?

a. Contact dermatitis

b. Pediculosis

c. Scabies

d. Tinea corporis

9. A patient is diagnosed with psoriasis after developing scales on the scalp, elbows, and behind the knees. The patient asks the nurse, "Where did I catch this from?" Which is the best response by the nurse?

a. Psoriasis is an inflammatory dermatosis that results from a superficial infection with *Staphylococcus aureus*.

b. Psoriasis comes from dermal abrasion.

c. Psoriasis is an inflammatory dermatosis that results from an overproduction of keratin.

d. Psoriasis results from excess deposition of subcutaneous fat.

10. The nurse is assessing a patient for psoriatic lesions after treatment with a nonsteroidal cream. Which characteristic is typical of a plaque psoriatic lesion?

a. Red, raised patch covered with silver scales

b. Cluster of pustules

c. Group of raised vesicles

d. Pattern of bullae that rupture and form a scaly crust

11. A patient is being treated for chronic venous stasis ulcers of the lower extremities. Which medication prescribed by the health care provider will increase peripheral blood flow by decreasing the viscosity of blood and assist with the healing of the ulcers?

    a. Heparin

    b. Warfarin

    c. Aspirin

    d. Pentoxifylline

12. A patient is diagnosed with seborrheic dermatitis on the face and is prescribed a corticosteroid preparation for use. Which will the nurse educate the patient about regarding use of the steroid on the face?

    a. Use very warm water to clean the face prior to applying the medication.

    b. Avoid using the medication around the eyelids because it may cause cataracts and glaucoma.

    c. Wash the face several times a day and reapply the medication.

    d. Scrape the scaly patches off prior to applying the medication.

13. A patient has developed a boil on the face, and the nurse observes the patient squeezing the boil. Which complication will the nurse discuss with the patient after encouraging them not to manipulate the boil?

    a. Scarring

    b. Brain abscess

    c. Erythema

    d. Cellulitis

14. The nurse is caring for a patient with extensive bullous lesions on the trunk and back. Prior to initiating skin care, which is a priority for the nurse to do?

    a. Wash the lesions vigorously.

    b. Rupture the bullous lesions.

    c. Administer analgesic pain medication.

    d. Apply cold compresses.

15. The nurse is assessing a patient with toxic epidermal necrolysis (TEN). Which assessment data will indicate that the patient may be progressing to keratoconjunctivitis? (Select all that apply.)

    a. Skin peeling on eyelids

    b. Pruritus of the eyes

    c. Burning of the eyes

    d. Dryness of the eyes

    e. Blurred optic discs

Management of Patients with Burn Injury

1. Identify the incidence and factors that affect severity of burn injury in the United States.
2. Describe the local and systemic effects of a major burn injury.
3. Use the nursing process as a framework for care of the patient in the emergent/resuscitative, acute/intermediate, and rehabilitation phases of a burn injury.
4. Compare priorities of care, including fluid replacement, wound management and psychosocial support, and potential complications for each phase of burn recovery.

SECTION I: ASSESSING YOUR UNDERSTANDING

Activity A *Fill in the blanks.*

1. The two age groups that have increased morbidity and mortality from burn injuries are _____ and _____.

2. Burns that exceed _____ of the total body surface area (TBSA) are considered major burn injuries and produce both local and systemic inflammatory response.

3. _____ is the immediate consequence of ensuing fluid loss and results in decreased perfusion and oxygen delivery.

4. Burn injuries are classified according to _____ and _____.

5. Two pulmonary complications that occur secondary to inhalation injuries are _____ and _____.

6. The leading cause of death in thermally injured patients is _____.

7. The resuscitation goal of fluid replacement therapy, postburn injury, is a urinary output of _____ to _____ for adults.

8. The three major bacteria responsible for infection in burn centers are _____, _____, and _____.

9. Three commonly used topical antibacterials for skin care are _____, _____, and _____.

10. Four signs of postburn sepsis include _____; _____; _____; and _____.

Activity B *Briefly answer the following.*

1. Which factors are instrumental in improving the survival rate for burn victims over the last 80 years?

_____

_____

_____

2. What are the three zones of burn injury and what areas are involved with each?

_____

_____

_____

3. What two detrimental effects does radiation injury have?

_____

_____

4. Explain the pathophysiology of carbon monoxide poisoning.

_____

_____

5. What types of general emergency procedures should be employed at the burn scene?

_____

_____

_____

6. What does the depth of burn injury depend on?

_____

_____

7. When a patient sustains inhalation injury below the vocal cords, what is the usual cause?

_____

_____

8. The nurse is performing a secondary survey for a patient who sustained severe burns. Which will the nurse include in this survey?

_____

_____

9. Describe the measures that can be taken to avoid the development of hypertrophic and keloid scars after a burn injury.

_____

_____

_____

_____

10. Discuss why congestive heart failure is a potential complication of an acute burn.

_____

_____

_____

Activity C *Match the term in Column I with the associated definition in Column II.*

Column I

____ **1.** Xenograft

____ **2.** Debridement

____ **3.** Eschar

____ **4.** Fasciotomy

____ **5.** Contracture

____ **6.** Homograft

____ **7.** Escharotomy

Column II

a. Graft transferred from one human (living or cadaveric) to another human; also called allograft

b. Graft obtained from an animal of a species other than that of the recipient (e.g., pigskin); also called a heterograft

c. Devitalized tissue resulting from a burn or wound

d. Shrinkage of burn scar through collagen maturation

e. Incision made through the fascia to release constriction of underlying muscle

f. Removal of foreign material and devitalized tissue until surrounding healthy tissue is exposed

g. Linear excision made through eschar to release constriction of underlying tissue

SECTION II: APPLYING YOUR KNOWLEDGE

Activity D *Consider the scenario and answer the questions.*

Brad Smith, age 22, sustained full-thickness burns on his anterior chest, face, and neck when he was trying to start a charcoal fire with lighter fluid to prepare dinner for his father. His father sprayed him with water from a hose and took him to a hospital emergency department 3 miles away. On arrival, Brad was semiconscious and in respiratory distress. Brad is determined to weigh 72 kg.

1. Upon arrival at the emergency department, which indicators does the nurse have that Brad may have an inhalation injury as well as severe burns?

   _____

   _____

   _____

2. What does the nurse prepare to assist with due to Brad's immediate condition?

   _____

   _____

3. According to the rule of 9's, Brad has been burned over 13.5% of his body. According to the American Burn Association (ABA) fluid resuscitation guide, how much fluid should he receive in the first 24 hours after the burn injury?

   _____

   _____

SECTION III: PRACTICING FOR NCLEX

Activity E *Answer the following questions.*

1. The nurse is caring for a patient with a full-thickness burn to the arm after being scalded with boiling water. Which indication does the nurse have for classifying the burns as full-thickness?
   a. Classification by the appearance of blisters
   b. Identification by the destruction of the dermis and epidermis
   c. Not associated with edema formation
   d. Usually very painful because of exposed nerve endings

2. The nurse is caring for a patient who sustained severe burns to 50% of the body 3 days previously. Which will the nurse report immediately to the health care provider when reviewing laboratory studies indicating massive cell destruction?
   a. Hypernatremia
   b. Hypokalemia
   c. Hyperkalemia
   d. Hypercalcemia

3. The nurse is reviewing the laboratory studies for a patient during fluid remobilization after a major burn. Which laboratory value reviewed by the nurse should be immediately reported?
   a. Hematocrit level of 45%
   b. A pH of 7.2, PaO_2 of 38 mm Hg, and bicarbonate level of 15 mEq/L
   c. Serum potassium level of 3.2 mEq/L
   d. Serum sodium level of 140 mEq/L

4. The nurse is caring for a patient with a major burn. Which serious gastrointestinal disturbance will the nurse monitor for that frequently occurs with a major burn?
   a. Diverticulitis
   b. Hematemesis
   c. Paralytic ileus
   d. Ulcerative colitis

5. The nurse is answering a phone call from a family member of a person that has sustained burns from a fire initiated by lighter fluid squirted into the flames. Which action will the nurse recommend while the patient is waiting for the ambulance?
   a. Be assisted into a bath of cool water while waiting for emergency personnel.
   b. Lie down, be covered with a blanket, and cover legs with petroleum jelly.
   c. Remove the burned pants so that the air can help cool the wound.
   d. Sit in a chair, elevate the legs, and have someone cut the pants off around the burned area.

6. The nurse in the emergency department receives a patient who sustained a severe burn injury. Which is the priority action by the nurse in this situation?

a. Establish a patent airway.

b. Insert an indwelling catheter.

c. Replace fluids.

d. Administer pain medication.

7. The nurse is administering fluid resuscitation using the Parkland formula for a 80 kg male with a 30% BSA burn. The patient should receive _____ mL in the first 8 hours.

8. The nurse is monitoring for fluid and electrolyte changes in the emergent phase of burn injury for a patient. Which will be an expected outcome? (Select all that apply.)

a. Base-bicarbonate deficit

b. Elevated hematocrit level

c. Potassium deficit

d. Sodium deficit

e. Magnesium deficit

9. The nurse is assessing a patient for signs of potassium shifting during the acute phase of burn injury. During which time frame should the nurse assess for signs of potassium shifting?

a. Within 24 hours

b. Between 24 and 48 hours

c. At the beginning of the third day

d. Beginning on day 4 or day 5

10. The nurse is planning the care of a patient with a major burn. Which outcome will be optimal during fluid replacement?

a. A urinary output of 10 mL/hr

b. A urinary output of 30 mL/hr

c. A urinary output of 80 mL/hr

d. A urinary output of 100 mL/hr

11. The nurse is monitoring a patient during the fluid remobilization phase of a burn injury. Which expected findings should the nurse monitor for? (Select all that apply.)

a. Hemodilution

b. Increased urinary output

c. Metabolic alkalosis

d. Sodium deficit

e. Hypoglycemia

12. The nurse is providing wound care for a patient with burns to the lower extremities. Which topical antibacterial agent carries a side effect of leukopenia that the nurse will monitor for within 48 hours after application?

a. Cerium nitrate solution

b. Gentamicin sulfate

c. Silver sulfadiazine

d. Mafenide

13. The nurse is providing burn care for a patient who has developed eschar over the burn site. Which topical antibacterial agent will the nurse recommend for use?

a. Acticoat

b. Mafenide acetate

c. Silver nitrate 0.5%

d. Silver sulfadiazine 1%

14. The nurse is applying an occlusive dressing to a burned foot. Which position will the foot be placed in after application of the dressing?

a. Adduction

b. Dorsiflexion

c. External rotation

d. Plantar flexion

15. The nurse is caring for a patient that is to receive biologic dressings from a cadaver. Which type of graft will the patient be educated about?

a. Autografts

b. Heterografts

c. Homografts

d. Xenografts

16. The nurse is administering an analgesic to a patient with major burns. Which is the recommended route for administration for this patient?

a. Intramuscular

b. Intravenous

c. Oral

d. Subcutaneous

17. To meet early nutritional demands for protein, a 198-lb (90-kg) burned patient will need to ingest a minimum of how much protein every 24 hours?

a. 90 g/day

b. 110 g/day

c. 180 g/day

d. 270 g/day

Sensory Function

CHAPTER 58

Assessment and Management of Patients with Eye and Vision Disorders

Learning Outcomes

1. Identify the major internal and external structures and function of the eye.
2. Specify assessment and diagnostic findings used in the evaluation of ocular disorders.
3. Describe assessment and management strategies for patients with low vision and blindness.
4. List the pharmacologic actions and nursing management of common ophthalmic medications.
5. Recognize the clinical features, assessment and diagnostic findings, as well as the medical or surgical management, and nursing management of the patient with glaucoma, cataracts, and other ocular disorders.

SECTION I: ASSESSING YOUR UNDERSTANDING

Activity A *Fill in the blanks.*

1. Normal intraocular pressure is _____.

2. The most common color vision test is performed using _____.

3. Two significant changes in the optic nerve that occur in patients with glaucoma are _____ and _____.

4. The most common laser surgeries for glaucoma are _____ and _____.

5. _____ is used to measure nerve fiber layer thickness and is an important indicator of glaucoma progression.

6. An initial treatment for a splash injury to the eye would be _____.

7. _____, _____, and _____ are the three organisms that most commonly cause bacterial conjunctivitis.

8. A characteristic sign of viral conjunctivitis is _____.

9. One of the most serious ocular consequences of diabetes is _____.

10. The most common cause of retinal inflammation in patients with acquired immune deficiency syndrome (AIDS) is _____.

11. _____, _____, and _____ are the three layers of a healthy tear.

12. The nurse is assessing a patient with a drooping eyelid and documents this as _____.

Activity B *Briefly answer the following.*

1. Describe how the nurse would assess a patient's visual acuity.

_____

_____

2. What should the nurse educate the patient about when performing tonometry?

_____

_____

3. When is the Amsler grid test used?

_____

_____

Activity C

PART I

Match the characteristic or function of the eye listed in Column II with its associated structure listed in Column I.

Column I

____ **1.** Choroid

____ **2.** Lens

____ **3.** Pupil

____ **4.** Retina

____ **5.** Vitreous humor

____ **6.** Cornea

____ **7.** Sclera

____ **8.** Iris

____ **9.** Uvea

____ **10.** Limbus

Column II

a. Maintains the form of the eyeball

b. Area where most of the blood vessels for the eye are located

c. Degree of convexity modified by contraction and relaxation of the ciliary muscles

d. Contractile membrane between the cornea and lens

e. Transparent part of the fibrous coat of the eyeball

f. Accommodates to the intensity of light by dilating or contracting

g. White part of the eye

h. The pigmented, vascular coating of the eye

i. The edge of the cornea where it joins the sclera

j. Contains nerve endings that transmit visual impulses to the brain

PART II

Match the term listed in Column II with its associated definition listed in Column I.

Column I

____ **1.** Excessive production of tears

____ **2.** Another term for an external hordeolum

____ **3.** Term for the right eye

____ **4.** A term used to describe an inflammatory condition of the uveal tract

____ **5.** Another term for nearsightedness

____ **6.** An inflammatory condition affecting the iris

____ **7.** Inflammation of the cornea

____ **8.** A loss of cornea substance or tissue as a result of inflammation

____ **9.** Abnormal sensitivity to light

____ **10.** Term for the left eye

____ **11.** Absence of the lens

____ **12.** Uneven curvature of the cornea

____ **13.** Drooping of the upper eyelid

____ **14.** A tear in the eye tissue

____ **15.** A condition in which one eye deviates from the object at which the person is looking

Column II

a. Iritis

b. Keratitis

c. Photophobia

d. Aphakia

e. Oculus dexter

f. Ptosis

g. Epiphora

h. Strabismus

i. Laceration

j. Ulcer

k. Oculus sinister

l. Uveitis

m. Astigmatism

n. Sty

o. Myopia

SECTION II: APPLYING YOUR KNOWLEDGE

Activity D *Consider the scenario and answer the questions.*

CASE STUDY: Cataract Surgery

Marcella Daniel is a 75-year-old with progressive diminished vision and increased difficulty with night driving. Her health care provider suspects that Mrs. Daniel has a cataract and does a complete eye examination and history.

1. During the health history, the nurse collects data that would indicate whether she has any common factors that contribute to cataract development. What would these factors be?

_____

_____

2. Mrs. Daniel informed the nurse of visual symptoms she has been having. Which symptoms would the nurse recognize as significant for cataracts?

_____

_____

3. It is determined that Mrs. Daniel has cataracts, and she has agreed to have surgery to remove them. When the nurse is providing postoperative education, what is important for the nurse to tell her about side-lying?

_____

_____

SECTION III: PRACTICING FOR NCLEX

Activity E *Answer the following questions.*

1. An older adult patient informs the nurse, "I don't see as well as I used to." What will the nurse educate the patient about regarding why vision becomes less efficient with age? (Select all that apply.)
   a. There is a decrease in pupil size.
   b. There is slowing of accommodation.
   c. There is an increase in lens opaqueness.
   d. Most older patients develop glaucoma.
   e. The optic nerve begins to degenerate.

2. During a routine eye examination, a patient reports being unable to read road signs at a distance when driving the car. Which will the patient be assessed for?
   a. Astigmatism
   b. Anisometropia
   c. Myopia
   d. Presbyopia

3. It is determined that a patient is legally blind and will be unable to drive any longer. Legal blindness refers to a best corrected visual acuity (BCVA) that does not exceed what reading in the better eye?
   a. 20/50
   b. 20/100
   c. 20/150
   d. 20/200

4. A patient is suspected of having glaucoma. Which reading of IOP would demonstrate an increase resulting from optic nerve damage?
   a. 0 to 5 mm Hg
   b. 6 to 10 mm Hg
   c. 11 to 20 mm Hg
   d. 21 mm Hg or higher

5. The nurse at the eye clinic is caring for a patient with suspected glaucoma. Which report by the patient would be significant for a diagnosis of glaucoma?
   a. A significant loss of central vision
   b. Diminished acuity
   c. Pain associated with a purulent discharge
   d. The presence of halos around lights

6. The nurse is performing an assessment of the visual fields for a patient with glaucoma. When assessing the visual fields in acute glaucoma, which will the nurse expect to find?
   a. Clear cornea
   b. Constricted pupil
   c. Marked blurring of vision
   d. Watery ocular discharge

7. The nurse is educating a patient with glaucoma about medications. Which medications will the nurse educate the patient about that decrease aqueous production? (Select all that apply.)
   a. Alpha-adrenergic agonists
   b. Carbonic anhydrase inhibitors
   c. Beta-blockers
   d. Miotics
   e. Calcium channel blockers

8. A patient has had cataract extractions and the nurse is providing discharge instructions. Which will the nurse encourage the patient to do at home after discharge?
   a. Maintain bed rest for 1 week.
   b. Lie on the stomach while sleeping.
   c. Avoid bending the head below the waist.
   d. Lift weights to increase muscle strength.

9. A patient is being seen in the ophthalmology clinic for a suspected detached retina. Which clinical manifestations does the nurse identify as significant for a retinal detachment? (Select all that apply.)
   a. A visual field of floating particles
   b. A definite area of blank vision
   c. Momentary flashes of light
   d. Pain
   e. Halos around the eyes

10. An older adult patient has noticed a significant amount of vision loss in the last few years. Which does the nurse recognize as the most common cause of visual loss in older adults?
    a. Macular degeneration
    b. Ocular trauma
    c. Retinal vascular disease
    d. Uveitis

11. A patient is brought into the emergency department with chemical burns to both eyes. Which is the priority action of the nurse for this patient's care?
    a. Administering local anesthetics and anti-bacterial drops for 24 to 36 hours
    b. Applying hot compresses at 15-minute intervals
    c. Flushing the lids, conjunctiva, and cornea with tap water or normal saline
    d. Cleansing the conjunctiva with a small cotton-tipped applicator

12. A patient comes to the clinic with a suspected eye infection. The nurse identifies that the patient most likely has conjunctivitis, as evidenced by which symptom?
    a. Blurred vision
    b. Elevated IOP
    c. A mucopurulent ocular discharge
    d. Severe pain

13. Which type of medication will the nurse use in combination with mydriatics to dilate the patient's pupil?
    a. Anti-infectives
    b. Corticosteroids
    c. Cycloplegics
    d. NSAIDs

14. A patient is to have an angiography done using fluorescein as a contrast agent to determine if the patient has macular edema. Which laboratory studies will the nurse monitor prior to the angiography?
    a. BUN and creatinine
    b. AST and ALT
    c. Hemoglobin and hematocrit
    d. Platelet count

15. The nurse is administering an ophthalmic ointment to a patient with conjunctivitis. Which disadvantage of the application of an ointment does the nurse explain to the patient?
    a. It does not work as rapidly as eye drops do.
    b. Blurred vision results after application.
    c. It has a lower concentration than eye drops.
    d. It has more side effects than eye drops.

CHAPTER 59

Assessment and Management of Patients with Hearing and Balance Disorders

Learning Outcomes

1. Describe the anatomy and physiology of the ear as well as the methods used to assess hearing and balance disorders.
2. List the manifestations that may be exhibited by a person with hearing and balance disorders.
3. Identify ways to communicate effectively with a person with a hearing disorder, incorporating the differences between Deaf culture and deafness.
4. Differentiate disorders of the external ear from those of the middle ear and inner ear.
5. Compare the various types of surgical procedures used for managing middle ear disorders and appropriate nursing care.
6. Use the nursing process as a framework for care of the patient undergoing mastoid surgery or of the patient with vertigo.
7. Recognize the different types of inner ear disorders, including the clinical manifestations, diagnosis, and management.

SECTION I: ASSESSING YOUR UNDERSTANDING

Activity A *Fill in the blanks.*

1. The organ of hearing is known as the _____.

2. Mechanical vibrations are transformed into neural activity so that sounds can be differentiated by the _____.

3. A sensorineural (perceptive) hearing loss results from impairment of the _____ cranial nerve.

4. The critical level of loudness that most people (without a hearing loss) are comfortable with is a decibel (dB) reading of _____ dB.

5. Severe hearing loss is associated with a decibel loss in the range of _____ to _____ dB.

6. A hearing loss that is a manifestation of an emotional disturbance is known as _____ hearing loss.

7. The minimum noise level known to cause noise-induced hearing loss, regardless of duration, is _____ to _____ dB.

8. It is projected that by 2050, _____% of people over age 55 will have some form of hearing loss.

9. A facial nerve neuroma is a tumor on the _____ nerve.

10. An acoustic neuroma is a benign tumor of the _____ nerve.

Activity B *Briefly answer the following.*

1. Describe how sound is conducted and transmitted.

_____

_____

_____

_____

2. What three tests are used to evaluate gross auditory acuity?

_____

_____

_____

3. When assessing hearing and balance, what will be included?

_____

_____

_____

4. Name the three characteristics that are essential when evaluating hearing.

_____

_____

_____

5. A patient is having a tympanogram. What is the significance of this test?

_____

_____

_____

Activity C *Match the term in Column I with the definition in Column II.*

Column I

____ 1. Dizziness

____ 2. Vertigo

____ 3. Exostoses

____ 4. Nystagmus

____ 5. Otalgia

____ 6. Otorrhea

____ 7. Otosclerosis

____ 8. Presbycusis

____ 9. Rhinorrhea

____ 10. Tinnitus

Column II

a. Illusion of movement in which the person or the surroundings are sensed as moving

b. Progressive hearing loss associated with aging

c. Sensation of fullness or pain in the ear

d. Drainage from the nose

e. Subjective perception of sound with internal origin; unwanted noises in the head or ear

f. A condition characterized by abnormal spongy bone formation around the stapes

g. Involuntary rhythmic eye movement

h. Altered sensation of orientation in space

i. Small, hard, bony protrusions in the lower posterior bony portion of the ear canal

j. Drainage from the ear

SECTION II: APPLYING YOUR KNOWLEDGE

Activity D *Consider the scenarios and answer the questions.*

CASE STUDY: Mastoid Surgery

Mrs. Amber is a 73-year-old scheduled for mastoid surgery to remove a cholesteatoma, a cystlike sac filled with keratin debris, which was large enough to occlude the ear canal.

1. The patient is informed that she will have a mastoid pressure dressing in place after surgery. When will the nurse inform her that the dressing will be removed?

_____

_____

_____

2. Although infrequent, what type of nerve damage will the nurse assess for and immediately report to the health care provider?

_____

_____

_____

3. What will the nurse inform the patient are indicators of an infection and are to be reported immediately to the health care provider?

_____

_____

_____

CASE STUDY: Ménière's Disease

David Wray is a 42-year-old lawyer who travels internationally. He has recently been diagnosed with Ménière's disease.

1. What does the nurse identify are classic symptoms that are diagnostic for Ménière's disease?

_____

_____

_____

2. The nurse is educating the patient with Ménière's disease about a dietary regimen. Which foods will the nurse include for the patient to avoid or limit?

_____

_____

_____

3. The nurse cautions Mr. Wray about taking certain medications that will increase the dizziness or tinnitus. Which medications will the nurse inform the patient should be avoided?

_____

_____

_____

SECTION III: PRACTICING FOR NCLEX

Activity E *Answer the following questions.*

1. The nurse is performing an assessment of a patient's ears. Which appearance of the tympanic membrane does the nurse document as normal?

   a. Pearly gray and translucent

   b. White and cloudy

   c. Pink with white exudate

   d. Dark yellow with cerumen

2. The nurse is assessing the auricles of a patient. When the left auricle is manipulated, the patient reports pain. Which is the significance of this finding?

   a. The patient may have seborrheic dermatitis.

   b. The patient may have an inner ear infection.

   c. The patient may have acute external otitis.

   d. The patient may have acute otitis media.

3. The nurse is examining the area behind the patient's auricle and sees a flaky scaliness. Which disorder does the nurse suspect the patient has?

   a. Sebaceous cysts

   b. Seborrheic dermatitis

   c. Tophi

   d. Acute external otitis

4. A nursing student is learning how to adequately use an otoscope to examine the ear. Which method should the instructor educate the student to use when examining with an otoscope?

   a. Otoscope should be held in the examiner's left hand, in a pencil-hold position, with the examiner's hand braced against the patient's face.

   b. Otoscope should be held in the examiner's left hand, with a full hand grasp to be able to guide the scope into the internal ear.

   c. Otoscope should be held in the examiner's right hand, with a full hand grasp to be able to guide the scope into the internal ear.

   d. Otoscope should be held in the examiner's right or left hand, with a full hand grasp to be able to guide the scope into the internal ear.

5. A patient comes to the clinic with some hearing loss. The health care provider is unable to observe the tympanic membrane due to the accumulation of cerumen. Which intervention will the nurse provide so that observation can be made?

   a. The nurse can remove the wax with a cerumen curette.

   b. The ear can be irrigated with cool water until all of the wax is removed.

   c. The nurse can instill a small amount of mineral oil into the canal and have the patient return for removal of the wax.

   d. The nurse can instill mineral oil into the canal and immediately irrigate to remove the adherent wax.

6. A patient is scheduled to have an auditory brain stem response in 2 days. What does the nurse instruct the patient to do in preparation for the test?

   a. Shave several areas on the scalp where the electrodes will be placed.

   b. Do not eat or drink 8 hours prior to testing.

   c. Wash and rinse hair before test but do not apply any other hair products.

   d. Omit daily medications prior to testing.

7. A patient with vertigo is scheduled to have an electronystagmography in 2 weeks. Which instructions will the nurse provide to the patient prior to the test?

   a. Withhold caffeine and alcohol 48 hours before the test.

   b. Withhold blood pressure medication 24 hours before the test.

   c. Withhold vestibular suppressants 48 hours before the test.

   d. Do not eat or drink anything 12 hours before testing.

8. A patient has been diagnosed with a fungal infection causing external otitis. Which is the most common fungal infection in the ear?

   a. *Staphylococcus aureus*

   b. *Aspergillus*

   c. *Pseudomonas*

   d. *Streptococcus*

9. A patient has been treated for external otitis for the second time during the summer months. Which education will be provided for the patient to reduce the risk of developing this problem? (Select all that apply.)

   a. Do not clean the external canal with cotton-tipped applicators.

   b. Irrigate the ears daily with a warm saline solution.

   c. Avoid getting the ear wet when swimming or showering.

   d. Use an antiseptic otic preparation after swimming, unless there is a history of tympanic membrane perforation.

   e. Ensure that cerumen is absent from the external canal by irrigating once a week after instilling mineral oil.

10. A patient has serous otitis media with significant hearing loss in the right ear. The patient states, "I have not been able to hear for 2 months." Which procedure does the nurse prepare the patient for?

    a. Irrigation of the ear

    b. Myringotomy

    c. Removal of cerumen with a cerumen curette

    d. Instillation of otic solution

11. The nurse is talking with a patient diagnosed with Ménière's disease about the patient's symptoms. Which symptom does the patient inform the nurse is the most problematic?

    a. Nausea

    b. Diarrhea

    c. Tinnitus

    d. Vertigo

12. The nurse is caring for a patient with Ménière's disease who is hospitalized with severe vertigo. Which medication will the nurse administer to shorten the attack?

    a. Meclizine

    b. Furosemide

    c. Cortisporin otic solution

    d. Gentamicin intravenously

13. A patient reports ringing in the left ear and hearing loss in the same ear, but does not have any associated dizziness or vertigo. Which condition will the patient be assessed for?

  a. Otitis media

  b. Acoustic neuroma

  c. Labyrinthitis

  d. Tinnitus

14. The nurse is talking to a family member of a hearing-impaired patient and the patient states, "I know you are talking about me. You are just whispering so that I will not hear what you are saying." Which is the significance of the statement made by the patient?

  a. False pride

  b. Indecision

  c. Insecurity

  d. Suspiciousness

15. The nurse is developing a plan of care for a patient with severe vertigo. Which expected outcome statement would be a priority for this patient?

  a. Patient will experience no falls due to balance disorder.

  b. Patient will take medications as prescribed.

  c. Patient will perform exercises as prescribed.

  d. Patient will have decreased fear and anxiety.

Neurologic Function

CHAPTER 60

Assessment of Neurologic Function

Learning Outcomes

1. Describe the structures and functions of the central and peripheral nervous systems.
2. Differentiate between pathologic changes that affect motor control and those that affect sensory pathways.
3. Compare and contrast the functioning of the sympathetic and parasympathetic nervous systems.
4. Explain the significance of physical assessment to the diagnosis of neurologic dysfunction.
5. Discuss diagnostic tests used for assessment of suspected neurologic disorders and the related nursing implications.

SECTION I: ASSESSING YOUR UNDERSTANDING

Activity A *Fill in the blanks.*

1. _____ is a neurotransmitter that helps control mood and sleep.

2. Parkinson's disease is caused by an imbalance in the neurotransmitter known as

   _____.

3. A person's personality and judgment are controlled by the area of the brain known as the _____ lobe.

4. The lobe of the cerebral cortex that is responsible for the understanding of language and music is the _____ lobe.

5. Voluntary muscle control is governed by a vertical band of "motor cortex" located in the _____ lobe.

6. The sleep–wake cycle regulator and the site of the hunger center is known as the _____.

7. The "master gland" is also known as the _____ gland.

8. The major receiving and communication center for afferent sensory nerves is the

   _____.

9. The normal adult produces about _____ mL of cerebrospinal fluid daily from the ventricles.

10. The preganglionic fibers of the sympathetic neurons are located in the segments of the spinal cord identified as _____ to _____.

11. The parasympathetic division of the autonomic nervous system yields impulses that are mediated by the secretion of _____, the dominant neurotransmitter in parasympathetic nervous system functions.

12. The brain center responsible for balancing and coordination is the _____.

Activity B *Briefly answer the following.*

1. What is the function of the blood–brain barrier?

_____

_____

2. Describe the role and functions of the autonomic nervous system.

_____

_____

_____

3. Name the principal signs of lower motor neuron disease.

_____

_____

4. What clinical manifestations occur when there is destruction or dysfunction in the basal ganglia?

_____

_____

Activity C

Neurotransmitters and Nervous System Response

Match the nervous system response listed in Column II with the neurotransmitter listed in Column I.

Column I

____ 1. Gamma-aminobutyric acid

____ 2. Enkephalin

____ 3. Norepinephrine

____ 4. Dopamine

____ 5. Acetylcholine

____ 6. Serotonin

Column II

a. Primarily excitatory; can produce vagal stimulation of heart

b. Inhibits pain pathways and can control sleep

c. Affects behavior, attention, and fine movement

d. Excitatory response, mostly affecting moods

e. Muscle and nerve inhibitory transmissions

f. Excitatory; inhibits pain transmission

Cranial Nerves

Next to each cranial nerve listed by number, write the appropriate corresponding terminology in Column I and a major associated function in Column II. The answers for the first cranial nerve are provided as an example.

Nerve No.	Column I	Column II
I	Olfactory	Smell
II		
III		
IV		
V		
VI		
VII		
VIII		
IX		
X		
XI		
XII		

SECTION II: APPLYING YOUR KNOWLEDGE

Activity D *Consider the scenario and answer the questions.*

CASE STUDY: Mental Status

Grace Bryan, age 82, is brought to the clinic by her son, who informs the nurse that his mother is not "as sharp" as she has been and has been forgetting to take some of her medication. The son asks that his mother be "checked out."

1. Which intervention is provided by the nurse when assisting Mrs. Bryan to change into a gown and to sit on the examining table?

_____

_____

2. After the health care provider examines Mrs. Bryan, laboratory studies and a CT scan of the brain are performed. When providing education to the patient and her son, how will the nurse ensure that the education provided is understood?

_____

_____

_____

_____

3. How would the nurse differentiate delirium from dementia in assessing Mrs. Bryan?

_____

_____

_____

_____

SECTION III: PRACTICING FOR NCLEX

Activity E *Answer the following questions.*

1. A patient arrives to have an MRI done in the outpatient department. Which information provided by the patient warrants further assessment to prevent complications related to the MRI?

   a. "I am trying to quit smoking and have a patch on."

   b. "I have been trying to get an appointment for so long."

   c. "I have not had anything to eat or drink for 3 hours."

   d. "My legs go numb sometimes when I sit too long."

2. A patient is scheduled for an electroencephalogram (EEG) in the morning. Which food on the patient's tray should the nurse remove prior to the test?

   a. Orange juice

   b. Toast

   c. Coffee

   d. Eggs

3. The nurse is assisting with a lumbar puncture and observes that when the health care provider obtains cerebrospinal fluid (CSF), it is clear and colorless. What is the significance of this finding?

   a. A subarachnoid hemorrhage

   b. Severe sepsis

   c. A normal finding; the fluid will be sent for testing to determine other factors

   d. Local trauma from the insertion of the needle

4. A patient had a lumbar puncture 3 days ago in the outpatient clinic and calls the nurse reporting a throbbing headache. Which education will the nurse provide to the patient regarding relief of the discomfort? (Select all that apply.)

   a. Limit the amount of fluid to decrease cerebral edema.

   b. Force fluids (unless contraindicated).

   c. Get plenty of bed rest.

   d. Take some over-the-counter analgesics.

   e. Walk around.

5. A patient is having a lumbar puncture and the health care provider has removed 20 mL of cerebrospinal fluid (CSF). Which nursing action is a priority after the procedure?

   a. Encourage the patient to ambulate immediately.

   b. Have the patient lie flat for 6 hours.

   c. Have the patient lie flat for 1 hour and then sit for 1 hour before ambulating.

   d. Have the patient lie in a semi-Fowler position with the head of the bed at 30 degrees.

6. The nurse is performing an assessment of cranial nerve function and asks the patient to cover one nostril at a time to see if the patient can smell coffee, alcohol, and mint. The patient is unable to smell any of the odors. Which cranial nerve does the nurse identify is not functioning as it should?

   a. CN I

   b. CN II

   c. CN III

   d. CN IV

7. The nurse obtains a Snellen eye chart when assessing cranial nerve function. Which cranial nerve is the nurse testing when using the chart?
   a. CN I
   b. CN II
   c. CN III
   d. CN IV

8. A patient is being tested for a gag reflex. When the nurse places the tongue blade to the back of the throat, there is no response elicited. Which dysfunction does the nurse identify the patient is experiencing?
   a. Dysfunction of the spinal accessory nerve
   b. Dysfunction of the acoustic nerve
   c. Dysfunction of the facial nerve
   d. Dysfunction of the vagus nerve

9. A patient sustained a head injury during a fall and has changes in personality and affect. Which part of the brain does the nurse identify has been affected in this injury?
   a. Frontal lobe
   b. Parietal lobe
   c. Occipital lobe
   d. Temporal lobe

10. A patient who has suffered a stroke is unable to maintain respiration and is intubated and placed on mechanical ventilator support. Which portion of the brain is most likely responsible for the inability to breathe?
    a. Frontal lobe
    b. Occipital lobe
    c. Parietal lobe
    d. Brain stem

11. A patient has expressive speaking aphasia after having a stroke. Which portion of the brain does the nurse identify has been affected?
    a. Temporal lobe
    b. Inferior posterior frontal areas
    c. Posterior frontal area
    d. Parietal–occipital area

12. The nurse is assessing the pupils of a patient who has had a head injury. Which parasympathetic effect does the nurse identify the patient is experiencing?
    a. Dilated pupils
    b. Constricted pupils
    c. One pupil is dilated and the opposite pupil is normal
    d. Roth spots

13. The nurse is caring for a patient who was involved in a motor vehicle injury and sustained a head injury. When assessing deep tendon reflexes (DTR), the nurse observes diminished or hypoactive reflexes. How will the nurse document this finding?
    a. 0
    b. 1+
    c. 2+
    d. 3+

14. The nurse is performing a neurologic assessment and requests that the patient stand with eyes open and then closed for 20 seconds to assess balance. Which type of test is the nurse performing?
    a. Weber test
    b. Rinne test
    c. Romberg test
    d. Watch-tick test

15. A patient comes to the emergency department with severe pain in the face that was stimulated by brushing the teeth. The nurse identifies which cranial nerve dysfunction is causing this pain?
    a. III
    b. IV
    c. V
    d. VI

Management of Patients with Neurologic Dysfunction

Learning Outcomes

1. Describe the causes, clinical manifestations, and medical management of various neurologic dysfunctions.
2. Use the nursing process as a framework for care of the patient with altered level of consciousness.
3. Identify the early and late clinical manifestations of increased intracranial pressure and apply the nursing process as a framework for are of the patient with increased intracranial pressure.
4. Compare and contrast the indications for intracranial or transsphenoidal surgery and use the nursing process as a framework for care of the patient undergoing intracranial or transsphenoidal surgery.
5. Explain the various types and causes of seizures and develop a plan of care for the patient experiencing seizures.
6. Recognize the causes, clinical manifestations, and medical and nursing management of the patient experiencing various types of headaches.

SECTION I: ASSESSING YOUR UNDERSTANDING

Activity A *Fill in the blanks.*

1. A patient has a lesion affecting the pons, resulting in paralysis and the inability to speak, but has vertical eye movements and lid elevation. This patient is suffering from _____.

2. Three major potential complications in a patient with a depressed level of consciousness (LOC) are _____, _____, and _____.

3. The earliest sign of increased ICP is _____ _____.

4. Three primary complications of increased ICP are _____, _____, and _____.

5. The primary, lethal complication of ICP is _____.

6. Nursing postoperative management includes detecting and reducing _____, relieving _____, preventing _____, and monitoring _____ and _____.

7. The leading cause of seizures in the older adult is _____.

8. A major potential complication of epilepsy is _____.

Activity B *Briefly answer the following.*

1. What is meant by an altered level of consciousness (LOC)?

_____

_____

_____

_____

2. List five potential collaborative problems for a patient with an altered LOC.

_____

_____

_____

3. When the nurse performs a neurologic examination, what will be included?

_____

_____

_____

_____

4. If a patient with an altered LOC requires suctioning, which intervention is a priority for the nurse to provide?

_____

_____

5. Which is the optimal way to determine the level of a patient's alertness?

_____

_____

_____

_____

Activity C *Match the neurologic dysfunction in Column II with its associated nursing intervention found in Column I. Some answers may be used more than once.*

Column I

____ 1. Assist with daily active or passive range of motion

____ 2. Elevate the head of the bed to 30 degrees

____ 3. Institute a bowel-training program

____ 4. Maintain dorsiflexion to affected area

____ 5. Place the patient in a lateral position

Column II

a. Footdrop

b. Incontinence

c. Impaired cough reflex

d. Keratitis

e. Paralyzed diaphragm

f. Paralyzed extremity

SECTION II: APPLYING YOUR KNOWLEDGE

Activity D *Consider the scenario and answer the questions.*

CASE STUDY: Optimizing Cerebral Perfusion Pressure

Alex Long, age 32, was riding his motorcycle without a helmet through the woods and hit a large log, ejecting him over the handlebars and into a tree. He was unconscious when his friends found him and called the rescue squad. He has had a craniotomy to relieve an epidural hematoma and is in the neurologic intensive care unit (ICU).

1. In order to optimize cerebral perfusion pressure (CPP) and decrease intracranial pressure (ICP), which position will the nurse maintain for Mr. Long?

_____

_____

_____

_____

2. Which action by the nurse can assist with avoiding Mr. Long performing the Valsalva maneuver?

_____

_____

_____

_____

3. When the nurse plans Mr. Long's care, how can his needs be met in order to prevent a rise in ICP and a decrease in CPP?

_____

_____

SECTION III: PRACTICING FOR NCLEX

Activity E *Answer the following questions.*

1. The nurse is caring for a patient with an altered level of consciousness (LOC). Which is the first priority of treatment for this patient?
   a. Assessment of pupillary light reflexes
   b. Determination of the cause
   c. Positioning to prevent complications
   d. Maintenance of a patent airway

2. A nurse assesses the patient's LOC using the Glasgow Coma Scale. Which score indicates severe impairment of neurologic function?
   a. 3
   b. 6
   c. 9
   d. 12

3. A patient has a severe neurologic impairment from a head trauma. Which does the nurse recognize is the type of posturing that occurs with the most severe neurologic impairment?
   a. Decerebrate
   b. Decorticate
   c. Flaccid
   d. Rigid

4. The nurse is caring for a patient in the neurologic ICU who sustained head trauma in a physical altercation. Which optimal range does the nurse identify for this patient?
   a. 8 to 15 mm Hg
   b. 0 to 10 mm Hg
   c. 20 to 30 mm Hg
   d. 25 to 40 mm Hg

5. A patient is admitted to the hospital with an ICP reading of 20 mm Hg and a mean arterial pressure of 90 mm Hg. Which is the calculated cerebral perfusion pressure?
   a. 50 mm Hg
   b. 60 mm Hg
   c. 70 mm Hg
   d. 80 mm Hg

6. A nurse caring for a patient with head trauma will be monitoring the patient for Cushing triad. Which are the identified symptoms associated with Cushing triad that the nurse documents? (Select all that apply.)
   a. Bradycardia
   b. Bradypnea
   c. Hypertension
   d. Tachycardia
   e. Pupillary constriction

7. The nurse is caring for a patient with a traumatic brain injury (TBI). Which does the nurse identify as the earliest sign of serious impairment of brain circulation related to increasing ICP?
   a. A bounding pulse
   b. Bradycardia
   c. Hypertension
   d. Lethargy and stupor

8. The nurse is caring for a patient with increased ICP. As the pressure rises, what osmotic diuretic does the nurse prepare to administer as prescribed?
   a. Glycerin
   b. Isosorbide
   c. Mannitol
   d. Urea

9. A nurse is assessing a patient's urinary output as an indicator of diabetes insipidus related to a traumatic brain injury. The nurse identifies that an hourly output of which volume over 2 hours may be a positive indicator?
   a. 50 to 100 mL/hr
   b. 100 to 150 mL/hr
   c. 150 to 200 mL/hr
   d. More than 200 mL/hr

10. When educating a patient about the use of anticonvulsant medication, what will the nurse inform the patient is a result of long-term use of the medication in women?

a. Anemia

b. Osteoarthritis

c. Osteoporosis

d. Obesity

11. The nurse is called to attend to a patient having a tonic-clonic seizure in the waiting area. Which nursing interventions are provided for this patient? (Select all that apply.)

a. Loosening constrictive clothing

b. Opening the patient's jaw and inserting a mouth gag

c. Positioning the patient on their side with head flexed forward

d. Providing for privacy

e. Restraining the patient to avoid self-injury

12. The nurse is educating a patient with a seizure disorder. Which nutritional approach for seizure management would be beneficial for this patient?

a. Low in fat

b. Restricts protein to 10% of daily caloric intake

c. High in protein and low in carbohydrate

d. At least 50% carbohydrate

13. The nurse is caring for a patient postoperatively after intracranial surgery for the treatment of a subdural hematoma. The nurse observes an increase in the patient's blood pressure from the baseline and a decrease in the heart rate from 86 to 54, and crackles in the bases of the lungs. Which situation does the nurse suspect is occurring?

a. Increased ICP

b. Exacerbation of uncontrolled hypertension

c. Infection

d. Increase in cerebral perfusion pressure

14. A patient 3 days postoperative from a craniotomy informs the nurse, "I feel something trickling down the back of my throat and I taste something salty." Which priority action does the nurse initiate?

a. Give the patient some mouthwash to gargle with.

b. Request an antihistamine for the postnasal drip.

c. Ask the patient to cough to observe the sputum color and consistency.

d. Notify the health care provider of a possible cerebrospinal fluid leak.

15. A patient had a small pituitary adenoma removed by the transsphenoidal approach and has developed diabetes insipidus. Which pharmacologic therapy will the nurse be administering to this patient as prescribed to control symptoms?

a. Mannitol

b. Furosemide (Lasix)

c. Vasopressin

d. Phenobarbital

Management of Patients with Cerebrovascular Disorders

Learning Outcomes

1. Describe the incidence of, risk factors and preventative measures for, and impact of cerebrovascular disorders.
2. Compare the various types of cerebrovascular disorders: their causes, clinical manifestations, and medical management.
3. Explain the principles of nursing management as they relate to the care of a patient in the acute stage of an ischemic stroke.
4. Use the nursing process as a framework for care of the patient recovering from an ischemic stroke or a hemorrhagic stroke.
5. Discuss essential elements for family education and preparation for home care of the patient who has had a stroke.

SECTION I: ASSESSING YOUR UNDERSTANDING

Activity A *Fill in the blanks.*

1. The primary cerebrovascular disorder in the United States is _____, which is also called a(n) _____ to emphasize the urgency of its occurrence.

2. Thrombolytic therapy with recombinant plasminogen activator (rt-PA) for ischemic stroke has significantly decreased post stroke symptoms. However, the treatment challenge is that the therapy has to be given within _____ hours.

3. As a cause of death in the United States, stroke currently ranks _____.

4. The main surgical procedure for managing transient ischemic attacks (TIAs) is
_____.

5. _____ is the most common cause of cerebrovascular disease.

6. The most common motor dysfunction of a stroke is _____.

7. Hemorrhagic strokes are caused by bleeding into _____, _____, or
_____.

8. Potential complications of a hemorrhagic stroke include _____,
_____, _____, or
_____.

9. The most common cause of intracerebral hemorrhage is _____.

10. _____ and _____ are the two categories of stroke.

Activity B *Briefly answer the following.*

1. A patient has a cardioembolic stroke. What is the most common cardiac arrhythmia that is observed on the monitor?

_____

2. Name the most common type of ischemic stroke.

_____

_____

_____

3. The risk of coronary heart disease and stroke has decreased in women on the Dietary Approaches to Stop Hypertension (DASH) diet. What does this dietary regimen consist of?

_____

_____

_____

4. Describe how thrombolytic agents treat ischemic stroke.

_____

_____

_____

Activity C *Match the clinical manifestations of specific neurologic deficits listed in Column II with the associated cause listed in Column I.*

Column I

_____ 1. Ataxia

_____ 2. Receptive aphasia

_____ 3. Dysphagia

_____ 4. Homonymous hemianopsia

_____ 5. Loss of peripheral vision

_____ 6. Expressive aphasia

_____ 7. Diplopia

_____ 8. Paresthesia

Column II

a. Difficulty judging distances

b. Unaware of the borders of objects

c. Double vision

d. Staggering, unsteady gait

e. Difficulty in swallowing

f. Difficulty with proprioception

g. Unable to form words that are understandable

h. Unable to comprehend the spoken word

SECTION II: APPLYING YOUR KNOWLEDGE

Activity D *Consider the scenario and answer the questions.*

Mrs. Lucy Coe, age 51, is brought into the emergency department by her partner. Her partner states, "She began slurring her words about 30 minutes ago, I noticed that her mouth was turned down on the left side." The partner recognized that she was exhibiting signs of a stroke and brought her in immediately for treatment.

1. Mrs. Coe was immediately taken for a CT scan of the brain and it was determined that she suffered an ischemic stroke. The health care provider prescribes t-PA. What will be done prior to initiating therapy?

_____

_____

2. Mrs. Coe weighs 72 kg. How much t-PA will the nurse give in the first minute as a bolus dose?

_____

_____

3. After the nurse gives the t-PA, what common side effect is it important that Mrs. Coe be monitored for?

_____

_____

_____

SECTION III: PRACTICING FOR NCLEX

Activity E *Answer the following questions.*

1. The nurse assesses that a patient is exhibiting symptoms associated with a Transient Ischemic Attack (TIA). After which period of time will the nurse monitor for these symptoms to subside?

   a. 1 hour

   b. 3 to 6 hours

   c. 12 hours

   d. 24 to 36 hours

2. A patient who had a stroke is experiencing memory loss and impaired learning capacity. In which lobe does the nurse determine that brain damage has most likely occurred?

   a. Frontal

   b. Occipital

   c. Parietal

   d. Temporal

3. A patient is brought to the emergency department with symptoms that indicate a possible stroke. Which initial diagnostic test for a stroke, usually performed in the emergency department, will the nurse prepare the patient for?

   a. 12-lead electrocardiogram

   b. Carotid ultrasound study

   c. Noncontrast computed tomography

   d. Transcranial Doppler flow study

4. The emergency department nurse is caring for a patient weighing 110 lb who is having a stroke. When administering recombinant rt-PA, which minimum dose will the patient receive?

   a. 50 mg

   b. 60 mg

   c. 85 mg

   d. 100 mg

5. A patient is exhibiting classic signs of a hemorrhagic stroke. Which report from the patient would be an indicator of this type of stroke?

   a. Numbness of an arm or leg

   b. Double vision

   c. Severe headache

   d. Dizziness and tinnitus

6. The nurse is caring for a patient having a hemorrhagic stroke. In which position in the bed will the nurse maintain this patient?

   a. High Fowler

   b. Prone

   c. Supine

   d. Semi-Fowler

7. A patient has had a large ischemic stroke and is hospitalized in the neurologic intensive care unit. Which interventions will be provided for this patient to decrease intracranial pressure? (Select all that apply.)

   a. Administer mannitol as prescribed.

   b. Maintain the partial pressure of arterial carbon dioxide ($PaCO_2$) within a range of 30 to 35 mm Hg.

   c. Administer heparin to induce anticoagulation.

   d. Administer supplemental oxygen if the oxygen saturation is below 88%.

   e. Elevate the head of the bed to 30 degrees and maintain in neutral position.

8. A patient having an acute stroke with no other significant medical disorders has a blood glucose level of 420 mg/dL. Which significance does the hyperglycemia have for this patient?

   a. The patient has new onset diabetes.

   b. This is significant for poor neurologic outcomes.

   c. The patient has developed diabetes insipidus due to the location of the stroke.

   d. The patient has liver failure.

9. A patient had a carotid endarterectomy yesterday and when the nurse arrives in the room to perform an assessment, the patient states, "All of a sudden, I am having trouble moving my right side." Which is a priority concern the nurse has related to this statement?

   a. A thrombus formation at the site of the endarterectomy

   b. This is a normal occurrence after an endarterectomy and not a concern

   c. Bleeding from the endarterectomy site

   d. Surgical wound infection

10. A patient is in the acute phase of an ischemic stroke. How long does the nurse determine that this phase may last?

    a. Up to 2 weeks

    b. Up to 1 week

    c. 1 to 3 days

    d. Up to 24 hours

11. A patient having an ischemic stroke is admitted to the acute care facility. When will the nurse plan the rehabilitation for this patient?

    a. The day before the patient is discharged

    b. After the patient has passed the acute phase of the stroke

    c. After the nurse has received the discharge orders

    d. The day the patient has the stroke

12. A patient who has had a stroke begins having complications regarding spasticity in the lower extremity. Which prescribed medication will the nurse administer as prescribed to help alleviate this issue?

    a. Diphenhydramine

    b. Lioresal

    c. Heparin

    d. Pregabalin

13. A patient having a stroke is having difficulty forming words. How will the nurse document this finding?

    a. Ataxia

    b. Arthralgia

    c. Dysphagia

    d. Dysarthria

14. After having a stroke, a patient has cognitive deficits. Which cognitive deficits does the nurse identify the patient has as a result of the stroke? (Select all that apply.)

    a. Poor abstract reasoning

    b. Decreased attention span

    c. Short- and long-term memory loss

    d. Expressive aphasia

    e. Paresthesias

15. A patient has had a right hemispheric stroke. Which clinical manifestations does the nurse identify to correlate with this type of stroke?

    a. Left visual field deficit

    b. Aphasia

    c. Slow, cautious behavior

    d. Altered intellectual ability

CHAPTER 63

Management of Patients with Neurologic Trauma

1. Describe the mechanisms of injury, clinical signs and symptoms, diagnostic testing, and treatment options for patients with traumatic brain and spinal cord injury.
2. Use the nursing process as a framework for care of the patient with traumatic brain injury.
3. Identify the population at risk for spinal cord injury and explain the clinical features and management of the patient with neurogenic shock.
4. Discuss the pathophysiology of autonomic dysreflexia and describe the appropriate nursing interventions.
5. Apply the nursing process as a framework for care of the patient with spinal cord injury and the patient with tetraplegia or paraplegia.

SECTION I: ASSESSING YOUR UNDERSTANDING

Activity A *Fill in the blanks.*

1. The cranial vault contains three main components: _____, _____, and _____.

2. According to the _____, the cranial vault is a closed system; and if one of the three components increases in volume, at least one of the other two must decrease in volume, or the pressure will increase.

3. Skull fractures are classified by type and location. Types include _____, _____, and _____ skull fractures, while location fractures include _____, _____, and _____ skull fractures.

4. A _____ is used to diagnose a skull fracture.

5. The most serious brain injury that can develop within the cranial vault is a _____.

6. The four signs of a rapidly expanding, acute subdural hematoma that would require immediate surgical intervention are _____, _____, _____, and _____.

7. The three cardinal signs of brain death are _____, _____, and _____.

8. A _____ after head injury is a temporary loss of neurologic function with no apparent structural damage.

9. The three criteria used to assess level of consciousness (LOC) using the Glasgow Coma Scale (GCS) are _____, _____, and _____.

10. Complications after traumatic head injuries can be classified according to _____, _____, and _____.

11. The five vertebrae most commonly involved in spinal cord injuries (SCIs) are the _____, _____, _____, _____, and _____.

Activity B *Briefly answer the following.*

1. Describe the characteristic clinical manifestations of Brown-Séquard syndrome.

_____

_____

2. Name the four most common causes of traumatic brain injury (TBI).

_____

_____

3. Compare and contrast primary and secondary brain injury.

_____

_____

_____

4. A patient sustains a grade 1 head injury. Describe the clinical manifestations that will be seen with this type of injury.

_____

_____

5. When a patient sustains a head injury and is admitted to the hospital for observation, what will be monitored?

_____

_____

Activity C *Match the segmental sensorimotor function in Column II with the injury level in Column I.*

Column I	Column II
____ **1.** C1	**a.** Full foot, leg, ankle control
____ **2.** C2–C3	**b.** Full elbow extension, wrist plantar flexion
____ **3.** C4	**c.** Requires continuous ventilation
____ **4.** C5	
____ **5.** C6	**d.** Knee flexion and ankle dorsiflexion
____ **6.** C7–C8	**e.** Full head and neck control
____ **7.** T1–T5	**f.** Independent of mechanical ventilation for short periods
____ **8.** T6–T10	**g.** Full hand and finger control
____ **9.** T11–L5	**h.** Good head and neck sensation and motor control
____ **10.** S1–S5	**i.** Fully innervated shoulder
	j. Abdominal muscle control, good balance

SECTION II: APPLYING YOUR KNOWLEDGE

Activity D *Consider the scenario and answer the questions.*

CASE STUDY: Spinal Cord Injury

Mr. Bill Mars, a 38-year-old man who was drinking heavily at a party, got into his car and drove home against the advice of friends. While driving, he crossed the opposite lane, swerved to get back into his lane, and hit a street sign. He was ejected from the vehicle and a passing motorist who witnessed the event called 911. After stabilization at the scene and transport to the emergency department, it was determined that Bill sustained a complete C6 fracture as well as a fractured left femur. He has been in the hospital for 3 weeks.

1. Mr. Mars states to the nurse, "I will never be able to do anything for myself anymore. I will have to live in a nursing home where someone will take care of me." What level of independence can the nurse expect that he will have after rehabilitation?

_____

2. When the nurse educates Mr. Mars about prevention of complications after going home, what does the nurse include?

_____

_____

_____

3. Which dietary information should Mr. Mars be educated about in order to maintain a healthy lifestyle and prevent complications?

_____

_____

_____

SECTION III: PRACTICING FOR NCLEX

Activity E *Answer the following questions.*

1. A patient sustained a head trauma in a diving injury and has a cerebral hemorrhage located within the brain. Which type of hematoma is this classified as?
   a. An epidural hematoma
   b. An extradural hematoma
   c. An intracerebral hematoma
   d. A subdural hematoma

2. A patient comes to the emergency department with a large scalp laceration after being struck in the head with a glass bottle. After assessment of the patient, which will the nurse do before the health care provider sutures the wound?
   a. Irrigate the wound to remove debris.
   b. Give an oral analgesic for pain.
   c. Give acetaminophen for headache.
   d. Shave the hair around the wound.

3. The nurse in the emergency department is caring for a patient brought in by the rescue squad after falling from a second-story window. The nurse assesses ecchymosis over the mastoid and clear fluid from the ears. Which type of skull fracture is this indicative of?
   a. Occipital skull fracture
   b. Temporal skull fracture
   c. Frontal skull fracture
   d. Basilar skull fracture

4. While riding a bicycle in a race, a patient fell into a ditch and sustained a head injury. Another cyclist found the patient lying unconscious in the ditch and called 911. Which type of concussion does the patient most likely have?
   a. Grade 1 concussion
   b. Grade 2 concussion
   c. Grade 3 concussion
   d. Grade 4 concussion

5. While stopped at a stop sign, a patient's car was struck from behind by another vehicle. The patient sustained a cerebral contusion and was admitted to the hospital. During which time period after the injury will the effects of injury peak?
   a. 6 to 8 hours
   b. 18 to 36 hours
   c. 12 to 24 hours
   d. 48 to 72 hours

6. A patient brought to the hospital after a skiing injury was unconscious for a brief period of time at the scene, then woke up disoriented and refused to go to the hospital for treatment. The patient became very agitated and restless, then quickly lost consciousness again. Which type of Traumatic Brain Injury (TBI) is suspected in this situation?
   a. Epidural hematoma
   b. Acute subdural hematoma
   c. Chronic subdural hematoma
   d. Grade 1 concussion

7. The nurse is caring for a patient in the emergency department with a diagnosed epidural hematoma. Which procedure will the nurse prepare the patient for?
   a. Hypophysectomy
   b. Application of halo traction
   c. Burr holes
   d. Insertion of Crutchfield tongs

8. A patient sustained a head injury and has been admitted to the neurosurgical intensive care unit (ICU). The patient began having seizures and was given a sedative–hypnotic medication that is ultra-short acting and can be titrated to patient response. What medication will the nurse be administering to control the seizures?
   a. Lorazepam
   b. Midazolam
   c. Phenobarbital
   d. Propofol

9. The nurse is planning the care of a patient with a Traumatic Brain Injury (TBI) in the neurosurgical ICU. In developing the plan of care, which interventions will be a priority? (Select all that apply.)

a. Making nursing assessments

b. Setting priorities for nursing interventions

c. Anticipating needs and complications

d. Initiating rehabilitation

e. Ensuring that the patient regains full brain function

10. The nurse is planning to provide education about prevention in the community YMCA due to the increase in number of spinal cord injuries (SCIs). Which predominant risk factors does the nurse address? (Select all that apply.)

a. Young age

b. Male gender

c. Older adult

d. Substance abuse

e. Low-income community

11. The nurse is caring for a patient with a spinal cord injury (SCI). What is the benefit of giving oxygen to maintain a high partial pressure of arterial oxygen (PaO_2)?

a. So that the patient will not have a respiratory arrest

b. Because hypoxemia can create or worsen a neurologic deficit of the spinal cord

c. To increase cerebral perfusion pressure

d. To prevent secondary brain injury

12. A patient was body surfing in the ocean and sustained a cervical spinal cord fracture. A halo traction device was applied. How will the patient benefit from the application of the halo device?

a. It is the only device that can be applied for stabilization of a spinal fracture.

b. It allows for stabilization of the cervical spine along with early ambulation.

c. It is less bulky and traumatizing for the patient to use.

d. The patient can remove it as needed.

13. A patient with a C7 spinal cord fracture informs the nurse, "My head is killing me!" The nurse assesses a blood pressure of 210/140 mm Hg, heart rate of 48, and observes diaphoresis on the face. Which is the first action by the nurse?

a. Place the patient in a sitting position.

b. Call the health care provider.

c. Assess the patient for a full bladder.

d. Assess the patient for a fecal impaction.

14. A patient has developed autonomic dysreflexia and all measures to identify a trigger have been unsuccessful. Which medication will the nurse administer as prescribed by the health care provider to decrease the blood pressure?

a. Nifedipine sublingual

b. Furosemide IV given rapidly

c. Hydralazine hydrochloride IV given slowly

d. Bumex rapid bolus IV

15. A patient has an S5 spinal fracture from a fall. Which type of assistive device will this patient require?

a. Voice or sip-and-puff controlled electric wheelchair

b. Electric or modified manual wheelchair, needs transfer assistance

c. Cane

d. The patient will be able to ambulate independently

Management of Patients with Neurologic Infections, Autoimmune Disorders, and Neuropathies

Learning Outcomes

1. Differentiate among the infectious disorders of the nervous system according to causes, manifestations, medical care, and nursing management.
2. Describe the pathophysiology, clinical manifestations, and medical and nursing management of multiple sclerosis, myasthenia gravis, and Guillain–Barré syndrome.
3. Use the nursing process as a framework for care of the patient with multiple sclerosis or Guillain–Barré syndrome.
4. Explain disorders of the cranial nerves, their manifestations, and indicated nursing interventions.
5. Apply the nursing process as a framework for care of the patient with a cranial nerve disorder.

SECTION I: ASSESSING YOUR UNDERSTANDING

Activity A *Fill in the blanks.*

1. The infectious disorders of the nervous system are _____, _____, _____, _____, and _____.

2. Classic clinical features of Guillain–Barré syndrome (GBS) are _____ and _____.

3. The most common cause of acute encephalitis in the United States is _____. The medication of choice for this disorder is _____.

4. The three diagnostic tests used to support diagnosis of Creutzfeldt–Jakob disease are _____, _____, and _____.

5. The primary pathology of multiple sclerosis (MS) is damage to the _____.

6. Disease-modifying therapies that are available to treat MS include _____ therapies and _____ agents.

7. Myasthenia gravis is considered an autoimmune disease in which antibodies are directed against _____.

8. The majority of patients with myasthenia gravis exhibit the clinical signs of _____ and _____.

9. _____ and _____ are the bacteria responsible for the majority of cases of bacterial meningitis in adults.

10. _____ with _____ is the clinical feature unique to the patient with St. Louis encephalitis.

Activity B *Briefly answer the following.*

1. The nurse is using a bedside risk scoring system for an adult patient with bacterial meningitis. Name five risks for an unfavorable outcome.

_____

_____

_____

2. Explain how *demyelination* correlates with a diagnosis of MS.

_____

_____

_____

3. Which strategies can the nurse educate the patient with MS about to avoid the disabling effects of fatigue?

_____

_____

_____

_____

Activity C *Match the cranial nerve listed in Column II with its associated clinical disorder listed in Column I. Answers may be used more than once.*

Column I

____ 1. Optic neuritis

____ 2. Pituitary tumor

____ 3. Brain stem ischemia

____ 4. Trigeminal neuralgia

____ 5. Bell palsy

____ 6. Herpes zoster

____ 7. Ménière's disease

____ 8. GBS

____ 9. Vagal body tumors

____ 10. Sinus tract tumor

Column II

a. I

b. II

c. IV

d. V

e. VI

f. VII

g. VIII

h. X

SECTION II: APPLYING YOUR KNOWLEDGE

Activity D *Consider the scenario and answer the questions.*

CASE STUDY: Multiple Sclerosis

Mrs. Bhani Singh, a 32-year-old mother of two, was diagnosed with multiple sclerosis (MS) 5 years ago. She is currently enrolled in a school of nursing. Her husband is supportive and assists with the care of their preschool sons. Mrs. Singh has been admitted to the acute care facility for diagnostic studies related to symptoms of a new onset of visual disturbances.

1. Mrs. Singh is enrolled full time in the nursing program and has classroom and clinical activities 4 days per week. What will the nurse educate Mrs. Singh about the cause of relapsing episodes of MS?

_____

_____

_____

_____

2. Mrs. Singh is prescribed IV prednisolone 1 g IV daily for 3 to 5 days, followed by an oral taper of prednisone. What will the nurse educate the patient about regarding the side effects of the medication?

_____

_____

3. The nurse is aware that MS may be affecting Mrs. Singh in other areas. Which will the nurse assess for during her hospitalization?

_____

_____

_____

_____

SECTION III: PRACTICING FOR NCLEX

Activity E *Answer the following questions.*

1. A college student goes to the infirmary with a fever, headache, and a stiff neck. The nurse suspects the student may have meningitis and has the student transferred to the hospital. If the diagnosis is confirmed, which will the nurse institute for those who have been in contact with this student? (Select all that apply.)

   a. Administration of rifampin

   b. Administration of ciprofloxacin hydrochloride

   c. Administration of ceftriaxone sodium

   d. Administration of amoxicillin

   e. Administration of rofecoxib

2. A patient has been diagnosed with meningococcal meningitis at a community living home. When will prophylactic therapy begin for those who have had close contact with the patient?

   a. Within 24 hours after exposure

   b. Within 48 hours after exposure

   c. Within 72 hours after exposure

   d. Therapy is not necessary prophylactically and should only be used if the person develops symptoms

3. The nurse caring for a patient with bacterial meningitis is giving dexamethasone that has been prescribed as an adjunct to antibiotic therapy. When does the nurse determine is the appropriate time to give this medication?

   a. 1 hour after the antibiotic has been infused and daily for 7 days.

   b. 15 to 20 minutes before the first dose of antibiotic and every 6 hours for the next 4 days.

   c. 2 hours prior to the administration of antibiotics for 7 days.

   d. It can be given every 6 hours for 10 days.

4. The nurse is caring for a patient admitted to the hospital with a brain abscess that developed from an untreated case of otitis media. Which assessment data is a priority to alert the nurse to changes in intracranial pressure?

   a. Level of consciousness

   b. Peripheral pulses

   c. Sensory perception

   d. Crackles bilaterally

5. The nurse is giving the IV antiviral medication ganciclovir to a patient with herpes simplex virus-1 (HSV-1) encephalitis. Which is the best way for the nurse to give the medication to avoid crystallization of the medication in the urine?

   a. Give the medication rapidly over 15 minutes with 100 mL of normal saline.

   b. Dilute the medicine in 500 mL of lactated Ringer solution.

   c. Give via slow IV over 1 hour.

   d. Give in a drip over 4 hours.

6. The nurse is volunteering for a Red Cross blood drive and is taking the history of potential donors. Which donor screened by the nurse will be unable to donate blood?

   a. A donor with a history of hypertension with a blood pressure of 140/90 mm Hg.

   b. A donor who is taking medication for benign prostatic hyperplasia.

   c. A donor who moved to the United States from Canada.

   d. A donor who was in college in England for 1 year.

7. A patient diagnosed with multiple sclerosis (MS) 2 years ago has been admitted to the hospital with another relapse. The previous relapse followed a complete recovery with the exception of occasional vertigo. Which type of MS does the nurse identify this patient most likely has?

   a. Benign

   b. Primary progressive

   c. Relapsing-remitting (RR)

   d. Disabling

8. The nurse is caring for a patient with multiple sclerosis (MS) having spasticity in the lower extremities, decreasing their physical mobility. Which interventions can the nurse provide to assist with relieving the spasms? (Select all that apply.)

   a. Have the patient take a hot tub bath to allow muscle relaxation.

   b. Demonstrate daily muscle stretching exercises.

   c. Apply warm compresses to the affected areas.

   d. Allow the patient adequate time to perform exercises.

   e. Assist with a rigorous exercise program to prevent contractures.

9. The nurse is assisting with administering a Tensilon test to a patient with ptosis. If the test is positive for myasthenia gravis, which outcome will the nurse observe?

   a. Thirty seconds after administration, the facial weakness and ptosis will be relieved for approximately 5 minutes.

   b. After administration of the medication, there will be no change in the status of the ptosis or facial weakness.

   c. The patient will have recovery of symptoms for at least 24 hours after the administration of the Tensilon.

   d. Eight hours after administration, the acetylcholinesterase begins to regenerate the available acetylcholine and will relieve symptoms.

10. During a Tensilon test to determine if a patient has myasthenia gravis, the patient reports cramping and becomes diaphoretic. Vital signs are BP 130/78, HR 42, and respiration 18. Which is the priority action by the nurse?

    a. Place the patient in the supine position.

    b. Give diphenhydramine for the allergic reaction.

    c. Give atropine to control the side effects of edrophonium.

    d. Call the rapid response team because the patient is preparing to arrest.

11. A patient with myasthenia gravis is in the hospital for treatment of pneumonia. The patient informs the nurse that it is very important to take pyridostigmine bromide on time. The nurse is busy and does not give the medication until after breakfast. Which outcome will the patient have related to this late dose?

    a. The muscles will become fatigued, and the patient will not be able to chew food or swallow pills.

    b. There should not be a problem, since the medication was only delayed by about 2 hours.

    c. The patient will go into cardiac arrest.

    d. The patient will require a double dose prior to lunch.

12. A patient suspected of having Guillain–Barré syndrome (GBS) has had a lumbar puncture for cerebrospinal fluid (CSF) evaluation. When reviewing the laboratory results, which will the nurse find that is diagnostic for this disease?

    a. Glucose in the CSF

    b. Elevated protein levels in the CSF

    c. Red blood cells present in the CSF

    d. White blood cells in the CSF

13. The nurse is caring for a patient with Guillain–Barré syndrome (GBS) in the intensive care unit and is assessing the patient for autonomic dysfunction. Which interventions will the nurse provide in order to determine the presence of autonomic dysfunction?

    a. Assess the respiratory rate and oxygen saturation.

    b. Assess the blood pressure and heart rate.

    c. Assess the peripheral pulses.

    d. Listen to the bowel sounds.

14. The nurse is caring for a patient in the emergency department reporting an onset of pain related to trigeminal neuralgia. Which subjective data stated by the patient does the nurse identify triggered the paroxysms of pain?

    a. "I was sitting at home watching television."

    b. "I was putting my shoes on."

    c. "I was brushing my teeth."

    d. "I was taking a bath."

15. A patient with Bell's palsy states to the nurse, "It doesn't hurt anymore to touch my face. How am I going to get muscle tone back so I don't look like this anymore?" Which interventions can the nurse suggest to the patient?

    a. Suggest massaging the face several times daily, using a gentle upward motion, to maintain muscle tone.

    b. Suggest applying cool compresses on the face several times a day to tighten the muscles.

    c. Inform the patient that the muscle function will return as soon as the virus dissipates.

    d. Tell the patient to smile every 4 hours.

Management of Patients with Oncologic or Degenerative Neurologic Disorders

Learning Outcomes

1. Describe brain and spinal cord tumors: their classification, pathophysiology, clinical manifestations, diagnosis, and medical and nursing management.
2. Use the nursing process as a framework for care of the patient with nervous system metastases or primary brain tumor.
3. Explain the pathophysiologic processes responsible for various neurodegenerative disorders.
4. Apply the nursing process as a framework for care of the patient with Parkinson's disease or the patient who has had a cervical discectomy.

SECTION I: ASSESSING YOUR UNDERSTANDING

Activity A *Fill in the blanks.*

1. The majority of metastatic lesions to the brain occur from the areas of _____, _____, _____, _____, _____, and _____.

2. The three most common systemic signs of increased intracranial pressure (ICP) are _____, _____, and _____.

3. The three common focal or localized symptoms of increased ICP are _____, _____, and _____.

4. A spinal cord tumor located within the spinal cord is classified as _____.

5. _____, _____, _____, _____, and _____ are five degenerative disorders of the central and peripheral nervous system.

6. The four cardinal signs of Parkinson's disease are _____, _____, _____, and _____.

7. The five chief symptoms of amyotrophic lateral sclerosis (ALS) are _____, _____, _____, _____, and _____.

8. Two common characteristics of muscular dystrophies are _____ and _____.

9. Cervical disc herniation usually occurs at the _____ or _____ interspaces.

10. Two major collaborative problems for patients with a cervical discectomy would be _____ and _____ .

1. Describe the physiologic changes that result from the infiltration of tissue subsequent to the growth of a brain tumor.

   _____

   _____

   _____

2. Describe the various classifications of brain tumors based on their pathophysiology.

   _____

   _____

   _____

3. Compare and contrast primary and secondary brain tumors.

   _____

   _____

   _____

4. Describe the process of stereotactic biopsy and its benefits in the diagnosis of brain tumors.

   _____

   _____

   _____

   _____

5. When a patient is assessed and determined to have Parkinson's disease, which clinical manifestation is most commonly present?

   _____

   _____

Activity C *Match the neurologic disorder listed in Column II with its associated description listed in Column I.*

Column I

____ 1. Impaired ability to execute voluntary movements

____ 2. Rapid, jerky, purposeless movements of extremities or facial muscles

____ 3. A sensation of "pins and needles"

____ 4. Restlessness and agitation

____ 5. Disease of the spinal nerve root

____ 6. Minute and illegible handwriting

____ 7. Very slow voluntary movements and speech

____ 8. Abnormal voice quality caused by incoordination of speech muscles

Column II

a. Akathisia

b. Bradykinesia

c. Chorea

d. Dyskinesia

e. Dysphonia

f. Micrographia

g. Paresthesia

h. Radiculopathy

SECTION II: APPLYING YOUR KNOWLEDGE

Activity D *Consider the scenarios and answer the questions.*

CASE STUDY: Parkinson's Disease

Charles Grimes is a 76-year-old retired professional golfer recently diagnosed with Parkinson's disease. He has tremors visible in both hands and stated that he noticed he is walking with a shuffling gait and that his friend has been telling him to "pick up your feet when you're walking."

1. Why is it important for the nurse to ensure that Mr. Grimes be started on an exercise regimen as part of his treatment plan?

   _____

   _____

   _____

   _____

2. Which types of exercises might the nurse recommend and why?

_____

_____

_____

3. Mr. Grimes will be started on a chemotherapy program using carbidopa/levodopa. What is the explanation of adding carbidopa to levodopa?

_____

_____

4. The nurse is developing a plan of care for Mr. Grimes. Which goals does the nurse set for him?

_____

_____

_____

CASE STUDY: Huntington Disease

Mike Carroll is a 49-year-old television producer who has been diagnosed as having Huntington disease. He lives alone in a penthouse apartment and is extremely busy and successful in his business. He has no living relatives. He is experiencing uncontrollable movements and has difficulty feeding himself. He recently started chemotherapy with haloperidol.

1. What does the nurse recognize as the most prominent features that he has related to the diagnosis of Huntington disease?

_____

_____

_____

2. Mr. Carroll has informed the nurse that he has no relatives or close friends who would be able to assist with his care. Which information will the nurse provide about the resources available to assist with his care?

_____

_____

3. Mr. Carroll has been prescribed a selective serotonin reuptake inhibitor (SSRI) included with other medications. What benefit will the SSRI have for him during his disease?

_____

_____

_____

SECTION III: PRACTICING FOR NCLEX

Activity E *Answer the following questions.*

1. A patient is diagnosed with an intracerebral tumor. The nurse identifies that the diagnosis may include which form(s) of tumor growth? (Select all that apply.)

    a. Astrocytoma

    b. Ependymoma

    c. Medulloblastoma

    d. Meningioma

    e. Acoustic neuroma

2. A patient is exhibiting seizurelike movements localized to one side of the body. Which type of brain tumor does the nurse determine the patient most likely has?

    a. A cerebellar tumor

    b. A frontal lobe tumor

    c. A motor cortex tumor

    d. An occipital lobe tumor

3. An older adult patient exhibiting clinical manifestations of a brain tumor is admitted to the hospital for testing. Which tumor type does the nurse identify is commonly seen in the older adult?

    a. Anaplastic astrocytoma

    b. Cerebral metastasis from other sites

    c. Glioblastoma multiforme

    d. Medulloblastoma

4. A patient with Parkinson's disease is exhibiting bradykinesia, rigidity, and tremors. These symptoms are directly related to which decreased neurotransmitter level?

   a. Acetylcholine

   b. Dopamine

   c. Serotonin

   d. Phenylalanine

5. The nurse is preparing to administer medications to a patient with Parkinson's disease. Which medication is administered that is considered the most effective drug currently given for the tremor of Parkinson's?

   a. Ropinirole

   b. Levodopa

   c. Amantadine

   d. Pergolide mesylate

6. A patient with a brain tumor reports headaches that are worse in the morning. Which is the best response by the nurse to explain the morning headaches?

   a. "You may have an increase in intracranial pressure."

   b. "You are most likely dehydrated."

   c. "You are probably experiencing migraine headaches."

   d. "The tumor is shrinking."

7. A patient diagnosed with a spinal cord tumor had a course of radiation and chemotherapy. Two months after the completion of the radiation, the patient reports severe pain in the back. Which does this indicate for the patient?

   a. Lumbar sacral strain

   b. Development of a skin ulcer from the radiation

   c. Hematoma formation

   d. Spinal metastasis

8. The nurse is performing an assessment for a patient in the clinic with Parkinson's disease. The nurse assesses that the patient's voice has changed since the last visit and is now more difficult to understand. How will the nurse document this finding?

   a. Dysphagia

   b. Dysphonia

   c. Hypokinesia

   d. Micrographia

9. A patient with Parkinson's disease is experiencing an on–off syndrome. Which assessment of the patient's clinical symptoms correlates with this syndrome?

   a. Unilateral resting tremors and then a period of no tremors present

   b. Slow, shuffling gait and then able to move at a faster pace

   c. A period when medication with levodopa will be unnecessary

   d. Periods of near immobility, followed by a sudden return of effectiveness of the medication

10. A patient with Parkinson's disease asks the nurse what can be done to prevent problems with bowel elimination. Which intervention will the nurse include when developing the plan of care to assist with a regular stool pattern?

    a. Take psyllium daily

    b. Take a laxative whenever bloating is experienced

    c. Adopt a diet with moderate fiber intake

    d. Adopt a high-fiber diet

11. The adult child of a patient with Huntington disease asks the nurse what the risk is of inheriting the disease. Which is the best response by the nurse?

    a. "The disease is not hereditary and therefore, there is no risk to you."

    b. "If one parent has the disorder, there is a 75% chance that you will inherit the disease."

    c. "If one parent has the disorder, there is a 50% chance that you will inherit the disease."

    d. "The disease is inherited and all offspring of a parent will develop the disease."

12. The nurse is caring for a patient with Huntington disease in the long-term care facility. Which most prominent symptom that correlates with this disease will the nurse document?

    a. Rapid, jerky, involuntary movements

    b. Slow, shuffling gait

    c. Dysphagia and dysphonia

    d. Dementia

13. A patient with Huntington disease is prescribed medication to reduce the chorea. Which medication will the nurse administer that is the only drug approved for the treatment of this symptom?

    a. Tetrabenazine

    b. Carbamazepine

    c. Phenobarbital

    d. Diazepam

14. A patient is diagnosed with amyotrophic lateral sclerosis (ALS). The nurse understands that the symptoms of the disease will begin in what way?

    a. Ascending paralysis

    b. Numbness and tingling in the lower extremities

    c. Weakness starting in the muscles supplied by the cranial nerves

    d. Jerky, uncontrolled movements in the extremities

15. A patient with amyotrophic lateral sclerosis (ALS) asks if the nurse has heard of a drug that will prolong the patient's life. Which is the best response to the patient's inquiry that may prolong life by 3 to 6 months?

    a. Baclofen

    b. Riluzole

    c. Dantrolene sodium

    d. Diazepam

Acute Community-Based Challenges

CHAPTER 66

Management of Patients with Infectious Diseases

Learning Outcomes

1. Differentiate between the concepts of colonization, infection, and disease.
2. Identify federal, state, and local resources available to the nurse seeking information about infectious diseases and discuss the benefits of recommended vaccines for health care workers and patients.
3. Compare and contrast standard and transmission-based precautions and discuss the elements of each of these prevention methods.
4. Describe the concept and the nursing management of patients with emerging infectious diseases.
5. Use the nursing process as a framework for care of the patient with sexually transmitted infections or with an infectious disease.

SECTION I: ASSESSING YOUR UNDERSTANDING

Activity A Fill in the blanks.

1. More than _____ vaccines are currently licensed in the United States (Centers for Disease Control and Prevention [CDC], 2016).

2. Health care workers should be immune to _____, _____, _____, _____, _____, _____, and _____.

3. The nurse should advise patients and parents of children receiving the measles, mumps, and rubella (MMR) vaccine that _____, _____, or _____ may occur following administration of the vaccine.

4. The two primary agencies involved in setting guidelines about infection prevention are the _____ and the _____.

5. Two bacteria that are part of normal skin flora are _____ and _____; _____ and _____, which are considered transient flora, have increased pathogenic potential.

6. The three primary organisms responsible for health care–associated infection (HAI) potential are _____, _____, and _____.

7. Immunosuppressed adults should be vaccinated for _____ and _____.

8. Portals of entry of STI-causing microorganisms and sites of infection include the _____, as well as the mucosal linings of the _____, _____, _____, _____, and _____.

Activity B *Briefly answer the following.*

1. Describe the chain of essential events necessary for an infection to occur.

_____

_____

_____

2. Compare and contrast an infectious disease and an infection.

_____

_____

3. What is the most frequent cause of bacterial infections in health care institutions?

_____

4. What is the most important aspect of reducing the risk of bloodborne infection?

_____

5. A patient has been admitted to the hospital with active tuberculosis infection. Which precautions will be provided for this patient?

_____

_____

_____

_____

Activity C *Match the disease or condition listed in Column II with its associated causative organism listed in Column I.*

Column I

___ 1. Varicella zoster

___ 2. *Neisseria gonorrhoeae*

___ 3. Hepatitis B virus

___ 4. *Staphylococcus aureus*

___ 5. Epstein–Barr virus

___ 6. *Salmonella* species

___ 7. *Streptococcus pneumoniae*

___ 8. *Microsporum* species

Column II

a. Chicken pox

b. Bloodborne hepatitis

c. Diarrheal disease

d. Gonorrhea

e. Impetigo

f. Mononucleosis

g. Pneumococcal pneumonia

h. Ringworm

SECTION II: APPLYING YOUR KNOWLEDGE

Activity D *Consider the scenario and answer the questions.*

Kallie Jackson, a 23-year-old woman, was informed by her boyfriend that he had been treated for gonorrhea (*Neisseria gonorrhoeae*) at the local clinic about 2 weeks ago but was reluctant to tell her. Kallie thought that she had a mild urinary tract infection because of burning when urinating.

1. Kallie goes to the clinic for diagnosis and treatment. Besides gonorrhea, what else will she be tested for?

_____

2. Kallie asks the nurse what would have happened if her boyfriend had not told her about the infection. Which complications of untreated gonorrhea should the nurse discuss with her?

_____

3. Which test will be performed to confirm a diagnosis of gonorrhea?

_____

4. Which education will the nurse provide to Kallie in order to prevent her from contracting another sexually transmitted infection (STI)?

_____

_____

SECTION III: PRACTICING FOR NCLEX

Activity E *Answer the following questions.*

1. The nurse is attempting to determine if a patient admitted to the hospital the previous day has a bacterial wound infection. Which laboratory study will the nurse review to obtain this information?

   a. The complete blood count (CBC)

   b. Culture and sensitivity

   c. MRI report

   d. Chemistry studies

2. The nurse is discussing childhood immunization recommendations with a pediatric patient's parent. Where would the nurse find the most current information on this topic?

   a. The World Health Organization (WHO)

   b. The Joint Commission

   c. Centers for Disease Control and Prevention (CDC)

   d. The Occupational Safety and Health Administration (OSHA)

3. After providing care for a patient with *Clostridium difficile,* the nurse is preparing to wash hands before leaving the room. Which is the best method of cleaning the hands in order to prevent spreading the bacteria?

   a. Remove gloves and wash the hands with soap and water.

   b. Remove gloves and use Hibiclens solution to wash hands.

   c. Remove gloves and use Betadine solution prior to washing hands with soap and water.

   d. Use an alcohol-based solution to clean hands.

4. The nurse is caring for a patient with a meningococcus infection. Which type of precautions will be used for this patient?

   a. Airborne

   b. Contact

   c. Droplet

   d. Standard

5. The nurse is providing an education program to reduce the incidence of infection currently on the rise in the community. Which areas will the nurse focus on when presenting this program? (Select all that apply.)

   a. Regulated health practices

   b. Sanitation techniques

   c. The use of antibiotics to prevent infections

   d. Immunization programs

   e. Swimming in the community pool

6. A patient who is 20-weeks pregnant asks the nurse if it is alright for her take the varicella immunization for entrance into nursing school. Which is the best response by the nurse?

   a. "If you will be working in the health care field, you must take the immunization."

   b. "It is not recommended that pregnant women take the live virus. You should wait until after your child is born."

   c. "It is not a live virus, so it should be fine."

   d. "You will have to delay entrance into the nursing program if they force you to take it."

7. A patient has developed chicken pox and asks the nurse what the incubation period would be. Which is the best response by the nurse?

   a. It is 24 to 48 hours

   b. It is 2 to 3 days

   c. It is 7 to 10 days

   d. It is 10 to 21 days

8. A patient is admitted with severe dehydration related to diarrhea. The patient was hiking in the mountains during a camping trip and drank water from a mountain stream without purifying. Which is the likely cause of this diarrhea?

   a. *Giardia lamblia*

   b. *Calicivirus*

   c. *Escherichia coli*

   d. *Shigella*

9. The nurse is admitting a patient with severe diarrhea. Which is the most important element of assessment for this patient?

   a. Stool color

   b. Hydration status

   c. Bowel sounds

   d. Appetite

10. A patient comes to the clinic reporting the presence of a painless sore on her lip 2 weeks after she had oral sex with her boyfriend. The nurse observes a chancre on the lips and the health care provider prescribes testing for syphilis. If results are positive, which is the likely stage the patient is in?

    a. Primary

    b. Secondary

    c. Latency

    d. Tertiary

11. The nurse has received several laboratory studies back at the clinic. Which of these results should be reported to the local health department?
    a. Wound infection with MRSA
    b. Positive influenza
    c. Positive gonorrhea
    d. Positive mononucleosis

12. An adolescent informs the school nurse that she is afraid of contracting an STI but her boyfriend does not want to use condoms. Which is the best response by the nurse?
    a. "You are too young to be having sex at all and should stop until you are older."
    b. "If he won't use a condom, then he doesn't care about you."
    c. "The use of condoms is one of the best ways to reduce the risk of acquiring an STI."
    d. "I can understand your concern and you should bring him here so that I can talk with him about STIs."

13. After attending a conference at a hotel for several days, a patient is having symptoms related to Legionnaires disease. When making a bed assignment for this patient, how will the assignment be made?
    a. Place in a private room on droplet precautions
    b. Place in a negative pressure room
    c. Place in a private room on airborne precautions
    d. Place in a semi-private room

14. The nurse has heard that there have been three cases of pertussis in the community and wants to make sure their inoculations are up-to-date. Which action should the nurse take?
    a. Have a single-dose Tdap given
    b. It is not necessary to be inoculated since there is a slim chance of acquiring the disease
    c. Take a series of three Tdap 3 months apart
    d. Have a Tdap given, and 6 months later have another

15. A family will be staying in a cabin by a lake and, upon arriving, observes rodent droppings on the floor in the kitchen. What is the best way for the family to clean up in order to avoid contracting hantavirus from the feces?
    a. Sweep up all of the droppings and then apply a bleach solution.
    b. Vacuum the droppings and then apply a bleach solution.
    c. Apply a bleach solution prior to sweeping or vacuuming the floor.
    d. Sweep the droppings in a pile and then vacuum them up.

Emergency Nursing

Learning Outcomes

1. Describe emergency care as a collaborative, holistic approach that ideally includes the patient, the family, and significant others.
2. Identify the priorities of care for the patient with an emergency disorder, particularly the patient with multiple system injuries.
3. Compare and contrast the emergency management of patients with heat stroke, frostbite, and hypothermia.
4. Specify the similarities and differences of the emergency management of patients with swallowed or inhaled poisons, skin contamination, and food poisoning.
5. Explain the emergency management of patients with drug overdose, those with acute alcohol intoxication, those who have been sexually assaulted, and those who have been victims of human trafficking.
6. Differentiate between the emergency care of patients who are overactive, those who are violent, those who are depressed, and those who are suicidal.

SECTION I: ASSESSING YOUR UNDERSTANDING

Activity A *Fill in the blanks.*

1. The _____ survey focuses on stabilizing life-threatening conditions.

2. According to the _____, every emergency department (ED) with a Medicare provider agreement must perform a medical screening examination on all patients arriving with an emergency medical complaint if their acute signs and symptoms could result in serious injury or death if left untreated.

3. A patient with a foreign body airway obstruction typically demonstrates the inability to _____, _____, or _____. With complete obstruction, permanent brain injury will occur in _____ minutes.

4. In the case of gunfire in the ED, _____ is a priority.

5. The cardinal manifestations of heat illness includes _____, particularly in the shoulders, abdomen, and lower extremities; _____, and _____ (ENA, 2020a).

6. Children under _____ years of age and those over the age of _____ have the highest risk of drowning.

7. The most common victims of snakebites are those between the ages of _____ and _____.

8. Antivenin to treat snakebites must be given within a time frame of _____ to _____ hours.

9. Depending on the severity of a snakebite, antivenin is diluted in _____ to _____ mL of _____.

Activity B *Briefly answer the following.*

1. Describe the indications for endotracheal intubation.

   _____

   _____

   _____

   _____

2. Why is lactated Ringer solution initially useful as fluid replacement for a patient experiencing hypovolemic shock?

   _____

   _____

   _____

   _____

3. When evaluating an older adult client, which risk factors of upper airway obstruction will the nurse carefully consider when performing the assessment?

   _____

   _____

   _____

   _____

4. When the nurse is performing a rapid neurologic assessment in the ED, what mnemonic is helpful?

   _____

   _____

   _____

   _____

5. Name and define the three categories commonly used in triage in the ED.

   _____

   _____

   _____

   _____

Activity C *Match the wound in Column I with the definition given in Column II.*

Column I

_____ **1.** Laceration

_____ **2.** Avulsion

_____ **3.** Abrasion

_____ **4.** Ecchymosis

_____ **5.** Hematoma

_____ **6.** Stab

_____ **7.** Cut

_____ **8.** Patterned

Column II

a. Incision of the skin with well-defined edges, usually caused by a sharp instrument; this type of wound is typically deeper than long

b. Denuded skin

c. Incision of the skin with well-defined edges, usually longer than deep

d. Tumorlike mass of blood trapped under the skin

e. Wound representing the outline of the object (e.g., steering wheel) causing the wound

f. Blood trapped under the surface of the skin

g. Skin tear with irregular edges and vein bridging

h. Tearing away of tissue from supporting structures

SECTION II: APPLYING YOUR KNOWLEDGE

Activity D *Consider the scenario and answer the questions.*

CASE STUDY: Heat Stroke

Carson Miller, age 42, was on a roof fixing several loose shingles in 95°F weather. His wife came outside to bring him something to drink and found him lying on the roof. When she called his name, he appeared not to understand her and lay there looking around. She immediately called the rescue squad and they were able to transport him to the hospital. He had a temperature of 106.2°F upon arrival to the ED.

1. Which other clinical manifestations does the nurse assess with Mr. Miller's diagnosis of heat stroke?

   _____

   _____

   _____

   _____

2. Which actions by the nurse may assist with preventing complications related to Mr. Miller's heat stroke?

   _____

   _____

   _____

   _____

3. Why is it important for the nurse to monitor his urine output at least every hour?

   _____

   _____

SECTION III: PRACTICING FOR NCLEX

Activity E *Answer the following questions.*

1. An adolescent is brought to the ED after a motor vehicle crash and is pronounced dead on arrival (DOA). When the parents arrive at the hospital, which is the priority action by the nurse?

   a. Ask them to sit in the waiting room until the nurse can spend time alone with them.

   b. Speak to both parents together and encourage them to support each other and express their emotions freely.

   c. Speak to one parent at a time in a private setting so that each can ventilate feelings of loss without upsetting the other.

   d. Ask the ED health care provider to medicate the parents so that they can handle their child's unexpected death quietly.

2. A triage nurse in the ED determines that a patient with dyspnea and dehydration is not in a life-threatening situation. Which triage category will the nurse choose?

   a. Delayed

   b. Emergent

   c. Immediate

   d. Urgent

3. The nurse in the ED is triaging patients during the shift. Which is the first priority by the nurse in treating any patient in the ED?

   a. Controlling hemorrhage

   b. Establishing an airway

   c. Obtaining consent for treatment

   d. Restoring cardiac output

4. The nurse is caring for a patient in the ED who is breathing but unconscious. In order to avoid an upper airway obstruction, the nurse is inserting an oropharyngeal airway. Which technique will the nurse use during insertion?

   a. At an angle of 90 degrees

   b. Upside down and then rotated 180 degrees

   c. With the concave portion touching the posterior pharynx

   d. With the convex portion facing upward

5. The nurse receives a patient from a motor vehicle crash who is hemorrhaging from a femoral wound. Which is the initial nursing action for the control of the hemorrhage?

   a. Apply a tourniquet

   b. Apply firm pressure over the involved area or artery

   c. Elevate the injured part

   d. Immobilize the area to control blood loss

6. The nurse is admitting a patient with a penetrating abdominal injury from a knife wound. Which are the priority actions by the nurse for this patient? (Select all that apply.)

   a. Assessing for manifestations of hemorrhage

   b. Covering any protruding viscera with sterile dressings soaked in normal saline solution

   c. Looking for any associated chest injuries

   d. Exploring the abdominal wound with a gloved finger

   e. Irrigating the wound with normal saline and a syringe

7. A patient sustains blunt force abdominal trauma during a motor vehicle crash and reports right upper quadrant abdominal pain. Which solid abdominal organ is of most concern to the nurse?

   a. Duodenum

   b. Large bowel

   c. Liver

   d. Pancreas

8. A patient is brought to the ED by a friend, who states that a tree fell on the patient's leg and crushed it while they were cutting firewood. Which priority actions will the nurse perform? (Select all that apply.)

   a. Applying a clean dressing to protect the wound

   b. Elevating the site to limit the accumulation of fluid in the interstitial spaces

   c. Inserting an indwelling catheter

   d. Splinting the wound in a position of rest to prevent motion

   e. Performing a fasciotomy

9. A patient has experienced multiple injuries. Which sequence of management would the nurse identify as a priority?

   a. Assess for head injuries, control hemorrhage, establish an airway, prevent hypovolemic shock

   b. Control hemorrhage, prevent hypovolemic shock, establish an airway, assess for head injuries

   c. Establish an airway, control hemorrhage, prevent hypovolemic shock, assess for head injuries

   d. Prevent hypovolemic shock, assess for head injuries, establish an airway, control hemorrhage

10. A female patient was sexually assaulted when leaving work. When assisting with the physical examination, which nursing actions are a priority? (Select all that apply.)

    a. Have the patient shower or wash the perineal area before the examination.

    b. Assess and document any bruises and lacerations.

    c. Record a history of the event, using the patient's own words.

    d. Label all torn or bloody clothes and place each item in a separate brown bag so that any evidence can be given to the police.

    e. Ensure that the police are present when the examination is performed.

11. A patient with frostbite to both lower extremities from exposure to the elements is preparing to have rewarming of the extremities. Which nursing actions will the nurse provide prior to rewarming of the extremities?

   a. Give an analgesic as prescribed.

   b. Massage the extremities.

   c. Elevate the legs.

   d. Apply a heat lamp.

12. A patient brought to the ED by the rescue squad after getting off a plane at the airport reports severe joint pain, numbness, and an inability to move the arms. The patient was on a diving vacation and went for a last dive this morning before flying home. Which is a priority action by the nurse?

   a. Ensure a patent airway and that the patient is receiving 100% oxygen.

   b. Send the patient for a chest x-ray.

   c. Send the patient to the hyperbaric chamber.

   d. Draw labs for a chemistry panel.

13. A nurse is working as a camp nurse during the summer. A camp counselor comes to the clinic after receiving a snakebite on the arm. Which is the first action by the nurse?

   a. Apply ice to the area.

   b. Apply a tourniquet to the arm above the bite.

   c. Have the patient lie down and place the arm below the level of the heart.

   d. Make an incision and suck the venom out.

14. The nurse is giving antivenin to a patient who was bitten on the arm by a poisonous snake. Which intervention provided by the nurse is required prior to the procedure and every 15 minutes after?

   a. Give diphenhydramine.

   b. Give cimetidine.

   c. Measure the circumference of the arm.

   d. Assess peripheral pulses.

15. A patient was bitten by a tick 3 months ago and is now having muscle aches as well as joint pain and swelling. The patient is having difficulty with self-care and requires assistance with activities of daily living (ADLs). Which stage of Lyme disease does the nurse recognize the patient is in?

   a. Stage I

   b. Stage II

   c. Stage III

   d. Stage IV

CHAPTER 68

Disaster Nursing

Learning Outcomes

1. Describe the types of disasters that the nurse may encounter as a member of the health care team.
2. Identify essential components of an emergency operations plan and disaster preparedness including personal protection and decontamination procedures.
3. Discuss how triage in a disaster differs from triage in an emergency department.
4. Explain clinical manifestations and treatment of injuries and illnesses resulting from natural disasters, from outbreaks, epidemics, and pandemics, and from various weapons of terror (blast, biologic, chemical, and radiologic events).

SECTION I: ASSESSING YOUR UNDERSTANDING

Activity A Fill in the blanks.

1. Natural disasters are caused by _____.

2. Federal agencies that may provide resources in response to an MCI or a disaster are _____, _____, and _____.

3. The _____ is responsible for ensuring that testing methods will provide both accurate and reliable results.

4. _____ is a key component of disaster management.

5. Two biologic agents most likely to be used during a terrorist attack are _____ and _____.

6. For patients who have been directly exposed to anthrax but have no signs and symptoms of disease, _____ or _____ is used for prophylaxis for 60 days.

7. Cremation is preferred for all deaths due to smallpox because the virus can survive in scabs for up to _____ years.

Activity B Briefly answer the following.

1. What role does Incident Command System (ICS) perform in the event of a specific local mass casualty incident (MCI)?

   _____

   _____

   _____

2. On April 8, 2020, the FEMA COVID-19 Supply Chain Task Force developed a four-step plan to preserve critical resources for medical use. List the four steps in the plan.

   _____

   _____

   _____

   _____

3. What will be included when documenting on the disaster tag for each patient?

_____

_____

_____

_____

4. Name at least four cultural variables that health care providers need to consider in any disaster situation in which a large number of diverse religious and ethnic groups of patients need to be treated.

_____

_____

_____

5. In which ways can the nurse assist victims of disaster?

_____

_____

_____

6. Describe the four levels of protective clothing and respiratory protection.

_____

_____

_____

Activity C

Triage Categories During a Mass Casualty Incident (MCI)

Match the color category in Column II with the condition in Column I. Colors may be used more than once.

Column I	Column II
____ **1.** Fractured humerus	**a.** Red
____ **2.** C-1 spinal transection	**b.** Yellow
____ **3.** Third-degree burns over 25% total body surface area (TBSA)	**c.** Green
	d. Black
____ **4.** Hemothorax	
____ **5.** Radiation exposure with seizures 24 hours after exposure	
____ **6.** Burn to hand	
____ **7.** Depression	
____ **8.** Maxillofacial wound without airway compromise	
____ **9.** Sucking chest wound	
____ **10.** Open femur fracture	
____ **11.** Third-degree burns over 75% TBSA	
____ **12.** Penetrating head wound with ice pick	
____ **13.** Stable abdominal wound without hemorrhage	
____ **14.** Soft-tissue injury of lower extremity with adequate collateral circulation	

SECTION II: APPLYING YOUR KNOWLEDGE

Activity D *Consider the scenario and answer the questions.*

A train derailment caused the injuries of 34 people, with injuries ranging from minor to critical. All patients have been brought to the local emergency department (ED) for treatment. Health care providers have been called from their offices to assist with caring for the wounded, and nurses have been called in to assist with the disaster.

1. What will the triage team be sure to do in order to ensure that all patients have been identified?

   _____

   _____

   _____

2. What does the nurse identify is the primary principle in a disaster when there are several critical patients?

   _____

   _____

   _____

3. What will the nurse ensure is in place in order to control the overload of patients, visitors, and EMS personnel in the ED?

   _____

   _____

SECTION III: PRACTICING FOR NCLEX

Activity E *Answer the following questions.*

1. The nurse is assisting in a disaster caused by an F-4 tornado that destroyed much of the community. This disaster will require statewide and federal assistance. Which classification would the disaster be?

   a. Level I

   b. Level II

   c. Level III

   d. Level IV

2. The Department of Homeland Security issues a code "blue" relative to a situation. What does this indicate to the nurse in the emergency department?

   a. Perceived low risk

   b. Guarded risk

   c. Possible risk but ill-defined

   d. High risk with no specific site

3. The nurse is triaging patients involved in a train derailment. A patient with survivable but life-threatening injuries will be tagged with which color?

   a. Black

   b. Green

   c. Red

   d. Yellow

4. The nurse is triaging people who have been involved in a bus accident. A triaged patient with psychological disturbances would be tagged with which color?

   a. Black

   b. Green

   c. Red

   d. Yellow

5. A triaged patient with a significant injury who can wait several hours for treatment would be assigned what priority?

   a. Priority 1

   b. Priority 2

   c. Priority 3

   d. Priority 4

6. Several patients who have been involved in a bombing are unlikely to survive. Which priority are these patients given during triage?

   a. Priority 1

   b. Priority 2

   c. Priority 3

   d. Priority 4

7. A patient was involved in an avalanche that illed many people on a ski trip, including the patient's brother. The nurse is educating the patient about recognition of stress reactions and ways to manage stress. Which type of process is the nurse introducing to the patient?

a. Defusing

b. Debriefing

c. Preparedness

d. Demobilization

8. The nurse receives a call from EMS personnel that they are bringing in eight patients who have been exposed to a chemical after a spill. The patients have been "washed off." After the initial assessment, which action will be taken?

a. Remove clothing and jewelry and rinse the patients off with water.

b. Have the patients wash with soap and water and then rinse.

c. Treat the patients for any burned areas from the chemical since they have already been decontaminated.

d. Start an IV with lactated Ringer solution at 125 mL/hr.

9. A patient was brought into the ED after sustaining injuries due to an explosion while welding. The patient is breathing but has an oxygen saturation of 90%, a respiratory rate of 32, and is coughing. Which is the priority action by the nurse?

a. Give oxygen at 2 L/min via nasal cannula.

b. Give oxygen with a nonrebreather mask.

c. Start an IV of normal saline solution at 125 mL/hr.

d. Obtain a chest x-ray.

10. A patient is suspected to have an air embolus after being in close proximity to an explosion at a sports arena. Which position will the nurse place the patient in to prevent migration of the embolus?

a. Supine with head of the bed at 30 degrees

b. High-Fowler position

c. Prone left lateral position

d. Lithotomy

11. A patient was suspected of being in direct contact with anthrax but is exhibiting no signs or symptoms. Which type of prophylaxis will the nurse educate the patient to take?

a. Penicillin G IM for 1 dose

b. Ceftriaxone IV for 7 days

c. Ciprofloxacin for 60 days

d. Erythromycin for 2 weeks

12. A patient is being brought into the ED, who is possibly infected with anthrax. The nurse will ensure which level of personal protective equipment to wear for everyone who will come in contact with the patient?

a. Level A

b. Level B

c. Level C

d. Level D

13. A soldier is preparing to enter an area in which there is a high risk for chemical exposure to a nerve agent. Which will the soldier be given prior to entering this area?

a. Mark I automatic injectors that contain 2 mg atropine and 600 mg pralidoxime chloride.

b. Mark I automatic injectors that contain an anticonvulsant medication such as carbamazepine.

c. Mark I automatic injector filled with morphine 10 mg.

d. Mark I automatic injector filled with cyanide.

14. A nuclear reactor overheated, releasing radiation throughout the plant. A worker close to reactor received at least 800 rads and has had an onset of vomiting, bloody diarrhea, and, when brought to the hospital, was in shock. Which is this patient's predicted survival?

a. Possible

b. Probable

c. Likely

d. Improbable

15. The nurse is triaging patients from a 10-car pileup on the interstate and assesses a patient with a sucking chest wound. Which category should this patient be placed in?

a. Priority 1

b. Priority 2

c. Priority 3

d. Priority 4

Answers

CHAPTER 1

SECTION I: ASSESSING YOUR UNDERSTANDING

Activity A

1. knowledge, skills, and attitudes (KSA)
2. cardiovascular disease, cancers, diabetes, and chronic lung diseases
3. interview, observation, and examination
4. veracity, fidelity, benevolence, wisdom, and moral courage

Activity B

1. the capacity to perform to the best of one's ability, the ability to adjust and adapt to varying situations, a reported feeling of well-being, and a feeling that everything is harmonious
2. Shifting population demographics; changing patterns of disease and wellness; advances in technology and genetics; emphasis on health care quality, costs, reform efforts, and interprofessional collaborative practices
3. Human responses requiring nursing intervention should include self-image changes, impaired ventilation, and anxiety and fear. Answer may also include pain and discomfort, grief, and impaired functioning in areas such as rest and sleep.
4. assessment, diagnosis, planning, implementation, and evaluation
5. In Maslow hierarchy of needs, needs are ranked as follows. Refer to Figure 1-1 in the textbook.

Need	Example
Physiologic	Food and water
Safety and security	Financial security
Belongingness and affection	Companionship
Esteem and self-respect	Recognition by society
Self-actualization	Achieved potential in an area
Self-fulfillment	Creativity (painting)
Knowledge and understanding	Information and explanation
Aesthetics	Attractive environment

6. caring and compassion
7. Nursing care must be culturally competent, appropriate, and sensitive to cultural differences.
8. Evidence-based practice is a best practice derived from valid and reliable research studies that also considers the health care setting, patient preferences and values, and clinical judgment.
9. When a nurse is faced with two conflicting alternatives, it is the nurse's moral responsibility to choose the lesser of the two evils. These situations often result in feelings of moral distress in the nurse who is obliged to make a choice.
10. Substance use disorders (SUDs), posttraumatic stress disorder (PTSD), traumatic brain injury (TBI), suicide, depression, hazardous substance exposure, and amputations
11. artificial intelligence, blockchain, cloud technology, disease management technology, and improved operability of electronic health records (EHRs)
12. clinical guidelines, algorithms, care mapping, multidisciplinary action plans (MAPs), and clinical pathways
13. communication and relationships, educational level, knowledge and ability to use critical thinking, familiarity with the environment and the context of care, experience and exposure to a variety of situations

SECTION II: APPLYING YOUR KNOWLEDGE

Activity C

1. c   2. a, b, c, d   3. b

SECTION III: PRACTICING FOR NCLEX

Activity D

1. d   2. a   3. d   4. b   5. a
6. d   7. a   8. b   9. d   10. c
11. a

CHAPTER 2

SECTION I: ASSESSING YOUR UNDERSTANDING

Activity A

1. Transitional care
2. cost, health care quality
3. ADLs and IADLs
4. cost-effectiveness, accountability, and quality care
5. Functional Independence Measure (FIM™)
6. Footdrop
7. Safety

Activity B

1. breakdowns in care transitions including during the discharge planning processes, as evidenced by patients' inability to manage their own care; and, as a result of poor communication between the hospital and the next level of care (e.g., home health facility, primary care office) regarding patients' needs and resources
2. helping the patient and the patient's family transition through different levels of care
3. adaptive devices and assistive devices
4. returning patients to optimal functionality through a holistic approach to care that is based on scientific evidence
5. Call the patient to obtain permission for a visit, schedule the visit, and verify the address.
6. During the initial home visit, the patient is evaluated, and a plan of care is established.
7. Refer to Table 2-1, Therapeutic Exercises, in the textbook.
8. reduction in reimbursement for costs associated with these readmissions
9. Medical-surgical nursing is a specialty area of practice that provides nursing services to patients from adolescence through the end of life in a variety of inpatient and outpatient clinical settings. Critical-care nursing is a specialty area of practice that provides nursing services to critically ill patients across the lifespan, traditionally delivered in acute care settings such as the hospital intensive care unit (ICU).
10. The development of a comprehensive discharge plan requires collaboration between professionals at the referring facility and the home care facility, as well as other community agencies that provide specific resources upon discharge.

SECTION II: APPLYING YOUR KNOWLEDGE

Activity C

CASE STUDY: Assessing the Need for a Home Visit

1. Refer to section "Home Health Visits" and Chart 2-3, Assessing the Home Environment, in the textbook to complete the case study.

SECTION III: PRACTICING FOR NCLEX

Activity D

1. b   2. c   3. a, c, d   4. b, c, d   5. a
6. b   7. c

CHAPTER 3

SECTION I: ASSESSING YOUR UNDERSTANDING

Activity A

1. Significant factors include the availability of health care outside the hospital setting, the employment of diverse health care providers to accomplish care management goals, and the increased use of alternative strategies other than the traditional approaches to care.
2. People with a chronic illness need as much health care information as possible to actively participate in and assume responsibility for the management of their own care. Health education can help the patient adapt to illness and cooperate with a treatment regimen. The goal of health education is to teach people to maximize their health potential.
3. Answer may include five of the following: medication adherence; maintaining a healthy diet; increasing daily exercise; self-monitoring for signs of illness; practicing good overall hygiene; seeking health screenings and evaluations; and performing therapeutic, preventive measures.
4. *Adherence* implies that a patient makes one or more lifestyle changes to carry out specific activities to promote and maintain health.
5. Factors influencing adherence include demographic variables such as age, gender, and education; illness variables such as the severity of illness and the effects of therapy; psychosocial variables such as intelligence and attitudes toward illness; financial variables; and therapeutic regimen variables.
6. Choice, establishment of agreed-upon goals, and the quality of the patient–provider relationship
7. Refer to the "Transtheoretical Model of Change" adapted from Miller (2015) and DiClemente (2007). Refer to Table 3-2, Stages in the Transtheoretical Model of Change, in the textbook.
8. The teaching–learning process requires the active involvement of teacher and learner, in an effort to reach the desired outcome: a change in behavior. The teacher serves as a facilitator of learning.
9. Answer may include six of the following: The older adult patient may have difficulty adhering to a therapeutic regimen because of increased sensitivity to medications, difficulty in adjusting to change and stress, financial constraints, forgetfulness, inadequate support systems, lifetime habits of self-medication, visual impairments, hearing deficits, and mobility limitations.

10. The desired outcomes and the critical time periods serve as a basis for evaluating the effectiveness of the teaching strategies.

11. The effects of a learning situation are influenced by a person's physical, emotional, and experiential readiness to learn. *Physical readiness* implies the physical ability of a person to attend to a learning situation. Basic physiologic needs are met so that higher-level needs can be addressed. *Emotional readiness* involves the patient's motivation to learn and can be encouraged by providing realistic goals that can be easily achieved so that self-esteem needs can be met. A person needs to be ready to accept the emotional changes (anxiety, stress) that accompany behavior modification resulting from the learning process. *Experiential readiness* refers to a person's past experiences that influence their approach to the learning process. Previous positive feedback and improved self-image reinforce experiential readiness.

12. Lecture method, group teaching, demonstrations, use of teaching aids, reinforcement, and follow-up

13. Refer to Chart 3-2.

14. self-responsibility, nutritional awareness, stress reduction and management, and physical fitness

15. Improves the function of the circulatory system and the lungs; decreases cholesterol and low-density lipoprotein levels; decreases body weight by increasing calorie expenditure; delays degenerative changes such as osteoporosis; and improves flexibility and overall muscle strength and endurance

Activity B

1. Health education is an <u>independent</u> function of nursing practice that is a primary responsibility of the nursing profession.

2. Although diseases in children and those of an infectious nature are of utmost concern, the largest groups of people today who need health education are those <u>with chronic illnesses and disabilities</u>.

3. Patients are encouraged to <u>adhere</u> to their therapeutic regimen. <u>Adherence</u> connotes <u>active, voluntary, and collaborative patient</u> *efforts*, whereas adherence is a more passive role.

4. Evaluation <u>should be continuous</u> throughout the teaching process so that the information gathered can be used to improve teaching activities.

5. The older adults <u>usually experience significant gains</u> from health promotion activities.

6. About <u>80%</u> of those older than 65 years of age have one or more chronic illnesses.

SECTION II: APPLYING YOUR KNOWLEDGE

Activity C

1. The variables of choice, establishment of mutual goals, and quality of the patient–provider relationship directly influence the behavioral changes that can result from patient education. These factors are directly linked to motivation for learning.

2. Using a learning contract or agreement can be a motivator for learning; positive reinforcement is provided as the person moves from one goal to the next.

SECTION III: PRACTICING FOR NCLEX

Activity D

1. b   **2.** a, b, e   **3.** a, b, e   **4.** b   **5.** a
6. a   **7.** a   **8.** a   **9.** b   **10.** a
11. a   **12.** c

CHAPTER 4

SECTION I: ASSESSING YOUR UNDERSTANDING

Activity A

1. obtaining a patient health history, performing a physical examination

2. Answer may include the following: patterns of sleep, exercise, nutrition, recreation, and personal habits such as smoking, the use of illicit drugs, alcohol, and caffeine.

3. heart disease, cancer, stroke

4. iron, folate, calcium

Activity B

1. The nurse needs to establish rapport, put the patient at ease, encourage honest communication, make eye contact, and listen carefully.

2. When an atmosphere of mutual trust and confidence exists between an interviewer and a patient, the patient becomes more open and honest, and is more likely to share personal concerns and problems.

3. Shared by members of the same cultural group. Includes an internal sense and external perception of distinctiveness. Influenced by specific conditions related to environmental and technical factors and to the availability of resources. Dynamic and ever changing.

4. Answer may include six of the following: cancer, hypertension, heart disease, diabetes, epilepsy, mental illness, tuberculosis, kidney disease, arthritis, allergies, asthma, alcoholism, and obesity.

5. United States, Great Britain, and Canada

6. The Mini-Nutritional Assessment (MNA)

7. Refer to Table 4-3, Factors Associated with Potential Nutritional Deficits, in the textbook.

Activity C

PART I

a. Inspection
b. Inspection
c. Palpation
d. Palpation
e. Percussion
f. Auscultation
g. Auscultation
h. Palpation

PART II

Refer to Table 4-2, Physical Indicators of Nutritional Status, in the textbook.

1. h   **2.** c   **3.** d   **4.** e   **5.** g
6. b

SECTION II: APPLYING YOUR KNOWLEDGE

Activity D

CASE STUDY: Estimate Ideal Body Weight

1. b, medium frame (her height-to-waist circumference ratio is 10:4)
2. 125 lb, lose, 50 lb (refer to Table 4-1, How Is BMI Calculated?, in the textbook)
3. 29, overweight

CASE STUDY: Cultural and Nutritional Assessment

1. Greet the patient using the last or complete name. Avoid being too casual or familiar. Point to yourself and say your name. Smile. Proceed in an unhurried manner. Pay attention to any effort by the patient or family to communicate. Speak in a low, moderate voice. Avoid talking loudly. Repeat and summarize frequently. Use audiovisual aids when feasible.
2. A patient who is Muslim does not eat pork or pork products.

SECTION III: PRACTICING FOR NCLEX

Activity E

1. b, d, e   **2.** a, c, d   **3.** d   **4.** b   **5.** b
6. c   **7.** b, c, d   **8.** a, b, c   **9.** b   **10.** a
11. d   **12.** a   **13.** a   **14.** a   **15.** a
16. d

CHAPTER 5

SECTION I: ASSESSING YOUR UNDERSTANDING

Activity A

1. challenging, damaging, threatening
2. dead, diseased, injured
3. hypothalamus
4. synthesize enzymes, transform energy, grow and reproduce
5. level of education
6. constancy, homeostasis, stress, and adaptation
7. blood pressure, acid–base balance, blood glucose levels, body temperature, fluid and electrolyte balance
8. redness, heat, swelling, pain, loss of function

Activity B

1. When the body suffers an injury, the response is *maladaptive* if the defense mechanisms have a negative effect on health.

2. *Hyperpnea* is the body's development of rapid breathing after intense exercise in response to an accumulation of lactic acid in muscle tissue and a deficit of oxygen.
3. Examples of acute, *time-limited* stressors may include taking an examination, giving a speech, or driving in a snowstorm. Examples of chronic, *enduring* stressors may include poverty, a handicap or disability, or living with an alcoholic.
4. **a.** Examples of day-to-day stressors may include traffic jam, sick child, missed appointment, car would not start, or train is late.
    b. Examples of major events affecting large groups of people could include earthquakes, wars, terrorism, or events of history.
    c. Examples of infrequent, significant events in a person's life would include marriage, birth, death, or retirement.
5. Adolph Meyer, in the 1930s, first showed a correlation between illness and critical life events. A Recent Life Changes Questionnaire (RLCQ) was developed by Holmes and Rahe (1967) that assigned numerical values to life events requiring a change in a person's life pattern. A correlation was seen between illness and the number of stressful events; the higher the numerical value, the greater the chance for becoming ill.
6. Internal cognitive appraisal refers to the evaluation of an event relative to what is at stake and what coping resources are available. External resources consist of money to purchase services and materials and social support systems that provide emotional and esteem support.
7. Hans Selye stated that "stress is essentially the rate of wear and tear on the body." He also defined stress as being a "nonspecific response" of the body regardless of the stimulus producing the response.
8. Answer should include six of the following: hypertension, diseases of the heart and blood vessels, kidney diseases, rheumatic and rheumatoid arthritides, inflammation of the skin and eyes, infections, allergic and hypersensitivity diseases, nervous and mental diseases, sexual dysfunction, digestive diseases, metabolic diseases, and cancer.
9. Answer can include anxiety, ineffective coping patterns, impaired thought processes, disrupted relationships, impaired adjustment, ineffective coping, social isolation, risk for spiritual distress, and decisional conflict.
10. People with positive energy and a healthy outlook on life typically perceive stressors as interesting, challenging, meaningful, and opportunities for change and growth.
11. Physical stressors include cold, heat, and chemical agents; physiologic stressors include pain and fatigue. An example of a psychosocial stressor is fear (e.g., fear of failing an examination, losing a job, waiting for a diagnostic test result).

Activity C
1. b   **2.** a   **3.** a   **4.** a   **5.** b
6. a   **7.** b   **8.** a

SECTION II: APPLYING YOUR KNOWLEDGE
Activity D
1. The goal of relaxation training is to produce a response that counters the stress response. When this goal is achieved, the action of the hypothalamus adjusts, decreasing sympathetic and parasympathetic nervous system activity.
2. Commonly used techniques include progressive muscle relaxation, the Benson relaxation response, and relaxation with guided imagery. Other relaxation techniques include meditation, breathing techniques, massage, Reiki, music therapy, biofeedback, and the use of humor.
3. The different relaxation techniques share four similar elements: (1) a quiet environment; (2) a comfortable position; (3) a passive attitude; and (4) a mental device (something on which to focus one's attention, such as a word, phrase, or sound).

SECTION III: PRACTICING FOR NCLEX
Activity E
1. b   **2.** c   **3.** a   **4.** a, c, d
5. a   **6.** a, b, c   **7.** b   **8.** d
9. c   **10.** a, c, d   **11.** d   **12.** a, c, d
13. b, c, d   **14.** a, b, d   **15.** a   **16.** d

CHAPTER 6

SECTION I: ASSESSING YOUR UNDERSTANDING
Activity A
1. genotype; phenotype
2. chromosomes; autosomes; sex chromosomes; X chromosomes; one X and one Y chromosome; one sex chromosome of each pair
3. 80, 50
4. Down syndrome
5. One in every 160, 50
6. Hemochromatosis (iron overload)
7. Genomics
8. 46
9. Sickle cell disease
10. Neural tube defects
11. heart disease, diabetes, arthritis

Activity B
1. *Genomic medicine* encompasses the recognition that multiple genes work in concert with environmental influences, resulting in the appearance and expression of disease.
2. See Chart 6-1, Essential Nursing Competencies for Genetics and Genomics.

3. Answer may include five of the following: heart disease, high blood pressure, cancer, osteoarthritis, neural tube defects, spina bifida, and anencephaly.
4. *Pharmacogenetics* involves the use of genetic testing to identify genetic variations that relate to the safety and efficacy of medications and gene-based treatments.
5. Nursing activities may include collecting and helping interpret relevant family and medical histories, identifying patients and families who need genetic evaluation and counseling, offering genetic information and resources, collaborating with the genetic specialist, and participating in management of patient care.

Activity C
PART I: Terminology
1. e   **2.** h   **3.** f   **4.** a   **5.** g
6. d   **7.** b   **8.** a

PART II: Adult-Onset Disorders
1. b   **2.** c   **3.** e   **4.** d   **5.** a
6. a   **7.** d   **8.** f

SECTION II: APPLYING YOUR KNOWLEDGE
Activity D
1. Maggie has an increased risk of pregnancy loss and of having children with an unbalanced chromosomal arrangement, which may result in physical or mental disabilities.
2. The nurse may suggest that Maggie and Josh explore prenatal counseling and testing.
3. FISH is used to detect small abnormalities and to characterize chromosomal rearrangements.

SECTION III: PRACTICING FOR NCLEX
Activity E
1. a   **2.** c   **3.** a   **4.** c   **5.** a
6. a   **7.** c   **8.** b   **9.** a   **10.** a

CHAPTER 7

SECTION I: ASSESSING YOUR UNDERSTANDING
Activity A
1. use of tobacco, use of alcohol, improper diet, physical inactivity
2. social, economic, environmental
3. obesity, hypertension, diabetes
4. developmental, acquired, age associated

Activity B
1. The presence of a prolonged course, the inability of a condition to resolve spontaneously, and the unlikely or rare possibility of a cure.
2. Refer to section "Implications of Managing Chronic Conditions" in the textbook.

3. Answers may include preventing the occurrence of other chronic conditions; alleviating and managing symptoms; preventing, adapting, and managing disabilities; preventing and managing crises and complications; adapting to repeated threats and progressive functional loss; and living with isolation and loneliness.

4. Promote hepatitis B immunization to prevent liver cancer and promote screening, and promote screening, immunization with the HPV vaccine, and early treatment of precancerous lesions to prevent cervical cancer.

5. A *disability* is an umbrella term for impairments, activity limitations, participation restrictions, and environmental factors. An *impairment* is a loss or abnormality in body structure or physiologic function.

6. Refer to section "Nursing Care of Patients with Chronic Conditions" in the textbook.

7. Refer to section "Federal Legislation" in the textbook.

Activity C

1. Explain that medical conditions are associated with psychological and social problems that can affect body image and alter lifestyles.

2. Explain that chronic conditions have acute, stable, and unstable periods; flare-ups; and remissions. Each phase requires different types of management.

3. Explain that complying with a therapeutic treatment plan requires time, knowledge, and a long-term commitment to prevent the incidence of complications.

4. Explain that the whole family experiences stress and caretaker fatigue. Social changes that can occur include loss of income, role reversals, and altered socialization activities.

SECTION II: APPLYING YOUR KNOWLEDGE

Activity D

1. Refer to section "Barriers to Health Care" in the textbook.

2. Refer to section "Federal Assistance Programs" in the textbook.

SECTION III: PRACTICING FOR NCLEX

Activity E

1. b	2. a	3. b	4. a	5. b
6. c	7. a	8. b	9. c	10. d

CHAPTER 8

SECTION I: ASSESSING YOUR UNDERSTANDING

Activity A

1. calcium
2. macular degeneration
3. thinking, problem solving; verbal
4. Depression
5. Falls
6. Medicare

Activity B

1. *Geriatric syndromes* refer to common conditions found in the older adult that tend to be multifactorial and do not fall under discrete disease categories, such as falls, delirium, frailty, dizziness, and urinary incontinence.

2. myocardial hypertrophy, fibrosis, valvular stenosis, decreased pacemaker cells, reduced stroke volume

3. Decreased cardiac output, and decreased perfusion of the liver.

4. pneumonia, urinary tract infections, tuberculosis, gastrointestinal infections, skin infections

5. *Continuing care retirement communities* (CCRCs) provide three levels of living arrangements and care and provide for "aging in place." CCRCs consist of independent single-dwelling houses or apartments for people who can manage all of their day-to-day needs; assisted living apartments for those who need limited assistance with their daily living needs; and skilled nursing services when continuous nursing assistance is required. CCRCs usually contract for a large down payment before the resident moves into the community. This payment gives a person or couple the option of residing in the same community from the time of total independence through the need for assisted or skilled nursing care. Decisions about living arrangements and health care can be made before any decline in health status occurs. CCRCs also provide continuity at a time in an older adult's life when many other factors, such as health status, income, and availability of friends and family members, may be changing.

6. Refer to section "Cognitive Aspects of Aging" in the textbook.

7. A comprehensive assessment that begins with a thorough medication history, including use of alcohol, recreational drugs, and OTC and herbal medications, is essential. It is best to ask the patient or reliable informants to provide all medications for review. Assessing the patient's understanding of when and how to take each medication as well as the purpose of each medication allows the nurse to assess the patient's knowledge about and compliance with the medication regimen. The patient's beliefs and concerns about the medications should be identified, including beliefs on whether a given medication is helpful.

8. Vascular dementia.

9. Refer to section "Social Services" in the textbook.

10. Refer to section "Health Care Costs of Aging" in the textbook.

11. Refer to section "Ethical and Legal Issues Affecting the Older Adult" in the textbook.

12. Refer to section "Ethical and Legal Issues Affecting the Older Adult" in the textbook.

SECTION II: APPLYING YOUR KNOWLEDGE

Activity C

CASE STUDY: Loneliness

1. A deterioration of self-concept, a loss of self-esteem, and extensive grief over frequently occurring losses.
2. Applying ointment to the skin several times a day, avoiding overexposure to the sun, and patting the skin dry instead of rubbing it with a towel.
3. The sense of smell diminishes as a result of neurologic changes and environmental factors such as smoking, medications, and vitamin B_{12} deficiencies. The ability to recognize sweet, sour, bitter, or salty foods diminishes over time, altering satisfaction with food. Salivary flow does not decrease in healthy adults, but about 30% of older adults may experience a dry mouth as a result of medications and diseases. Difficulties with chewing and swallowing are generally associated with lack of teeth and disease.
4. 60 g.
5. Keep personal items stored at a level between the hips and eyes, make certain that all shoes fit securely, avoid climbing and bending.

CASE STUDY: Alzheimer's Disease

1. Providing a calm and predictable environment.
2. Maintaining personal dignity and autonomy is still an important part of Mr. Thomas's life.
3. Alzheimer's support groups are available. Socializing with old friends may be comforting. Alzheimer's disease does not eliminate the need for intimacy.
4. Pneumonia, malnutrition, and dehydration.

CASE STUDY: Dehydration

1. Make sure that the environmental temperature is adequate, palpate Mrs. Vega's skin periodically to assess for warmth, and place extra blankets at her bedside in case she becomes cold, especially in the evening.
2. Offer the patient the use of the bedpan or bedside commode frequently. Immediately change wet pads and use skin barrier cream to avoid redness and breakdown.
3. Sitting in a rocking chair discourages hypostatic pulmonary congestion, increases pulmonary ventilation, and improves venous return through contraction of the calf muscles.

SECTION III: PRACTICING FOR NCLEX

Activity D

1. a	**2.** a, c, d	**3.** a	**4.** c	**5.** a
6. b	**7.** c	**8.** a	**9.** c	**10.** b, d, e

CHAPTER 9

SECTION I: ASSESSING YOUR UNDERSTANDING

Activity A

1. duration, location, etiology
2. Acute, chronic (nonmalignant), cancer related
3. pain threshold; pain tolerance
4. longer than 6 months
5. respiratory depression; 24; 6 and 12
6. enkephalin

Activity B

1. Refer to Chart 9-2, Patient Education: Educating Patients and Their Families How to Use a Pain Rating Scale, in the textbook.
2. The suppression of immune function that promotes tumor growth
3. histamine, bradykinin, acetylcholine, serotonin, substance P
4. past experiences with pain, anxiety, culture, age, gender, genetics, expectations about pain relief
5. intensity, timing, location, quality, personal meaning of pain, aggravating and alleviating factors, pain behaviors
6. tachycardia, hypertension, tachypnea, pallor, diaphoresis, mydriasis, hypervigilance, increased muscle tone
7. *Balanced analgesia* refers to the use of more than one form of analgesia concurrently to obtain more pain relief with fewer side effects.
8. A *placebo effect* occurs when a person responds to a medication or treatment because of an expectation that the treatment will work rather than the treatment's actual effectiveness.
9. Answer may include massage, thermal therapies, transcutaneous electrical, distraction, relaxation techniques, guided imagery, and music therapy.
10. Acute pain lasts from seconds to 3 to 6 weeks (e.g., appendectomy, ankle sprain). Chronic, persistent, nonmalignant pain lasts 6 months or longer (e.g., rheumatoid arthritis, fibromyalgia). Cancer-related pain can be directly associated with the cancer and/or the result of cancer treatment (e.g., ovarian and lung cancer).
11. Refer to Chart 9-5, Use of Opioids, in the textbook.
12. See the section "Opioid Analgesic Agents" in the textbook.
13. Refer to section "Patient-Controlled Analgesia" in the textbook.
14. Distraction, which involves focusing the patient's attention on something other than the pain, reduces the perception of pain by stimulating the descending control system. This results in the transmission of fewer painful stimuli to the brain.

Activity C

1. f	**2.** j	**3.** a	**4.** h	**5.** b
6. g	**7.** c	**8.** i	**9.** e	**10.** d

SECTION II: APPLYING YOUR KNOWLEDGE

Activity D

CASE STUDY: Pain Experience

1. It will be brief in duration.
2. Muscle tension.
3. Promoting relaxation, playing music or watching a video, using cutaneous stimulation.
4. Clarify that Courtney knows what type of pain signals a problem, remind her that acute pain may persist for several days, review methods of pain management.

SECTION III: PRACTICING FOR NCLEX

Activity E

1. b	**2.** b	**3.** c	**4.** a	**5.** a
6. a	**7.** c	**8.** c	**9.** b	**10.** b
11. d	**12.** c, d, e	**13.** d	**14.** c	**15.** c
16. d	**17.** d	**18.** c	**19.** a	

CHAPTER 10

SECTION I: ASSESSING YOUR UNDERSTANDING

Activity A

1. 66%, potassium; intravascular, interstitial, transcultural; sodium; 50%, 6, plasma. (Refer to Table 13-1, Concentrations of Extracellular and Intracellular Electrolytes in Adults, in the textbook.)
2. bones; soft tissue
3. 7.35 to 7.45
4. 6.8 on the lower range, 7.8 on the upper range
5. 1.5
6. 8
7. 95%
8. osmolality, affects the movement of water between fluid compartments
9. thirst, antidiuretic hormone, renin–angiotensin–aldosterone
10. muscle contraction and the transmission of nerve impulses
11. bicarbonate–carbonic acid buffer system
12. tetany

Activity B

PART I

1. *Osmotic pressure* is the amount of hydrostatic pressure needed to stop the flow of water by osmosis. It is primarily determined by the concentration of solutes.
2. *Urine specific gravity* measures the kidney's ability to excrete or conserve water. *Blood urea nitrogen,* made up of urea, is an end product of protein (muscle and dietary) metabolism by the liver. *Creatinine,* as the end product of muscle metabolism, is a better indicator of renal function than blood urea nitrogen.

3. *Baroreceptors,* which are responsible for monitoring the circulating volume, are small nerve receptors that detect changes in pressure within blood vessels. *Osmoreceptors* sense changes in sodium concentration.
4. Calcium levels are primarily regulated by the combined actions of parathyroid hormone and vitamin D.
5. Metastatic calcification of soft tissue, joints, and arteries.
6. Na $\times$ 2 = glucose divided by 18 + BUN divided by 3.
7. Intense supervision is required because only small volumes are needed to elevate the serum sodium from dangerously low levels.
8. Answer may include dyspnea, cyanosis, a weak pulse, hypotension, unresponsiveness, and pain (chest, shoulder, low back).

PART II

1.

a. Low	**b.** Low	**c.** High	**d.** High	**e.** High
f. Low	**g.** High	**h.** Low	**i.** Low	**j.** High
k. High	**l.** Low			

2.

a. Low	**b.** High	**c.** Low	**d.** Low	**e.** High
f. Low	**g.** Low	**h.** Low	**i.** Low	**j.** High
k. Low	**l.** High			

3.

a. High	**b.** Low	**c.** High	**d.** High	**e.** Low
f. High	**g.** Low	**h.** Low		

4.

a. Low	**b.** High	**c.** Low	**d.** Low	**e.** Low

5.

a. Low	**b.** High	**c.** Low	**d.** Low	**e.** High

6.

a. R-ACID	**b.** M-ACID	**c.** M-ACID	**d.** R-ACID
e. R-ALKA	**f.** R-ACID	**g.** M-ACID	**h.** M-ALKA
i. M-ALKA	**j.** R-ALKA		

Activity C

1. f	**2.** d	**3.** c	**4.** b	**5.** a
6. e				

SECTION II: APPLYING YOUR KNOWLEDGE

Activity D

CASE STUDY: Extracellular Fluid Volume Deficit

1. A drop in postural blood pressure.
2. The nurse should obtain orthostatic vital signs to include blood pressure and pulse with the patient lying down, then sitting up, and then standing.
3. Monitoring urinary output to assess kidney perfusion, positioning the patient flat in bed with legs elevated to maintain adequate circulating volume, teaching leg exercises to promote venous return and prevent orthostatic hypotension when the patient stands.

CASE STUDY: Congestive Heart Failure

1. A full pulse, edema, and neck vein distention.
2. Rapid weight gain.
3. Auscultating for abnormal breath sounds, inspecting for leg edema, and weighing the patient daily.

CASE STUDY: Diabetes

1. Metabolic acidosis.
2. Hypertension, lethargy, and hypokalemia.
3. Hyperkalemia.
4. Sodium bicarbonate.

CASE STUDY: Intravenous Therapy

1. Air embolism, febrile reaction, and circulatory overload.
2. Subclavian or internal jugular.
3. Total volume divided by the total time equals the mL/h.

SECTION III: PRACTICING FOR NCLEX

Activity E

1. a	**2.** c	**3.** c	**4.** b	**5.** c
6. a	**7.** b	**8.** b, c, e	**9.** a, c, d	**10.** c
11. a, c, d	**12.** a	**13.** c	**14.** a	**15.** c
16. a	**17.** b	**18.** c	**19.** b	**20.** d
21. c				

CHAPTER 11

SECTION I: ASSESSING YOUR UNDERSTANDING

Activity A

1. inadequate tissue perfusion; poor oxygen and nutrient delivery, cellular starvation, cell death, organ dysfunction leading to organ failure, eventual death
2. glucose; adenosine triphosphate (ATP)
3. blood volume, cardiac pump, vasculature
4. stroke volume, heart rate; diameter of the arterioles
5. carotid sinus, aortic arch; aortic arch, carotid arteries
6. cellular, tissue
7. lactated Ringer solution, 0.9% sodium chloride solution (normal saline solution)
8. B-type natriuretic peptide (BNP)

Activity B

1. *Mean arterial pressure (MAP)* is the average pressure at which blood flows through the vasculature. MAP must exceed 65 mm Hg.
2. Limit additional myocardial damage, increase cardiac contractility, and decrease ventricular afterload.
3. Loss of sympathetic tone and release of biochemical mediators from cells.
4. Spinal cord injury, spinal anesthesia, the depressant action of medications, and glucose deficiency.

Activity C

1. c	**2.** a	**3.** a	**4.** e	**5.** f
6. d	**7.** c	**8.** b	**9.** b	**10.** e

SECTION II: APPLYING YOUR KNOWLEDGE

Activity D

CASE STUDY: Hypovolemic Shock

1. 700 to 1500 mL of blood.
2. In the compensatory stage of shock, the BP remains within normal limits. Vasoconstriction, increased heart rate, and increased contractility of the heart contribute to maintaining adequate cardiac output.
3. Output <30 mL/h.
4. Colloids, Ringer lactate, and normal saline.

CASE STUDY: Septic Shock

1. Temperature >38.3°C (>101°F) or <36°C (<96.8°F), tachycardia, tachypnea, and a white blood cell (WBC) count >12,000 cells/mm^3, <4000 cells/mm^3, or >10% immature WBC (bands).
2. Lactic acidosis, oliguria, altered level of consciousness, thrombocytopenia, and altered hepatic function.
3. Urine, blood, sputum, and wound drainage.
4. Cardiovascular overload and pulmonary edema.

SECTION III: PRACTICING FOR NCLEX

Activity E

1. b, c, d	**2.** c	**3.** d	**4.** b	**5.** a, d, e
6. a, b, c	**7.** c	**8.** d	**9.** d	**10.** d
11. a	**12.** a, b, c	**13.** b	**14.** b	**15.** c
16. d	**17.** d	**18.** b	**19.** d	**20.** d

CHAPTER 12

SECTION I: ASSESSING YOUR UNDERSTANDING

Activity A

1. lung, prostate, colorectal area; breast, lung, colorectal area.
2. Carcinoembryonic antigen (CEA), prostate-specific antigen (PSA)
3. lymph, blood
4. 75%
5. tobacco
6. Cabbage, broccoli, cauliflower. Fats, alcohol, salt-cured and smoked meats (ham), nitrite/nitrate-containing foods (bacon and red and processed meats)
7. nausea, vomiting
8. leukopenia, neutropenia, anemia, thrombocytopenia; infection, bleeding
9. cisplatin, methotrexate, mitramycin

Activity B

1. Cancer begins when an abnormal cell, after being transformed by the genetic mutation of DNA, forms a clone and begins to proliferate abnormally, ignoring growth-regulating signals.

2. Breast and ovarian cancer syndrome (*BRCA1* and *BRCA2*), and multiple endocrine neoplasia syndrome (*MEN1* and *MEN2*)

3. Answer should include four of the following: mouth, pharynx, larynx, esophagus, liver, colorectum, and breast.

4. Antibodies produced by B-lymphocytes, lymphokines, macrophages, natural killer (NK) cells, and T-lymphocytes

5. Answer should include three from each of the following choices:
   a. Skin: alopecia, erythema, desquamation
   b. Oral mucosal membrane: xerostomia, stomatitis, decreased salivation, loss of taste
   c. Stomach or colon: anorexia, nausea, vomiting, diarrhea
   d. Bone marrow–producing sites: anemia, leukopenia, and thrombocytopenia

6. Answer should include five of the following: redness; pain; swelling; a mottled appearance; phlebitis; loss of blood return; resistance to flow; tissue necrosis; or damage to underlying tendons, nerves, and blood vessels.

Activity C

PART I

1. a	**2.** b	**3.** f	**4.** e	**5.** d
6. g	**7.** h	**8.** c		

PART II

1. b	**2.** a	**3.** a	**4.** b	**5.** b

PART III

Refer to Table 12-7, Select Antineoplastic Agents, in the textbook.

1. a; bone marrow suppression
2. c; nausea, vomiting, and diarrhea
3. f; masculinization and feminization
4. a; bone marrow suppression
5. b; delayed and cumulative myelosuppression
6. d; bone marrow suppression
7. a; nausea, vomiting, and cystitis
8. c; proctitis, stomatitis, and renal toxicity
9. e; neuropathies
10. h; bone marrow suppression
11. g; hepatotoxicity

SECTION II: APPLYING YOUR KNOWLEDGE

Activity D

CASE STUDY: Cancer of the Breast

1. Genetics.
2. Attitudes toward her body image, feelings of self-esteem, and social and sexual values.
3. Denial.
4. Tissue manipulation during surgery, apprehension regarding the prognosis of her condition, and anger stemming from her change in body image.
5. Her lungs may possibly produce more mucus, the skin at the treatment area may become red and inflamed, she may tire more easily and require additional rest periods.
6. Handle the area gently, avoid irritation with soap and water, wear loose-fitting clothing.
7. Bone marrow depression, altered nutrition, leukopenia.

CASE STUDY: Cancer of the Lung

1. Denial.
2. Answer questions and concerns, identify resources and support people, communicate and share concerns, help frame questions for the primary provider.
3. Weight loss.
4. Elevated white blood cell count.

SECTION III: PRACTICING FOR NCLEX

Activity E

1. a	**2.** a, b, c	**3.** c	**4.** a	**5.** c
6. b	**7.** c	**8.** b	**9.** a	**10.** d
11. b	**12.** b	**13.** a	**14.** d	**15.** a
16. a				

CHAPTER 13

SECTION I: ASSESSING YOUR UNDERSTANDING

Activity A

1. Kübler-Ross, *On Death and Dying*
2. Hospice
3. Interdisciplinary collaboration
4. Palliative Performance Scale
5. bronchodilators, corticosteroids
6. Complicated or prolonged grief

Activity B

1. Structure and process, physical aspects, psychological and psychiatric, social, cultural, care of the imminently dying, ethical and legal, and spiritual/religious/existential.
2. *Palliative care* and *hospice care* involve coordinated programs of interdisciplinary services provided by professional caregivers and trained volunteers to patients with serious, progressive illnesses who are not responsive to curative treatments. However, palliative care does not focus primarily on preparation for death, as does hospice care.
3. dyspnea, cough, anxiety, and delirium
4. Durable power of attorney for health care—a legal document through which the signer appoints and authorizes another person to make medical decisions on the signer's behalf when the signer is no longer able to speak for themselves. This is also known as a health care power of attorney or a proxy directive. Living will—a type of advance directive in which the person documents treatment preferences. It provides instructions for care in the event that the signer is terminally ill and not able to communicate their wishes directly and often is

accompanied by a durable power of attorney for health care. This is also known as a medical directive or treatment directive.

5. Cancer (26%), cardiac diseases (15%), pulmonary conditions (9%), neurologic diagnoses (9%), and infectious causes (7%)

SECTION II: APPLYING YOUR KNOWLEDGE
Activity C

1. Refer to the section "Anorexia and Cachexia at the End of Life" in the textbook.
2. The nurse can make a referral to hospice.

SECTION III: PRACTICING FOR NCLEX
Activity D

1. b	**2.** c	**3.** c	**4.** d	**5.** d
6. a	**7.** d	**8.** d	**9.** c	**10.** a, b, c

CHAPTER 14

SECTION I: ASSESSING YOUR UNDERSTANDING
Activity A

1. when the decision to do surgery is made, is transferred onto the operating room table
2. is transferred to the operating room table, the patient is admitted to the PACU
3. the number and severity of coexisting health problems, the nature and duration of the operative procedure
4. respiratory, cardiac
5. hypoglycemia, hyperglycemia, acidosis, glucosuria
6. 7 to 10; inhibiting platelet aggregation

Activity B

1. it is invasive, it requires sedation or anesthesia, it involves radiation, and/or it has more than a slight risk of potential harm
2. dehydration, hypovolemia, electrolyte imbalances
3. improve circulation, prevent venous stasis, promote optimal respiratory function
4. Refer to Chart 14-3, Selected Risk Factors: Surgical Complications, in the textbook.

Activity C

Refer to Table 14-2, Nutrients Important for Wound Healing, in the textbook.

1. d	**2.** a	**3.** e	**4.** c	**5.** b

Activity D

Medication Administration

Refer to Table 14-3, Examples of Medications with the Potential to Affect the Surgical Experience, in the textbook.

Preoperative Nursing

A wide range of interventions is used to prepare the patient physically and psychologically and to maintain safety. Beginning with the nursing history and physical examination, listing of medications taken routinely, allergies, surgical and anesthetic histories, the patient's overall health status, and level of experience and understanding may be established. For more information, refer to section "Preoperative Nursing Interventions" in the textbook.

SECTION II: APPLYING YOUR KNOWLEDGE
Activity E

1. Instruct the patient about diaphragmatic breathing, coughing, leg exercises, turning to the side, and how to get out of the bed. For more information, see Chart 14-5, Patient Education: Preoperative Instructions to Prevent Postoperative Complications, in the textbook.
2. Ingesting even moderate amounts of alcohol prior to surgery can weaken a patient's immune system and increase the likelihood of developing postoperative infections. In addition, the use of illicit drugs and alcohol may impede the effectiveness of some medications. People who abuse drugs or alcohol frequently deny or attempt to hide it. In such situations, the nurse who is obtaining the patient's health history needs to ask frank questions with patience, care, and a nonjudgmental attitude. See Chapter 4 for an assessment of alcohol and drug use.
3. Patients who smoke are urged to stop 4 to 8 weeks before surgery to significantly reduce pulmonary and wound healing complications. Preoperative smoking cessation interventions can be effective in changing smoking behavior and reducing the incidence of postoperative complications. Patients who smoke are more likely to experience poor wound healing, a higher incidence of surgical site infection, and complications that include venous thromboembolism and pneumonia.

SECTION III: PRACTICING FOR NCLEX
Activity F

1. c	**2.** b	**3.** a	**4.** c	**5.** a
6. a	**7.** a	**8.** c	**9.** a	**10.** b
11. a	**12.** a, b, c	**13.** d	**14.** a	**15.** a
16. c, d, e	**17.** d	**18.** c	**19.** d	**20.** c

CHAPTER 15

SECTION I: ASSESSING YOUR UNDERSTANDING
Activity A

1. warning signs
2. smoke evacuator
3. the subarachnoid space at the lumbar level (usually between L4 and L5)
4. epidural
5. 104°F or 42°C
6. quiet environment
7. sodium citrate/citric acid

Activity B

1. *Restricted zone*: area in the operating room where scrub attire and surgical masks are required; includes operating room and sterile core areas. *Semirestricted zone*: area in the operating room where scrub attire is required; may include areas where surgical instruments are processed. *Unrestricted zone*: area in the operating room that interfaces with other departments; includes patient reception area and holding area.
2. Anesthesia is reduced with age because the percentage of fatty tissue increases as one gets older. Fatty tissue has an affinity for anesthetic agents.
3. Handling tissue, providing exposure at the operative field, suturing, maintaining hemostasis
4. Answer may include five of the following: exposure to blood and body fluids, hazards associated with laser beams, exposure to latex and adhesive substances, exposure to radiation and toxic agents, faulty equipment, improper use of equipment, surgical plume (smoke generated by electrosurgical cautery), cuts, needlestick injuries.
5. Complete return of sensation in the patient's toes, in response to a pinprick, indicates recovery.
6. nausea and vomiting, anaphylaxis, hypoxia, hypothermia, malignant hypothermia
7. Refer to section "Types of Anesthesia and Sedation" in the textbook.
8. Refer to Chart 18-1, Potential Adverse Effects of Surgery and Anesthesia, in the textbook.
9. The older adults have a variety of age-related cardiovascular and pulmonary changes as well as changes in the liver and kidneys. Refer to section "Gerontologic Considerations" in the textbook.
10. Refer to section "Health Hazards Associated with the Surgical Environment" in the textbook.
11. *Anesthesia awareness* is a condition in which patients are partially awake while under general anesthesia. Cardiac, obstetric, and major trauma patients are most at risk.

Activity C

Inhalation Anesthetic Agents

Refer to Table 15-1, Inhalation Anesthetic Agents, in the textbook.
1. d   2. b   3. a   4. c   5. e

Common Intravenous Medications

Refer to Table 15-2, Commonly Used Intravenous Medications, in the textbook.
1. d   2. b   3. a   4. c   5. e

SECTION II: APPLYING YOUR KNOWLEDGE

Activity D

CASE STUDY: General Anesthesia

1. fast recovery, low incidence of respiratory depression, rapid induction and recovery, not explosive or flammable

2. It may produce hypoxia
3. Respiratory depression, ECG abnormalities

CASE STUDY: Moderate Sedation

1. Moderate sedation involves the IV administration of sedatives or analgesic medications to reduce patient anxiety and control pain during diagnostic or therapeutic procedures.
2. The continual assessment of the patient's vital signs, level of consciousness, and cardiac and respiratory function is an essential component of moderate sedation. Pulse oximetry, ECG monitor, and frequent measurement of vital signs are used to monitor the patient.
3. The goal is to depress a patient's level of consciousness to a moderate level to enable surgical, diagnostic, or therapeutic procedures to be performed while ensuring the patient's comfort and cooperation during the procedure.

SECTION III: PRACTICING FOR NCLEX

Activity E

1. b	**2.** a	**3.** c	**4.** a, b, c	**5.** b
6. c	**7.** c	**8.** a	**9.** b, c, d	**10.** a, b, c
11. b	**12.** b	**13.** d	**14.** b	**15.** b
16. c	**17.** a	**18.** c	**19.** a	

CHAPTER 16

SECTION I: ASSESSING YOUR UNDERSTANDING

Activity A

1. respiratory function (ventilation); hypoxemia and hypercapnia
2. hypotension, shock, hemorrhage, hypertension, arrhythmias
3. respiratory
4. paralytic ileus and intestinal obstruction
5. bowel sounds, the passage of flatus
6. the stress response; muscle tension and local vasoconstriction
7. sympathetic activity; myocardial demand, oxygen consumption
8. blood viscosity, platelet aggregation; phlebothrombosis, pulmonary embolism

Activity B

1. The answer should include five of the following: medical diagnosis; type of surgery performed; patient's general condition, including age, airway patency, vital signs; anesthetic and other medications used; any intraoperative problems that might influence postoperative care (shock, hemorrhage, cardiac arrest); any pathology encountered; fluid given; patent IV site; blood loss and replacement; tubing, drains, catheters, or other supportive aids; and specific information about which surgeon or anesthesiologist wishes to be notified.

2. To monitor for cardiovascular stability, the nurse assesses the patient's level of consciousness; vital signs; cardiac rhythm; skin temperature, color, and moisture; and urine output. The nurse also assesses the patency of all IV lines.
3. Patient-controlled analgesia refers to self-administration of pain medication by way of intravenous or epidural routes within prescribed time/dosage limits.
4. Atelectasis and hypostatic pneumonia are reduced with early ambulation because ventilation is increased and the stasis of bronchial secretions in the lungs is reduced.
5. Wound *dehiscence* refers to the disruption of the wound or surgical incision. Wound *evisceration* refers to the protrusion of wound contents.
6. Pallor; cool, moist skin; tachypnea; cyanosis (lips, gums, tongue); rapid, weak, and thready pulse; narrowing pulse pressure; hypotension; and concentrated urine.
7. Refer to section "Managing Potential Complications" in the textbook.
8. Refer to Figure 16-3 and section "Determining Readiness for Postanesthesia Care Unit Discharge" in the textbook.
9. The respiratory depressive effects of opioids, decreased lung expansion secondary to pain, and decreased mobility are three conditions that put patients at risk for atelectasis, pneumonia, and hypoxemia.
10. See Table 16-3, Factors Affecting Wound Healing, and section "Caring for Wounds" in the textbook.

SECTION II: APPLYING YOUR KNOWLEDGE
Activity C
CASE STUDY: Hypopharyngeal Obstruction
1. The primary objective in the immediate postoperative period is to maintain ventilation and thus prevent hypoxemia and hypercapnia.
2. The signs of occlusion include choking; noisy and irregular respirations; decreased oxygen saturation scores; and within minutes, a blue dusky color of the skin.
3. The treatment of hypopharyngeal obstruction involves tilting the head back and pushing forward on the angle of the lower jaw, as if to push the lower teeth in front of the upper teeth. This maneuver pulls the tongue forward and opens the air passages.

CASE STUDY: Wound Healing
1. Surgical wound healing occurs in three phases: first-, second-, and third-intention wound healing.
2. Ongoing assessment of the surgical site involves inspection for approximation of wound edges, integrity of sutures or staples, redness, discoloration, warmth, swelling, unusual tenderness, or drainage. Inspect for a reaction to tape or trauma from tight bandages.

3. Pain, redness, and warmth.
4. Encouraging coughing and deep breathing to enhance pulmonary and cardiovascular function.

SECTION III: PRACTICING FOR NCLEX
Activity D
1. c	**2.** d	**3.** b	**4.** a	**5.** b, c, d
6. d	**7.** a	**8.** d	**9.** a	**10.** c
11. b	**12.** c	**13.** d	**14.** d	**15.** a
16. c	**17.** a, b, d	**18.** a	**19.** d	**20.** d

CHAPTER 17

SECTION I: ASSESSING YOUR UNDERSTANDING
Activity A
1. the *apneustic center* in the lower pons, the *pneumotaxic center* in the upper pons
2. 50
3. pleura
4. one less lobe
5. lobar bronchi, segmented bronchi, subsegmented bronchi, bronchioles
6. Type II cells
7. respiration
8. inspiratory reserve volume
9. 500
10. diffusion
11. low-pressure system
12. PaO_2

Activity B
1. *Ventilation* refers to the movement of air in and out of the airways, whereas *respiration* refers to gas exchange between atmospheric air and blood and between the blood and the cells of the body.
2. The epiglottis is a flap of cartilage that covers the opening of the larynx during swallowing.
3. Low or decreased compliance occurs with certain pathology. Answer should include four of the following: morbid obesity, atelectasis, pneumothorax, hemothorax, pulmonary fibrosis or edema, pleural effusion, ARDS.
4. *Partial pressure* is the pressure exerted by each type of gas (e.g., oxygen, carbon dioxide) in a mixture of gases.
5. Answer should include six of the following: dyspnea, cough, sputum production, chest pain, wheezing and hemoptysis, tachypnea, hypoxia.
6. Wheezing
7. Cheyne–Stokes respirations are characterized by alternating episodes of apnea (cessation of breathing) and periods of deep breathing. It is usually associated with heart failure and damage to the respiratory center.
8. Cilia move the mucus back to the larynx.

9. Contraction of bronchial smooth muscle, thickening of bronchial mucosa, airway obstruction, and loss of lung elasticity
10. Diffusion is the exchange of oxygen and carbon dioxide at the air–blood interface. Pulmonary perfusion is the actual flow of blood through the pulmonary circulation.

SECTION II: APPLYING YOUR KNOWLEDGE

Activity C

CASE STUDY: Bronchoscopy

1. Supplying information about the procedure, withholding food and fluids for at least 6 hours, ensuring that informed consent is obtained
2. Aspiration, infection, and pneumothorax
3. Monitor the patient's respiratory status and observe for hypoxia, hypotension, tachycardia, arrhythmias, hemoptysis, and dyspnea.
4. Offer ice chips and eventually fluids after the gag and cough reflex return.

CASE STUDY: Thoracentesis

1. Informing Mrs. Lomar about pressure sensations that will be experienced during the procedure, making sure that chest roentgenograms prescribed in advance have been completed, seeing that the consent form has been explained and signed
2. Sitting on the edge of the bed with the patient's feet supported and arms and head on a padded overbed table
3. Second and third intercostal space
4. Blood-tinged mucus, signs of hypoxemia, and tachycardia.

SECTION III: PRACTICING FOR NCLEX

Activity D

1. a	2. c, d, e	3. c	4. d	5. c, d, e
6. d	7. a	8. a	9. c	10. c
11. b	12. b	13. a, c, d	14. c	15. a, b, c
16. b	17. a	18. c	19. b	20. d

CHAPTER 18

SECTION I: ASSESSING YOUR UNDERSTANDING

Activity A

1. viral; hoarseness, aphonia, severe cough
2. symptom relief
3. Antihistamines
4. acute, subacute, chronic
5. Peritonsillar abscess
6. hemorrhage

Activity B

1. Rhinitis causes the nasal passages to become inflamed, congested, and edematous. The swollen conchae block the sinus openings and cause sinusitis.

2. *Streptococcus pneumoniae, Haemophilus influenzae, Staphylococcus aureus, Moraxella catarrhalis*
3. Answer should include four of the following: severe orbital cellulitis, subperiosteal abscess, cavernous sinus thrombosis, meningitis, encephalitis, and ischemic infarction.
4. Refer to section "The Patient with Upper Airway Infection" in the textbook.
5. Complications may include sepsis, a peritonsillar abscess, otitis media, sinusitis, and meningitis.
6. Obstructive sleep apnea is defined as frequent loud snoring and breathing cessation for 10 seconds or longer with five or more episodes per hour. This is followed by awakening abruptly with a loud snort when the blood oxygen level drops.
7. esophageal speech, an artificial larynx, tracheoesophageal puncture

Activity C

1. b	2. e	3. c	4. a	5. d

SECTION II: APPLYING YOUR KNOWLEDGE

Activity D

CASE STUDY: Tonsillectomy and Adenoidectomy

1. Bleeding from the surgical site.
2. Hemorrhage.
3. In the immediate postoperative period, the most comfortable position is prone, with the patient's head turned to the side to allow drainage from the mouth and pharynx.
4. Offer her soft foods for several days to minimize local discomfort and supply her with necessary nutrients.

CASE STUDY: Epistaxis

1. Gilberta should sit upright with her head tilted forward to prevent swallowing and aspiration of blood. She should also pinch the soft outer portion of the nose against the midline spectrum for 5 to 10 continuous minutes.
2. Application of nasal decongestants (phenylephrine, one or two sprays) to act as vasoconstrictors may be necessary.
3. The packing may remain in place for 3 to 4 days if necessary to control bleeding.

CASE STUDY: Cancer of the Larynx

1. Palpation of the neck for swelling.
2. "You will most likely have radiation or surgery."
3. A complete dental examination is performed to rule out any oral disease.

CASE STUDY: Laryngectomy

1. Supraglottic laryngectomy.
2. The nurse should inform him that there are ways he will be able to carry on a conversation without his voice, making sure that he knows he will require a permanent tracheal stoma, and reminding him that he will not be able to sing, whistle, or laugh.

3. One week.
4. The nurse should inform him that the laryngecto-my tube will be removed when the stoma is well healed.

SECTION III: PRACTICING FOR NCLEX

Activity E

1. b, c, d	**2.** a	**3.** a	**4.** c, d, e	**5.** a
6. a, b, c	**7.** a, b, d	**8.** c	**9.** a	**10.** b
11. c	**12.** d	**13.** d	**14.** b	**15.** a

CHAPTER 19

SECTION I: ASSESSING YOUR UNDERSTANDING

Activity A

1. 48
2. rifampin, pyrazinamide, ethambutol, isoniazid
3. empyema
4. Tachypnea, dyspnea, mild to moderate hypoxemia
5. silent aspiration
6. *Streptococcus pneumoniae, Haemophilus influenzae, Staphylococcus aureus*
7. alcoholism, chronic obstructive pulmonary disease (COPD), acquired immune deficiency syndrome (AIDS), diabetes, heart failure
8. hypotension, shock, respiratory failure
9. impaired central nervous system (CNS) function, neuromuscular, musculoskeletal, pulmonary dysfunction
10. ARDS

Activity B

1. Refer to Figure 19-1 and section "Atelectasis" in the textbook.
2. Dyspnea, cough, sputum production, tachycardia, tachypnea, pleural pain, and central cyanosis
3. Frequent turning, early mobilization, deep breath-ing maneuvers, assistance with the use of spirome-try, suctioning, postural drainage, aerosol nebulizer treatments, and chest percussion
4. *Superinfection* is suspected when a subsequent infection occurs with another bacterium during antibiotic therapy.
5. Hypoxemia that does not respond to supplemental oxygen
6. Enlargement of the right ventricle of the heart because of diseases affecting the structure or functions of the lung
7. Refer to Chart 19-9, Risk Factors for Acute Respiratory Distress Syndrome, in the textbook.

Activity C

1. d	**2.** c	**3.** f	**4.** b	**5.** a
6. e				

SECTION II: APPLYING YOUR KNOWLEDGE

Activity D

CASE STUDY: Community-Acquired Pneumonia

1. Provide Theresa with fluids, at least 1 L/day.
2. Fever, stabbing or pleuritic chest pain, tachypnea
3. Bronchospasm causes alveolar collapse, which decreases the surface area necessary for perfusion. Mucosal edema occludes the alveoli, thereby producing a drop in alveolar oxygen; venous blood is shunted from the right to the left side of the heart.
4. Atelectasis, hypotension and shock, and pleural effusion.

CASE STUDY: Tuberculosis

1. He has been exposed to *Mycobacterium tuberculosis* or has been vaccinated with BCG.
2. Sputum culture.
3. Rifampin.

CASE STUDY: Acute Respiratory Distress Syndrome

1. Arrhythmias and hypotension, contraction of the accessory muscles of respiration, tachypnea, and tachycardia.
2. Drowsiness, irritability, and confusion.
3. 44%.

CASE STUDY: Pulmonary Embolism

1. "Most of the time, the clots form from venous stasis due to immobility."
2. Dyspnea.
3. Cardiac output.

SECTION III: PRACTICING FOR NCLEX

Activity E

1. a, b, c	**2.** a	**3.** c	**4.** d	**5.** a
6. c	**7.** d	**8.** a	**9.** c	**10.** b
11. a	**12.** b	**13.** d	**14.** a	**15.** d
16. c	**17.** a, b, d, e	**18.** a	**19.** b	**20.** b

CHAPTER 20

SECTION I: ASSESSING YOUR UNDERSTANDING

Activity A

1. Cor pulmonale
2. Smoking
3. cigarette smoking
4. Spirometry
5. bullectomy
6. cessation of smoking
7. tracheobronchial infection, air pollution

8. *Streptococcus pneumoniae, Haemophilus influenzae*
9. allergy; cough, wheezing, dyspnea
10. status asthmaticus, respiratory failure, pneumonia, atelectasis
11. Chest physiotherapy

Activity B

1. Chronic inflammation results in the following: increased goblet cells and enlarged submucosal glands (proximal airways), inflammation and airway narrowing (peripheral airways), and narrowing of the airway lumen.
2. In the panlobular (panacinar) type of emphysema, there is destruction of the respiratory bronchiole, alveolar duct, and alveolus. All airspaces within the lobule are essentially enlarged, but there is little inflammatory disease. A hyperinflated (hyperexpanded) chest, marked dyspnea on exertion, and weight loss typically occur. In the centrilobular (centroacinar) form, pathologic changes take place mainly in the center of the secondary lobule, preserving the peripheral portions of the acinus (i.e., the terminal airway unit where gas exchange occurs). Frequently, there is a derangement of ventilation–perfusion ratios, producing chronic hypoxemia, hypercapnia, polycythemia (i.e., an increase in red blood cells), and episodes of right-sided heart failure. This leads to central cyanosis and respiratory failure. The patient also develops peripheral edema.
3. reduce symptoms, improve quality of life, and increase physical and emotional participation in everyday activities.
4. Chronic cough, sputum production, and dyspnea on exertion.
5. Answer should include five of the following: history of cigarette smoking, passive smoking exposure, age, rate of decline of FEV_1, hypoxemia, weight loss, reversibility of airflow obstruction, pulmonary artery pressure, and resting heart rate.
6. Alter smooth muscle tone, reduce airway obstruction, and improve alveolar ventilation

Activity C

1. f   **2.** c   **3.** e   **4.** d   **5.** b   **6.** a

SECTION II: APPLYING YOUR KNOWLEDGE

Activity D

CASE STUDY: Emphysema

1. "Air trapping" in the lungs
2. Dyspnea
3. Respiratory acidosis
4. Arrhythmias, central nervous system excitement, and tachycardia
5. Decreased respiratory rate, increased alveolar ventilation, and reduction of functional residual capacity
6. A Venturi mask that delivers a predictable oxygen flow at about 24%

SECTION III: PRACTICING FOR NCLEX

Activity E

1. b	**2.** a	**3.** b	**4.** a, b, c	**5.** b
6. d	**7.** a	**8.** c	**9.** d	**10.** d
11. c	**12.** a, c, d	**13.** a	**14.** c	**15.** c

CHAPTER 21

SECTION I: ASSESSING YOUR UNDERSTANDING

Activity A

1. 20, 10
2. Cholesterol, triglycerides, lipoproteins
3. atherosclerosis
4. size, contour, position
5. 2, 6
6. preload, afterload, contractility
7. hyperlipidemia, hypertension, diabetes
8. <70 mg/dL; <140/90 mm Hg; <110 mg/day; 18.5 to 24.9 kg/m^2
9. creatine kinase (CK), isoenzyme CK-MB; troponins T and I, myoglobin

Activity B

1. hypertension, CAD, heart failure, stroke, congenital cardiovascular defects
2. The atrioventricular (AV) valves separate the atria from the ventricles. The tricuspid separates the right atrium and ventricle; the bicuspid separates the left atrium and ventricle. The AV valves permit blood to flow from the atria into the ventricles. The semilunar valves are situated between each ventricle and its corresponding artery. The pulmonic valve is between the right ventricle and the pulmonary artery; the aortic valve is between the left ventricle and the aorta. These valves permit blood to flow from the ventricles into the arteries.
3. Depolarization is said to have occurred when the electrical difference between the inside and the outside of the cell is reduced. The inside of the cell becomes less negative, membrane permeability to calcium is increased, and muscle contraction occurs.
4. Cardiac output (stroke volume × heart rate) would equal 5320 mL.
5. Starling law of the heart refers to the relationship between increased stroke volume and increased ventricular end-diastolic volume for a given intrinsic contractility.
6. Physiologic effects of the aging process may include reduction in the size of the left ventricle, decreased elasticity and widening of the aorta, thickening and rigidity of cardiac valves, and increased connective tissue in the sinoatrial and atrioventricular nodes and bundle branches.

7. below the fifth intercostal space and lateral to the midclavicular line
8. Cardiac catheterization is used most frequently to assess the patency of the patient's coronary arteries and to determine readiness for coronary bypass surgery. It is also used to measure pressures in the various heart chambers and to determine oxygen saturation of the blood by sampling specimens.
9. Selective angiography refers to the technique of injecting a contrast medium into the vascular system to outline a particular heart chamber or blood vessel.
10. A lowered central venous pressure reading indicates that the patient is hypovolemic. Serial measurements are more reflective of a patient's condition and should be correlated with the patient's clinical status.
11. Answer should include any four of the following: infection, pulmonary artery rupture, pulmonary thromboembolism, pulmonary infarction, catheter kinking, arrhythmias, and air embolism.

Activity C

PART I

1. c   2. e   3. a   4. d   5. b
6. f

PART II

1. d   2. g   3. a   4. f   5. i
6. k   7. b   8. j   9. c   10. h
11. e

Activity D

	Pericarditis	Musculoskeletal Disorders
Duration of pain	Intermittent	Hours to days
Precipitating events and aggravating factors	Sudden onset; pain increases with inspiration, coughing, and trunk rotation	Most often follows respiratory tract infection with significant coughing, vigorous exercise, or posttrauma
		Some cases are idiopathic
		Exacerbated by deep inspiration, coughing, sneezing, and movement of upper torso or arms
Alleviating factors	Sitting upright, antispasmodic agents, and anti-inflammatory agents	Rest, ice, or heat

Analgesic or anti-inflammatory medications |

SECTION II: APPLYING YOUR KNOWLEDGE

Activity E

CASE STUDY: Cardiac Assessment for Chest Pain

1. Peripheral cyanosis
2. d
3. c
4. 45 degrees
5. Fifth intercostal space

SECTION III: PRACTICING FOR NCLEX

Activity F

1. a   2. c   3. d   4. a   5. b
6. c   7. d   8. d   9. c   10. a
11. a   12. b   13. c   14. b   15. a, b, c

CHAPTER 22

SECTION I: ASSESSING YOUR UNDERSTANDING

Activity A

1. arrhythmic
2. automaticity
3. conductivity
4. depolarization
5. diastole
6. Ablation
7. QT interval
8. 0.12, 0.20 seconds
9. premature atrial complex
10. atrial flutter
11. 100 bpm

Activity B

1. Atria, atrioventricular node or junction, sinus node, and ventricles.
2. Electrical conduction through the heart begins in the sinoatrial node (SA), travels across the atria to the atrioventricular node (AV), and then travels down the right and left bundle branches and Purkinje fibers to the ventricular muscle.
3. Answer should include five of the following: fever, hypovolemia, anemia, exercise, pain, congestive heart failure, anxiety, and sympathomimetic or parasympatholytic drugs.
4. Ventricular tachycardia occurs when there are more than three premature ventricular contractions (PVCs) in a row and the rate exceeds 100 bpm.
5. A thromboembolic event, heart failure, and cardiac arrest.
6. The difference is in the timing of the electrical current. With cardioversion, the current is synchronized with the patient's electrical events; with defibrillation, the current is unsynchronized and immediate.

7. The standard procedure is to place one paddle to the right of the upper sternum below the right clavicle and the other paddle just to the left of the cardiac apex.

8. An on-demand pacemaker is set for a specific rate and stimulates the heart when normal ventricular depolarization does not occur; the fixed-rate pacemaker stimulates the ventricle at a preset constant rate, independently of the patient's rhythm.

9. Small incisions are made throughout the atria so that scar tissue forms and prevents reentry conduction of the electrical impulse.

Activity C

1. b	**2.** d	**3.** f	**4.** h	**5.** g
6. e	**7.** c	**8.** a		

SECTION II: APPLYING YOUR KNOWLEDGE

Activity D

Graph Analysis

1.
   a. T wave
   b. PR interval
   c. P wave
   d. QRS complex
   e. ST segment
2.
   a. Q wave is larger.
   b. ST segment is elevated.
   c. T wave is inverted.

Graphic Recordings

1. P waves come early in cycle and close to T wave of previous heartbeat.
2. QRS complex is bizarre. P waves are hidden in QRS complexes.
3. Three or more PVCs in a row, occurring at a rate of 100 bpm.

Activity E

CASE STUDY: Permanent Pacemaker

1. Yes. Heart rate can vary as much as 5 bpm faster or slower than the preset rate.
2. Bleeding, hematoma formation, and infection.
3. Dislodgment of the pacing electrode.
4. The pacemaker model, date and time of insertion, location of pulse generator, stimulation threshold, pacer settings
5. Nursing interventions would include the education of the patient and sterile wound care. Expected outcomes are that Mr. Woo will be free from infection, adhere to a self-care program, maintain pacemaker function, understand signs and symptoms of infection and when to seek medical attention, assess pulse rate at regular intervals, and experience no abrupt changes in pulse rate or rhythm.

SECTION III: PRACTICING FOR NCLEX

Activity F

1. d	**2.** c	**3.** b	**4.** a	**5.** c
6. a	**7.** d	**8.** a	**9.** c	**10.** d
11. a, b, c	**12.** b	**13.** d	**14.** a	**15.** c

CHAPTER 23

SECTION I: ASSESSING YOUR UNDERSTANDING

Activity A

1. acute MI, sudden death
2. smoking
3. Oral contraceptive
4. 130/80
5. supplemental oxygen, aspirin, nitroglycerin, morphine
6. cardiovascular disease
7. atherosclerosis
8. chest pain referred to as *angina pectoris*
9. C-reactive protein
10. less than 200 mg/dL; 3.5:1.0; less than 100 mg/dL; greater than 40 mg/dL for males, 50 mg/dL for females; 150 mg/dL
11. focused
12. an elevated ST segment in two contiguous leads
13. greater saphenous vein
14. the formation of a thrombus

Activity B

1. Answer should include four of the following: hyperlipidemia, cigarette smoking, obesity, hypertension, diabetes, metabolic syndrome, and physical activity.
2. insulin resistance, central obesity, dyslipidemia, hypertension (>130/85 mm Hg), increased levels of C-reactive protein (proinflammation), and elevated fibrinogen levels (prothrombotic)
3. Answer should include three of the following: acute coronary syndrome or MI, arrhythmias, cardiac arrest, heart failure, and cardiogenic shock.
4. Answer should include four of the following: fever, pericardial pain, pleural pain, dyspnea, pericardial effusion, pericardial friction rub, and arthralgia.
5. An atheroma, also called plaque, is a fibrous cap of smooth muscle cells that form over lipid deposits within the arterial vessels, protrude and narrow the lumen, and then obstruct blood flow.
6. improve blood flow within a coronary artery by compressing the atheroma

Activity C

1. f	**2.** e	**3.** b	**4.** c	**5.** d
6. a				

SECTION II: APPLYING YOUR KNOWLEDGE

Activity D

CASE STUDY: Angina Pectoris

1. "There is not enough blood flow in your coronary arteries to get adequate oxygen to the heart muscle."
2. It is relieved by rest and is predictable.
3. Causing venous pooling throughout the body, dilating the coronary arteries to increase the oxygen supply, lowering systemic blood pressure.

4. Administer a third nitroglycerin and give her oxygen at 2 L/min via nasal cannula.

CASE STUDY: Decreased Myocardial Tissue Perfusion

1. The first hour after symptoms begin.
2. Enlarged T wave.
3. Elevations in troponin levels, CK-MB, and myoglobin.
4. Cardiogenic shock.

SECTION III: PREPARING FOR NCLEX

Activity E

1. a	**2.** c	**3.** a	**4.** c	**5.** b
6. a	**7.** b, c, d	**8.** b, c, d	**9.** b	**10.** c
11. c	**12.** a, b, c	**13.** c	**14.** a	**15.** a, b, c

CHAPTER 24

SECTION I: ASSESSING YOUR UNDERSTANDING

Activity A

1. systolic click
2. left ventricle; left atrium
3. stenosis
4. Commissurotomy
5. chordotomy
6. caffeine, alcohol, cigarettes
7. at the third and fourth intercostal spaces at the left sternal border; a blowing diastolic murmur
8. prophylactic antibiotics
9. penicillin therapy; rheumatic fever
10. streptococci, enterococci, pneumococci, staphylococci
11. digitalis; digitalis toxicity

Activity B

1. MVP is usually an inherited connective tissue disorder that causes enlargement of both mitral valve leaflets. Usually there are no symptoms. It can result in valve incompetency and regurgitation. As valve dysfunction progresses, symptoms of heart failure ensue.
2. Answer should include four of the following: congestive heart failure, ventricular arrhythmias, atrial arrhythmias, cardiac conduction defects, pulmonary or cerebral embolism, and valvular dysfunction.
3. Cardiomyopathy, ischemic heart disease, valvular disease, rejection of previously transplanted hearts, and congenital heart disease
4. An inflamed endothelium causes a fibrin clot to form (vegetation), which converts to scar tissue that thickens, contracts, and causes deformities. The result is leakage or valvular regurgitation and stenosis.
5. Myocarditis is an inflammatory process that usually results from an infection. The infectious process can cause heart dilation, thrombi formation, infiltration of blood cells around the coronary vessels and between the muscle fibers, and eventual degeneration of the muscle fibers themselves.
6. Listen at the left sternal edge of the thorax in the fourth intercostal space where the pericardium comes in contact with the left chest wall.
7. Answer should include six of the following: idiopathic, infection, disorders of connective tissue, sarcoidosis, hypersensitivity states, disorders of adjacent structures, neoplastic disease, radiation therapy of chest and upper torso, trauma, kidney failure, and uremia.

Activity C

1. a	**2.** e	**3.** d	**4.** b	**5.** c

SECTION II: APPLYING YOUR KNOWLEDGE

Activity D

CASE STUDY: Infective Endocarditis

1. Roth spots
2. The nurse should report headache; temporary or transient cerebral ischemia; and strokes, which may be caused by emboli to cerebral arteries. Embolization may be a presenting symptom; it may occur at any time and may involve other organ systems.
3. Five days

CASE STUDY: Acute Pericarditis

1. Pain may be relieved with a forward-leaning or sitting position.
2. Determine the cause, administer therapy for treatment and symptom relief, and detect early signs and symptoms of cardiac tamponade. When cardiac output is impaired, the patient should be placed on bed rest until fever, chest pain, and friction rub have subsided.
3. Left sternal edge in the fourth intercostal space.

SECTION III: PRACTICING FOR NCLEX

Activity E

1. a	**2.** a	**3.** c	**4.** b	**5.** d
6. b	**7.** c	**8.** c	**9.** b	**10.** a
11. a	**12.** b	**13.** b	**14.** a	**15.** b

CHAPTER 25

SECTION I: ASSESSING YOUR UNDERSTANDING

Activity A

1. venous return, ventricular compliance; the diameter/distensibility of the great vessels, the opening/competence of the semilunar valves
2. jugular venous distention, mean arterial blood pressure, a positive hepatojugular test
3. pulmonary embolism

4. dry and nonproductive
5. coronary artery disease, cardiomyopathy, hypertension, valvular disorders
6. dilated, hypertrophic, restrictive; dilated
7. dyspnea, cough, pulmonary crackles, low oxygen saturation, extra heart sound (ventricular gallop)
8. dependent edema, hepatomegaly, ascites, anorexia, nausea, weakness, weight gain (fluid retention)
9. Angiotensin-converting enzyme (ACE) inhibitors, beta-blockers, diuretics
10. hypoxia, acidosis, the accumulation of lactic acid

Activity B

1. Cardiac output equals the heart rate times the stroke volume (the amount of blood pumped out with each contraction).
2. Preload is the amount of myocardial stretch created by the volume of blood within the ventricle before systole. Afterload refers to the amount of resistance to the ejection of the blood from the ventricle.
3. Answer should include four of the following: symptomatic hypotension, hyperuricemia, ototoxicity, electrolyte imbalances, dizziness, and balance problems.
4. Older adults may not always detect or accurately interpret common symptoms of HF such as shortness of breath, or they may have atypical symptoms such as weakness and somnolence. Decreased renal function can make the older patient resistant to diuretics and more sensitive to changes in volume.
5. Atropine

Activity C

1. a	**2.** b	**3.** a	**4.** b	**5.** b
6. a	**7.** a	**8.** b	**9.** a	**10.** b

SECTION II: APPLYING YOUR KNOWLEDGE

Activity D

CASE STUDY: Pulmonary Edema

1. Rest decreases blood pressure, increases the heart reserve, and reduces the work of the heart.
2. The patient should maintain an upright position with the feet and legs dependent to reduce left ventricular workload.
3. Symptoms of toxicity include anorexia, bradycardia and tachycardia, nausea and vomiting. Mr. Wolman should call his doctor if any of these symptoms occur.
4. Bananas, raisins, and orange juice.

SECTION III: PRACTICING FOR NCLEX

Activity E

1. b	**2.** d	**3.** b	**4.** c	**5.** c
6. c, d, e	**7.** a	**8.** a	**9.** c	**10.** d
11. d	**12.** a, b, c, d	**13.** a	**14.** a	**15.** b

CHAPTER 26

SECTION I: ASSESSING YOUR UNDERSTANDING

Activity A

1. resistance vessels
2. intermittent claudication
3. C-reactive protein
4. edema, altered pigmentation, pain, stasis dermatitis
5. the use of tobacco products

Activity B

1. Pain, pallor, pulselessness, paresthesia, poikilothermia (coldness), and paralysis.
2. Venous stasis, vessel wall injury, and altered blood coagulation.
3. The rate of blood flow through a vessel is determined by dividing the pressure difference (ΔP) (arterial and venous) by the resistance to flow (R).
4. The pain in intermittent claudication is caused by the inability of the arterial system to provide adequate blood flow to the tissues in the phase of increased demands for oxygen and nutrients during exercise.
5. Refer to section "Thoracic Aortic Aneurysm."
6. Refer to Chart 26-6, Home Care Checklist: Foot and Leg Care in Peripheral Vascular Disease.
7. Chronic venous occlusion, pulmonary emboli from dislodged thrombi, valvular destruction, and venous obstruction.

Activity C

1. a	**2.** b	**3.** a	**4.** a	**5.** b
6. b	**7.** a	**8.** a		

SECTION II: APPLYING YOUR KNOWLEDGE

Activity D

CASE STUDY: Peripheral Arterial Occlusive Disease

1. Intermittent claudication.
2. The first step in determining the ABI is to have the patient rest in a supine position (not seated) for approximately 5 minutes. An appropriate-sized blood pressure cuff (typically, a 10-cm cuff) is applied to the patient's ankle above the malleolus. After identifying an arterial signal at the posterior tibial and dorsalis pedis arteries, the systolic pressures are obtained in both ankles while listening to the Doppler signal at each artery. Diastolic pressures in the ankles cannot be measured with Doppler. If pressure in these arteries cannot be measured, then pressure can be measured in the peroneal artery, which can also be assessed at the ankle.
3. A planned program involving systematic lowering of the extremity below heart level, Buerger–Allen exercises, and graded extremity exercises.

4. The examiner should use light touch and avoid using only the index finger for palpation, because this finger has the strongest arterial pulsation of all the fingers. The thumb should not be used for the same reason.

SECTION III: PRACTICING FOR NCLEX

Activity E

1. d	2. a, c, d	3. b	4. a, b, c	5. a, b, c
6. a	7. b	8. c	9. d	10. a
11. d	12. d	13. a, b, d	14. d	15. c
16. b				

CHAPTER 27

SECTION I: ASSESSING YOUR UNDERSTANDING

Activity A

1. cardiac output; peripheral resistance
2. heart rate; stroke volume
3. White Coat Hypertension
4. 130/80 mm Hg
5. vasoconstriction, high blood pressure, thrombosis, fibrosis, and inflammation
6. hypotension
7. rebound hypertension
8. Hypertensive emergency, hypertensive urgency

Activity B

1. Cigarette smoking does not cause high blood pressure; however, if a person with hypertension smokes, that person's risk of dying from heart disease or related disorders increases significantly.
2. Nonadherence with recommended therapeutic regimen.
3. Hypertension that has been poorly controlled, undiagnosed hypertension, and patients who have abruptly discontinued their medications.
4. Weight reduction, DASH diet, dietary sodium restriction, increasing physical activity, and moderation of alcohol consumption.
5. A diet rich in fruits, vegetables, and low-fat dairy products with a reduced content of saturated fats and total fat.

Activity C

1. d	2. b	3. f	4. a	5. c
6. e				

SECTION II: APPLYING YOUR KNOWLEDGE

Activity D

CASE STUDY: Secondary Hypertension

1. Releasing renin in response to decreased renal perfusion.
2. An eye examination with an ophthalmoscope is particularly important because retinal blood vessel damage indicates similar damage elsewhere in the vascular system. The patient is questioned about blurred vision, spots in front of the eyes, and diminished visual acuity.

3. Blocks reabsorption of sodium, chloride, and water in the kidneys.
4. Adhere to dietary regimens, become involved with a regular exercise program, and take her medication as prescribed.

SECTION III: PRACTICING FOR NCLEX

Activity E

1. a	2. d	3. a, b	4. b	5. c
6. b	7. a	8. c	9. d	10. a, c, d
11. a	12. c	13. b	14. a	15. d

CHAPTER 28

SECTION I: ASSESSING YOUR UNDERSTANDING

Activity A

1. 5 to 6
2. bone marrow
3. ribs, vertebrae, pelvis, sternum
4. hemoglobin; transport oxygen between the lungs and the tissues
5. 15
6. 2 mg
7. C
8. albumin, globulins
9. the sternum, the iliac crest

Activity B

1. An intricate clotting mechanism is activated when necessary to seal any leak in the blood vessels. Excessive clotting is equally dangerous, because it can obstruct blood flow to vital tissues. To prevent this, the body has a thrombolytic (fibrinolytic) mechanism that eventually dissolves clots formed within blood vessels.
2. The stroma is important in an indirect manner, in that it produces the colony-stimulating factors needed for hematopoiesis.
3. Iron, vitamin B_{12}, folic acid, pyridoxine, protein, and other factors are required. A deficiency of these factors during erythropoiesis can result in decreased red cell production.
4. An increased number of band cells is sometimes called a left shift or shift to the left. A shift to the left indicates that more immature cells are present in the blood than normal.
5. NK cells accumulate in the lymphoid tissues (especially spleen, lymph nodes, and tonsils), where they mature. When activated, they serve as potent killers of virus-infected and cancer cells. They also secrete chemical messenger proteins, called cytokines, to mobilize the T and B cells into action.
6. Knowledge of correct administration techniques and possible complications is required. It is very important to be familiar with the facility's policies and procedures for transfusion therapy.

Activity C

1. e	**2.** j	**3.** g	**4.** o	**5.** a
6. p	**7.** f	**8.** b	**9.** q	**10.** h
11. k	**12.** c	**13.** r	**14.** g	**15.** n
16. d	**17.** m	**18.** i		

SECTION II: APPLYING YOUR KNOWLEDGE

CASE STUDY: Blood Transfusion

Activity D

1. Check for the abnormal presence of gas bubbles and cloudiness in the blood bag; check that the blood has been typed and cross-matched and that the recipient's blood numbers match the donor's blood numbers.
2. Determine any history of previous transfusions as well as previous reactions to transfusion. The history should include the type of reaction, its manifestations, the interventions required, and whether any preventive interventions were used in subsequent transfusions.
3. The nurse knows that reactions are usually mild and should respond to an antihistamine such as diphenhydramine.

SECTION III: PRACTICING FOR NCLEX

Activity E

1. d	**2.** b	**3.** a	**4.** a	**5.** a
6. c	**7.** d	**8.** d	**9.** b, c, d, e	**10.** b, c, d
11. a	**12.** c, d, e	**13.** a	**14.** b	**15.** a

CHAPTER 29

SECTION I: ASSESSING YOUR UNDERSTANDING

Activity A

1. Anemia
2. 50%
3. heart failure, paresthesias, delirium
4. 4% to 6%, 13% to 14%
5. neurologic
6. Antacids, dairy products
7. Aplastic anemia
8. Proton pump inhibitors (PPIs), metformin
9. skin, mucous membranes, tongue
10. Sickle cell disease
11. Heparin infusion

Activity B

1. Factors include the rapidity with which the anemia has developed, the duration of the anemia, the metabolic requirements of the patient, other concurrent disorders or disabilities, and complications or concomitant features of the condition that produced the anemia.
2. Correcting or controlling the cause of the anemia.

3. Answer may include decreased mobility, increased depression, increased risk for falling, and delirium. The heart rate and cardiac output do not increase as quickly; thus fatigue, dyspnea, and confusion may be seen more readily in the anemic older adult.
4. Dietary teaching sessions should be individualized, involve family members, and include cultural aspects related to food preferences and food preparation. Additional amounts of iron, up to 2 mg daily, must be absorbed by women of childbearing age to replace that lost during menstruation.
5. Bleeding from ulcers, gastritis, inflammatory bowel disease (IBD), or gastrointestinal (GI) tumors
6. Chemical agents potentially responsible for bone marrow aplasia include benzene and benzene derivatives such as airplane glue, paint remover, and dry-cleaning solutions. Certain toxic materials—such as inorganic arsenic, glycol ethers, plutonium, and radon—have also been implicated as potential causes.
7. The patient with sickle cell trait usually has a normal hemoglobin level, a normal hematocrit, and a normal blood smear. In contrast, the patient with sickle cell disease has a low hematocrit and sickled cells on the smear. The diagnosis is confirmed by hemoglobin electrophoresis.
8. Answer may include the following: in an acute exacerbation of anemia, in the prevention of severe complications from anesthesia and surgery, in improving the response to infection, in the case of acute chest syndrome and multiorgan failure, in thwarting the evolution of a stroke or an acute neurologic defect, and in diminishing episodes of sickle cell crisis in pregnant women.
9. Sepsis, trauma, cancer, shock, abruption placentae, toxins, and allergic reactions

Activity C

1. c	**2.** a	**3.** b	**4.** a	**5.** c
6. b				

SECTION II: APPLYING YOUR KNOWLEDGE

Activity D

1. The patient is experiencing DIC.
2. If possible, the nurse should avoid administering medications that interfere with platelet function, such as aspirin, nonsteroidal anti-inflammatory drugs (NSAIDs), and beta-lactam antibiotics.
3. Neurologic checks, hemodynamics, abdominal girth, urine output, and amount of external bleeding.
4. Heparin.

SECTION III: PRACTICING FOR NCLEX

Activity E

1. b	**2.** a	**3.** c	**4.** c	**5.** c
6. a	**7.** d	**8.** c	**9.** d	**10.** b
11. a	**12.** b	**13.** a, b, c	**14.** c	**15.** a

CHAPTER 30

SECTION I: ASSESSING YOUR UNDERSTANDING

Activity A

1. assess, monitor, educate, intervene
2. cells
3. B lymphocyte
4. leukemias
5. lymphoid, myeloid
6. acute, chronic
7. 55, 67
8. bleeding, infection
9. stem cell
10. dysplasia

Activity B

1. The signs and symptoms result from insufficient production of normal blood cells.
2. The results will show an excess of immature blast cells, which is the hallmark of the diagnosis.
3. The goal of treatment is to obtain remission without excess toxicity and with a rapid hematologic recovery so that additional therapy can be administered if needed.
4. Because the illness is unpredictable.
5. See Chart 12-4 in Chapter 12, which lists long-term potential complications associated with chemotherapy or radiation therapy.

Activity C

1. h	2. c	3. d	4. g	5. a
6. e	7. f	8. i	9. b	

SECTION II: APPLYING YOUR KNOWLEDGE

Activity D

Case Study: Multiple Myeloma

1. The classic presenting symptom of multiple myeloma is bone pain, usually in the back or ribs. The bone pain usually increases with movement and decreases with rest; he may report less pain when awakening but more during the day.
2. As more and more malignant plasma cells are produced, the marrow has less space for erythrocyte production, and anemia may develop. It is also caused by a diminished production of erythropoietin by the kidney.
3. Chemotherapy.
4. NSAIDs can cause gastritis and renal dysfunction, so renal function must be carefully monitored and patients assessed for gastritis; many patients are unable to use NSAIDs due to concurrent renal insufficiency.

SECTION III: PRACTICING FOR NCLEX

Activity E

1. a	2. b	3. c	4. d	5. a
6. a	7. b	8. d	9. b	10. c
11. d	12. a, c, d	13. a, b, c	14. a	15. c

CHAPTER 31

SECTION I: ASSESSING YOUR UNDERSTANDING

Activity A

1. bone marrow, lymphoid tissue, white blood cells
2. bone marrow
3. thymus
4. lymphocytes
5. neutrophils
6. monocytes
7. phagocytic immune response
8. lymphocytes
9. protein
10. natural deficiency
11. proliferation

Activity B

1. Activation of complement, arrival of killer T cells, and attraction of macrophages.
2. By altering the antigen's cell membrane, causing cellular lysis, and producing lymphokines, which destroy invading organisms.
3. Disorders arise from excesses or deficiencies of immunocompetent cells, alterations in cellular functioning, immunologic attack on self-antigens, and inappropriate or exaggerated responses to specific antigens.
4. Natural immunity, which is nonspecific, is present at birth. Acquired immunity is more specific and develops throughout life. Active acquired immunity refers to defenses developed by the person's own body. Passive acquired immunity is a temporary immunity transmitted from another source that has developed immunity through previous disease or immunization.
5. Complement is a term used to describe circulating plasma proteins that are made in the liver and activated when an antibody couples with an antigen. Complement defends the body against bacterial infection, bridges natural and acquired immunity, and disposes of immune complexes and by-products associated with inflammation.
6. BRMs suppress antibody production and cellular immunity.
7. See Table 31-4, Age-Related Changes in Immunologic Function, in the textbook.
8. See Table 31-5, Select Medications and Effects on the Immune System, in the textbook.

Activity C

Immunoglobulins

1. d	2. e	3. c	4. d	5. a
6. b	7. a			

Medications

1. d	2. b	3. a	4. c	5. b
6. a	7. e			

SECTION II: APPLYING YOUR KNOWLEDGE

Activity D

1. The first line of defense, the *phagocytic immune response,* primarily involves the WBCs (granulocytes and macrophages), which have the ability to ingest foreign particles and destroy the invading agent; eosinophils are only weakly phagocytic. Phagocytes also remove the body's own dying or dead cells. Dying cells in necrotic tissue release substances that trigger an inflammatory response.
2. A second protective response, the *humoral immune response* (sometimes called the *antibody response*), begins with the B lymphocytes, which can transform themselves into plasma cells that manufacture antibodies. These antibodies are highly specific proteins that travel in the bloodstream and attempt to disable invaders.
3. The third mechanism of defense, the *cellular immune response,* also involves the T lymphocytes, which can turn into special cytotoxic (or killer) T cells that can attack the pathogens.

SECTION III: PRACTICING FOR NCLEX

Activity E

1. a	**2.** c	**3.** a, b, c	**4.** c	**5.** a, b, d
6. b, c, d	**7.** b	**8.** b	**9.** a	**10.** d
11. d	**12.** d	**13.** a, b, c, d	**14.** b	**15.** b

CHAPTER 32

SECTION I: ASSESSING YOUR UNDERSTANDING

Activity A

1. severe infections, autoimmunity, cancer
2. humoral immunity, T-cell defects, combined B- and T-cell defects, phagocytic disorders, complement production
3. CD4$^+$ count
4. 36%, 76%
5. Immune reconstitution inflammatory syndrome (IRIS)

Activity B

1. Complete blood count with manual differential should always be analyzed first.
2. Live vaccines are contraindicated in patients with antibody deficiency disorders because the patient is incapable of generating antibodies, and the live substance in the vaccine can cause disease.
3. The two major components of ART resistance are transmission of drug resistant HIV at the time of initial infection and selective drug resistance in patients who are receiving nonsuppressive regimens.
4. Patients with neutropenia are at increased risk for developing severe infections.
5. The most common manifestations of PCP are subacute onset of progressive dyspnea, fever, nonproductive cough, and chest discomfort that worsens within days to weeks. In mild cases, pulmonary examination usually is normal at rest. With exertion, tachypnea, tachycardia, and diffuse dry (cellophane) rales may be auscultated. Oral thrush is a common coinfection. Fever is apparent in most cases and may be the predominant symptom. Hypoxemia is the most characteristic laboratory abnormality, along with elevated lactate dehydrogenase levels.

Activity C

1. f	**2.** d	**3.** e	**4.** a	**5.** c
6. b				

SECTION II: APPLYING YOUR KNOWLEDGE

Activity D

1. Human immune deficiency virus type 1 (HIV-1) is transmitted in body fluids (blood, seminal fluid, vaginal secretions, amniotic fluid, and breast milk) that contain infected cells.
2. While behavioral interventions such as encouraging the use of condoms are highly effective in reducing the transmission of HIV, the person that is HIV-negative must be motivated and have the freedom to choose to use the method.
3. **Pre-exposure prophylaxis (PrEP)** might be appropriate. PrEP involves taking one pill containing two HIV medications (tenofovir disoproxil fumarate 300 mg and emtricitabine 200 mg) daily in order to avoid the risk of sexual HIV acquisition in adults and adolescents of age 12 and older (CDC, 2019c). HIV status should be checked every 3 months to be sure that the person has not become infected. The ultimate goal of PrEP is to reduce the acquisition of HIV infection with its resulting morbidity, mortality, and cost to individuals and society (CDC, 2019c).

SECTION III: PRACTICING FOR NCLEX

Activity E

1. c	**2.** b	**3.** b	**4.** a	**5.** b, d, e
6. d	**7.** a	**8.** a	**9.** b	**10.** d
11. c	**12.** b	**13.** a	**14.** a	**15.** a

CHAPTER 33

SECTION I: ASSESSING YOUR UNDERSTANDING

Activity A

1. neutralizing toxic antigens, precipitating the antigens out of solution, coating the surface of the antigens
2. IgE
3. immunoglobulins
4. the pain and fever seen with inflammatory responses

5. Answer should include two of the following: systemic lupus erythematosus, rheumatoid arthritis, serum sickness, certain types of nephritis, and some types of bacterial endocarditis.
6. contact dermatitis, latex allergy
7. penicillin
8. epinephrine, in a 1:1000 dilution given subcutaneously
9. 4 to 10

Activity B

1. An allergic reaction occurs when the body is invaded by an *antigen,* usually a protein that the body recognizes as foreign. The body responds in an effort to destroy the invading antigen. *Antibodies* (protein substances) are produced. When an interaction between the antigen and antibody results in tissue injury, an allergic reaction occurs and chemical mediators are released into the body.
2. Refer to section "Histamine" in the textbook.
3. Anaphylactic (Type I) Hypersensitivity, Cytotoxic (Type II) Hypersensitivity, Immune Complex (Type III) Hypersensitivity, Delayed-Type (Type IV) Hypersensitivity.
4. The three types of allergy tests are skin testing (including skin prick tests, scratch tests, and intradermal skin testing), which entails the intradermal injection or superficial application (epicutaneous) of solutions at several sites; provocative testing, which involves the direct administration of the suspected allergen to the sensitive tissue, such as the conjunctiva, nasal or bronchial mucosa, or gastrointestinal tract (by ingestion of the allergen), with observation of target organ response; and radioallergosorbent testing (RAST), in which a sample of the patient's serum is exposed to a variety of suspected allergen particle complexes. Refer to the sections "Skin Tests," "Provocative Testing," and "Serum-Specific IgE Test" in the textbook for more information.
5. Refer to section "Allergic Disorders" in the textbook.
6. The systemic reactions of flushing, warmth, and itching rapidly progress to bronchospasm, laryngeal edema, severe dyspnea, cyanosis, and hypotension. Cardiac arrest and coma can occur. Onset can begin within 2 hours post exposure.
7. Refer to section "Anaphylaxis."
8. Refer to Table 33-4, Types, Testing, and Treatment of Contact Dermatitis in the textbook.

Activity C

1. c   2. b   3. d   4. a   5. e

SECTION II: APPLYING YOUR KNOWLEDGE

Activity D

CASE STUDY: Allergic Rhinitis

1. Breathing difficulties, pruritus, and tingling sensations.
2. Hoarseness, a rash or hives, and wheezing.

3. Information about reducing exposure to allergens, desensitization procedures, and the correct use of medications.

CASE STUDY: Latex Allergy

1. Irritant contact dermatitis, a nonimmunologic response, may be caused by mechanical skin irritation or an alkaline pH associated with latex gloves.
2. These symptoms can be eliminated by changing glove brands or by using powder-free gloves.
3. Use of hand lotion before donning latex gloves can worsen the symptoms, because lotions may leach latex proteins from the gloves, increasing skin exposure and the risk of developing true allergic reactions.
4. Sensitization is detected by skin testing, RAST, EIA, ELISA or level of Hevea latex-specific IgE antibody in the serum. Testing for the chemicals used in latex rubber production is performed using the patch test. Skin patch testing is the preferred method for patients with contact allergies.

SECTION III: PRACTICING FOR NCLEX

Activity E

1. a	**2.** b	**3.** d	**4.** a	**5.** a
6. a	**7.** b	**8.** d	**9.** a, b, c	**10.** c
11. b	**12.** c	**13.** d	**14.** c	**15.** a

CHAPTER 34

SECTION I: ASSESSING YOUR UNDERSTANDING

Activity A

1. pain
2. T lymphocytes
3. milky, cloudy, dark yellow
4. collagen
5. synovial tissue

Activity B

1. One theory of *degradation* is that genetic or hormonal influences, mechanical factors, and prior joint damage cause cartilage failure. Degradation of cartilage ensues, and increased mechanical stress on bone ends causes stiffening of bone tissue. Another theory is that bone stiffening occurs and results in increased mechanical stress on cartilage, which in turn initiates the processes of degradation. For more information, refer to section "Rheumatic Diseases" in the textbook.
2. *Exacerbation* is a period of time when the symptoms of a disorder occur or increase in intensity and frequency. *Remission* is a period of time when symptoms are reduced or absent.
3. In *inflammatory* rheumatic disease, the inflammation occurs as the result of an immune response. Newly formed synovial tissue is infiltrated with

inflammatory cells (pannus formation), and joint degeneration occurs as a secondary process. In *degenerative* rheumatic disease, synovitis results from mechanical irritation. A secondary inflammation occurs.

4. Refer to Table 34-2, Management Goals and Strategies for Rheumatic Diseases, in the textbook.
5. Range-of-motion (ROM), isometric, dynamic, aerobic, and pool exercises are used to promote mobility for patients with rheumatic diseases. For more information, including the purpose of and precautions for each type of exercise, refer to Table 34-3, Exercise to Promote Mobility, in the textbook.
6. synovitis, polyarthritis, and spondylitis
7. Refer to Table 34-2, Select Medications Used in Rheumatic Diseases, in the textbook.
8. Manifestations of gout include acute gouty arthritis (recurrent attacks of severe articular and periarticular inflammation), tophi (crystalline deposits accumulating in articular tissue, osseous tissue, soft tissue, and cartilage), gouty nephropathy (renal impairment), and uric acid urinary calculi. For more information, refer to section "Gout" in the textbook.
9. Nurses need to pay special attention to supporting patients with fibromyalgia and providing encouragement as they begin their program of therapy. Patient support groups may be helpful. Careful listening to patients' descriptions of their concerns and symptoms is essential to help them make the changes that are necessary to improve their quality of life. Refer to section "Fibromyalgia" in the textbook.

Activity C

1. c	**2.** d	**3.** e	**4.** a	**5.** f
6. b	**7.** h	**8.** g		

SECTION II: APPLYING YOUR KNOWLEDGE

Activity D

CASE STUDY: Diffuse Connective Tissue Disease

1. Symmetric joint pain, swelling, warmth, erythema, and lack of function are classic symptoms of RA.
2. Rheumatoid factor is present in about 80% of patients with RA, but its presence alone is not diagnostic of RA, and its absence does not rule out the diagnosis.
3. Two to 6 weeks after treatment begins.
4. Research suggests that methotrexate combined with low-dose prednisone improves patient outcome, compared to use of methotrexate alone for early RA.

CASE STUDY: Systemic Lupus Erythematosus (SLE)

1. Cardiovascular assessment includes auscultation for pericardial friction rub, possibly associated with myocarditis and accompanying pleural effusions.

2. The mainstay of SLE treatment is based on pain management and nonspecific immunosuppression. Therapy includes NSAIDs, corticosteroids, antimalarials, and cytotoxic agents. Each of these medications has potentially serious side effects, including organ damage.
3. One of the most important risk factors associated with corticosteroid usage in SLE is osteoporosis and fractures. Osteopenia is reported in 25% to 74% and osteoporosis in 1.4% to 68% of SLE patients.

SECTION III: PRACTICING FOR NCLEX

Activity E

1. a, b, d	**2.** d	**3.** b	**4.** d	**5.** b
6. c	**7.** a	**8.** a	**9.** a	**10.** b
11. a, b, c	**12.** b	**13.** a	**14.** c	**15.** d

CHAPTER 35

SECTION I: ASSESSING YOUR UNDERSTANDING

Activity A

1. arthritis
2. 98%
3. 206
4. 1000 to 1200
5. sternum, ilium, vertebrae, ribs
6. parathyroid hormone, calcitonin
7. Crepitus

Activity B

1. The musculoskeletal system provides protection for vital organs, including the brain, heart, and lungs; provides a sturdy framework to support body structures; and makes mobility possible.
2. *Osteoblasts* function in bone formation by secreting bone matrix. The matrix consists of collagen and ground substances (glycoproteins and proteoglycans) that provide a framework in which inorganic mineral salts are deposited. These minerals are primarily composed of calcium and phosphorus. *Osteocytes* are mature bone cells involved in bone maintenance; they are located in lacunae (bone matrix units). *Osteoclasts,* located in shallow Howship lacunae (small pits in bones), are multinuclear cells involved in dissolving and resorbing bone.
3. Vitamin D increases calcium in the blood by promoting calcium absorption from the gastrointestinal tract and by accelerating the mobilization of calcium from the bone.
4. The sex hormones testosterone and estrogen have important effects on bone remodeling. Estrogen stimulates osteoblasts and inhibits osteoclasts; therefore, bone formation is enhanced and resorption is inhibited. Testosterone has both direct and indirect effects on bone growth and formation. It directly causes skeletal growth in adolescence and

has continued effects on skeletal muscle growth throughout the lifespan.

5. Phase I, reactive phase; phase II, reparative phase; phase III, remodeling phase.

6. During isometric contraction, almost all of the energy is released in the form of heat; during isotonic contraction, some of the energy is expended in mechanical work. In some situations (i.e., shivering), the need to generate heat is the primary stimulus for muscle contraction.

7. Refer to Table 35-1, Age-Related Changes of the Musculoskeletal System, in the textbook.

8. **kyphosis:** increase in the convex curvature of the thoracic spine, **lordosis:** increase in concave curvature of the lumbar spine, **scoliosis:** lateral curving of the spine.

See Chart 35-3, Assessment—Assessing for Peripheral Nerve Function, in the textbook.

Activity C

1. c   2. a   3. d   4. b   5. e

SECTION II: APPLYING YOUR KNOWLEDGE

Activity D

1. If joint motion is compromised or the joint is painful, the joint is examined for *effusion* (excessive fluid within the capsule), swelling, and increased temperature that may reflect active inflammation. An effusion is suspected if the joint is swollen and the normal bony landmarks are obscured. The most common site for joint effusion is the knee. If large amounts of fluid are present in the joint spaces beneath the patella, it may be identified by assessing for the balloon sign and for ballottement of the knee (see Fig. 35-5 in the textbook).

2. Jewelry, hair clips, hearing aids, credit cards with magnetic strips, and other metal-containing objects must be removed before the MRI is performed; otherwise, they can become dangerous projectile objects or cause burns. Credit cards with magnetic strips may be erased, and nonremovable cochlear devices can become inoperable. Also, transdermal patches (e.g., nicotine patch [NicoDerm], nitroglycerin transdermal [Transderm-Nitro], scopolamine transdermal [Transderm Scop], clonidine transdermal [Catapres-TTS]) that have a thin layer of aluminized backing must be removed before MRI because they can cause burns. The primary provider should be notified before the patches are removed.

3. Arthrocentesis.

SECTION III: PRACTICING FOR NCLEX

Activity E

1. a   2. b   3. c   4. b   5. c
6. d   7. a   8. d   9. c   10. b
11. a, b, c   12. d   13. a, c, d

CHAPTER 36

SECTION I: ASSESSING YOUR UNDERSTANDING

Activity A

1. bone fracture
2. 45 and 55, after menopause
3. a deficiency in activated vitamin D (calcitriol)
4. bisphosphonates, plicamycin
5. L4, L5, S1
6. ingrown toenail
7. diabetes, peripheral vascular disease
8. 1000 to 1500
9. calcium intake, muscular activity, weight bearing
10. osteochondroma

Activity B

1. Answer should include five of these conditions: acute lumbosacral strain, unstable lumbosacral ligaments, weak lumbosacral muscles, osteoarthritis of the spine, spinal stenosis, intervertebral disc problems, and unequal leg length.

2. Refer to section "Bursitis and Tendonitis" in the textbook.

3. Impingement syndrome is a general term that describes impaired movement of the rotator cuff of the shoulder. Impingement usually occurs from repetitive overhead movement of the arm or from acute trauma resulting in irritation and eventual inflammation of the rotator cuff tendons or the subacromial bursa as they grate against the coracoacromial arch.

4. Tinel sign may be elicited in patients with carpal tunnel syndrome by percussing lightly over the median nerve, located on the inner aspect of the wrist. If the patient reports tingling, numbness, and pain, the test for Tinel sign is considered positive.

5. Refer to Chart 36-7 in the textbook.

6. The patient with acute septic arthritis presents with a warm, painful, swollen joint with decreased range of motion (ROM). Systemic chills, fever, and leukocytosis are sometimes present. Although any joint may be infected, 50% of cases involve a knee.

Activity C

1. c   2. b   3. d   4. a   5. e
6. f

SECTION II: APPLYING YOUR KNOWLEDGE

Activity D

CASE STUDY: Osteoporosis

1. Patient education focuses on factors influencing the development of osteoporosis, interventions to arrest or slow the process, and measures to relieve symptoms. The nurse emphasizes that people of any age need sufficient calcium, vitamin D, and weight-bearing exercise to slow the progression of

osteoporosis. Patient education related to medication therapy as described previously is important. Patients must understand that having one fracture increases the probability of sustaining another.
2. Women have a lower peak bone mass than men, and estrogen loss affects the development of the disorder.
3. Refer to section "Risk Factors" under "Osteoporosis" in the textbook.
4. 1000 to 1500 mg

SECTION III: PRACTICING FOR NCLEX

Activity E

1. b	**2.** b	**3.** c	**4.** c	**5.** c
6. c	**7.** b	**8.** d	**9.** a, b, c	**10.** b
11. c, d, e	**12.** d	**13.** c	**14.** a	**15.** b

CHAPTER 37

SECTION I: ASSESSING YOUR UNDERSTANDING

Activity A

1. strain
2. neck
3. osteomyelitis, tetanus, gas gangrene
4. Colles fracture
5. deep vein thrombosis
6. atelectasis, pneumonia
7. abduction, external rotation, flexion
8. flexion contracture of the hip
9. 10, 4
10. tibial shaft

Activity B

1. AVN is tissue death due to anoxia and diminished blood supply.
2. The sensation is caused by the rubbing of bone fragments against each other; the nurse would document it as crepitus.
3. Early: Answer should include three of the following: shock, fat embolism, compartment syndrome, deep vein thrombosis, thromboembolism, DIC, and infection. Delayed: Answer should include three of the following: delayed union and nonunion, avascular necrosis of bone, reaction to internal fixation devices, complex regional pain syndrome (CRPS), and heterotopic ossification.
4. Stabilizing the fracture to prevent further hemorrhage, restoring blood volume and circulation, relieving the patient's pain, providing proper immobilization, and protecting against further injury.
5. Deep vein thrombosis, thromboembolism, and pulmonary embolus.
6. With an open fracture, the wound is covered with a sterile dressing to prevent contamination of deeper tissues. No attempt is made to reduce the

fracture, even if one of the bone fragments is protruding through the wound. Splints are applied for immobilization.
7. Closed reduction is performed without a surgical incision and can be done when there is a dislocation of a fracture. Cast may be applied after the procedure. Open reduction is usually performed with plate and screws to provide mobilization of the bone, especially if there is displacement of the fracture.
8. See Chart 37-2, Factors That Inhibit Fracture Healing.

Activity C

PART I

1. c	**2.** a	**3.** b	**4.** e	**5.** d

PART II

1. c	**2.** b	**3.** a	**4.** d	**5.** e

SECTION II: APPLYING YOUR KNOWLEDGE

Activity D

CASE STUDY: Above-the-Knee Amputation

1. Color and temperature, palpable responses, and palpable pulses
2. The circulatory status of the affected limb, the type of prosthesis to be used, and the ability to understand and use the prosthetic device
3. Triceps brachii.
4. "This is referred to as phantom limb pain. Sensations may be felt even after the limb is removed."
5. Monitoring vital signs to detect any indication of bleeding, placing the residual limb in an extended position with brief periods of elevation, and keeping a tourniquet nearby in case of hemorrhage.
6. Abduction deformities of the hip, flexion deformities, and nonshrinkage of the residual limb
7. Begin vertical turns on the anterior surface of the residual limb.

SECTION III: PRACTICING FOR NCLEX

1. b	**2.** d	**3.** b	**4.** c	**5.** a, b, c
6. a	**7.** b	**8.** d	**9.** a	**10.** d
11. b	**12.** a, b, c	**13.** a	**14.** a, b, e	**15.** c

CHAPTER 38

SECTION I: ASSESSING YOUR UNDERSTANDING

Activity A

1. trypsin, amylase, lipase
2. mixed waves that move the intestinal contents back and forth in a churning motion; a movement that propels the contents of the small intestine toward the colon.
3. 4; 12

4. decreased motility and emptying, weakened gag reflex, decreased resting pressure of the lower sphincter
5. cardiac sphincter
6. ptyalin
7. 1.0
8. B_{12}
9. secretin
10. Bile
11. cardia, fundus, body, pylorus
12. glucose

Activity B

1. Both the sympathetic and parasympathetic portions of the autonomic nervous system innervate the GI tract. In general, sympathetic nerves exert an inhibitory effect on the GI tract, decreasing gastric secretion and motility, and causing the sphincters and blood vessels to constrict. Parasympathetic nerve stimulation causes peristalsis and increases secretory activities. The sphincters relax under the influence of parasympathetic stimulation, except for the sphincter of the upper esophagus and the external anal sphincter, which are under voluntary control.
2. Obstruction of the GI tract increases the force of intestinal contraction. Distention occurs above the point of obstruction, causing pain and a sense of bloating.
3. 16 to 20 inches
4. The nurse will educate the patient to avoid ingesting red meats, aspirin, and nonsteroidal anti-inflammatory drugs for 72 hours prior to the study because it is thought that these factors are associated with false-positive results; likewise, patients are advised to avoid ingesting vitamin C from supplements or foods, because it is believed that this is associated with false-negative results.
5. MRI is contraindicated when the patient has any of the following: permanent pacemakers, artificial heart valves, and implanted insulin pumps.
6. Intrinsic factor, also secreted by the gastric mucosa, combines with dietary vitamin B_{12} so that the vitamin can be absorbed in the ileum. In the absence of intrinsic factor, vitamin B_{12} cannot be absorbed, and pernicious anemia results.

Activity C

1. f   2. a   3. e   4. c   5. b
6. d

SECTION II: APPLYING YOUR KNOWLEDGE

Activity D

1. Adequate colon cleansing provides optimal visualization and decreases the time needed for the procedure.
2. Colonoscopy is performed while the patient is lying on the left side with the legs drawn up toward the chest. The patient's position may be changed during the test to facilitate advancement of the scope.

3. The patient's cardiac and respiratory function and oxygen saturation are monitored continuously, with supplemental oxygen used as necessary.
4. Complications during and after the procedure can include cardiac arrhythmias and respiratory depression resulting from the medications administered, vasovagal reactions, and circulatory overload or hypotension resulting from overhydration or underhydration during bowel preparation.

SECTION III: PRACTICING FOR NCLEX

Activity E

1. c   2. b   3. a   4. a   5. c
6. d   7. c   8. c   9. a, b, c   10. b
11. c   12. a   13. d   14. d   15. b

CHAPTER 39

SECTION I: ASSESSING YOUR UNDERSTANDING

Activity A

1. mouth
2. cigarette smoking
3. aphthous stomatitis
4. sugar
5. 5 years
6. parotid
7. Xerostomia
8. *Clostridium difficile* (*C. difficile*) colitis

Activity B

1. Tooth decay is an erosive process that begins with the action of bacteria on fermentable carbohydrates in the mouth, which produces acids that dissolve tooth enamel.
2. Measures used to prevent and control dental caries include practicing effective mouth care, reducing the intake of starches and sugars (refined carbohydrates), applying fluoride to the teeth or drinking fluoridated water, refraining from smoking, controlling diabetes, and using pit and fissure sealants. Regular dental visits are an important method of preventive dental maintenance.
3. In the early stages of an infection, a dentist or oral surgeon may perform a needle aspiration or drill an opening into the pulp chamber to relieve pressure and pain, and to provide drainage.
4. Sialadenitis is an inflammation of the salivary gland; sialolithiasis are calculi in the submandibular gland.
5. Hemorrhage, chyle fistula, and nerve injury.
Refer to Table 39-1, Disorders of the Lips, Mouth, and Gums, in the textbook.

Activity C

1. f   2. g   3. e   4. a   5. d
6. b   7. c   8. h

SECTION II: APPLYING YOUR KNOWLEDGE

Activity D

CASE STUDY: Radical Neck Dissection

1. Shoulder drop and poor cosmesis (visible neck depression).
2. Altered respiratory status, wound infection, and hemorrhage.
3. Fowler position.
4. Stridor.
5. Hypoglossal nerve.
6. Referral for a home health nurse to visit and educate the wife about the care of the patient.

CASE STUDY: Mandibular Fracture

1. On his side with his head slightly elevated to prevent aspiration.
2. Nasogastric suctioning is needed to remove stomach contents, thereby reducing the danger of aspiration.
3. A wire cutter or scissors.
4. Clear liquids.

CASE STUDY: Cancer of the Mouth

1. The typical lesion is a painless, indurated (hardened) ulcer with raised edges.
2. Pain.
3. A sore, roughened area that has not healed in 3 weeks; minor swelling in an area adjacent to the lesion; numbness in the affected area in the mouth.

SECTION III: PRACTICING FOR NCLEX

Activity E

1. a	**2.** b	**3.** a, c, d	**4.** b	**5.** c
6. a	**7.** a	**8.** a	**9.** b, c, d	**10.** b
11. c	**12.** d	**13.** d	**14.** b	**15.** a

CHAPTER 40

SECTION I: ASSESSING YOUR UNDERSTANDING

Activity A

1. duodenum
2. type O
3. ibuprofen and aspirin
4. hemorrhage
5. Upper endoscopy
6. *Helicobacter pylori*
7. Hemorrhage, perforation, penetration, pyloric obstruction
8. Gastric secretory studies

Activity B

1. Dilute and neutralize the offending agent. To neutralize a corrosive acid, use common antacids such as milk and aluminum hydroxide. To neutralize an alkali, use diluted lemon juice or diluted vinegar.

2. Patients with gastritis due to a vitamin deficiency exhibit antibodies against intrinsic factor, which interferes with vitamin B_{12} absorption.
3. Hypersecretion of acid pepsin and a weakened gastric mucosal barrier predispose to peptic ulcer development.
4. Hypersecretion of gastric juice, multiple duodenal ulcers, hypertrophied duodenal glands, and gastrinomas (islet cell tumors) in the pancreas.
5. A stress ulcer refers to acute mucosal ulceration of the duodenal or gastric area that occurs after a stressful event.
6. Cushing's ulcers, which are common in patients with brain trauma, usually occur in the esophagus, stomach, or duodenum. Curling's ulcers occur most frequently after extensive burns and usually involve the antrum of the stomach and duodenum.
7. The objective of the ulcer diet is to avoid oversecretion and hypermotility in the gastrointestinal tract. Extremes of temperature should be avoided, as well as overstimulation by meat extractives, coffee (including decaffeinated), alcohol, and diets rich in milk and cream. Current therapy recommends three regular meals per day if an antacid or histamine blocker is taken.
8. When peptic ulcer perforation occurs, the patient experiences severe upper abdominal pain, vomiting, fainting, and an extremely tender abdomen that can be boardlike in rigidity; signs of shock will be present (hypotension and tachycardia).
9. There are few clinical manifestations that differentiate gastric ulcers from duodenal ulcers; however, classically, the pain associated with gastric ulcers most commonly occurs immediately after eating, whereas the pain associated with duodenal ulcers most commonly occurs 2 to 3 hours after meals. In addition, approximately 50% to 80% of patients with duodenal ulcers awake with pain during the night, whereas 30% to 40% of patients with gastric ulcers voice this type of complaint. Patients with duodenal ulcers are more likely to express relief of pain after eating or after taking an antacid than patients with gastric ulcers.

Activity C

Pharmacologic Therapy for Peptic Ulcer Disease and Gastritis

1. b	**2.** a	**3.** d	**4.** e	**5.** c

SECTION II: APPLYING YOUR KNOWLEDGE

Activity D

CASE STUDY: Gastric Cancer

1. Ascites and hepatomegaly.
2. Esophagogastroduodenoscopy and barium x-ray of the upper gastrointestinal tract; endoscopic ultrasound; computed tomography.
3. Wide resection of the middle and distal portions of the stomach (removal of about 75% of the stomach).
4. 5-Fluorouracil (5-FU).

SECTION III: PRACTICING FOR NCLEX

Activity E

1. a, b, c	**2.** b	**3.** b	**4.** a, b, c	**5.** c
6. a	**7.** b, c, d	**8.** a	**9.** a	**10.** d
11. c	**12.** c	**13.** a	**14.** c, d	**15.** d

CHAPTER 41

SECTION I: ASSESSING YOUR UNDERSTANDING

Activity A

1. Anorectal manometry
2. Megacolon
3. metabolic acidosis
4. adhesions, hernias, neoplasms
5. adenocarcinoid tumors
6. Zollinger-Ellison syndrome
7. vitamin B_{12}
8. abdominal CT scan
9. abdominal pain, diarrhea
10. 2 to 3

Activity B

1. Peritonitis, abscess formation, fistulas, and bleeding
2. *Escherichia coli, Klebsiella, Proteus,* and *Pseudomonas*
3. Answer should include six of the following: increasing age; family history of colon cancer (Lynch syndrome) or polyps (familial adenomatous polyposis [FAP]); previous colon cancer or adenomatous polyps; high consumption of alcohol; cigarette smoking; obesity; history of gastrectomy; history of IBD; high-fat, high-protein (with high intake of beef), low-fiber diet; genital cancer (e.g., endometrial cancer, ovarian cancer) or breast cancer (in women).
4. Forcible exhalation against a closed glottis followed by a rise in intrathoracic pressure and subsequent possible dramatic rise in arterial pressure.
5. The four classifications for constipation are:
   * Functional constipation, which involves normal transit mechanisms of mucosal transport. This type of constipation is most common and can be successfully treated by increasing intake of fiber and fluids.
   * Slow-transit constipation, which is caused by inherent disorders of the motor function of the colon (e.g., Hirschsprung disease), and is characterized by infrequent bowel movements.
   * Defecatory disorders, which are caused by dysfunctional motor coordination between the pelvic floor and anal sphincter. Dyssynergic constipation is a common cause of chronic constipation and is caused by an inability to coordinate the abdominal, pelvic floor, and rectoanal muscles to defecate. *Anismus* is a term used to describe pelvic floor dysfunction and constipation. This can cause not only constipation but also fecal incontinence.

   * Opioid-induced constipation, which includes new or worsening symptoms that occur when opioid therapy is initiated, changed, or increased and must include two or more symptoms of functional constipation.
6. Although no anatomic or biochemical abnormalities have been found that account for its common symptoms, various factors are associated with the syndrome: heredity, psychological stress or conditions such as depression and anxiety, a diet high in fat and stimulating or irritating foods, alcohol consumption, and smoking.
7. The hallmarks of malabsorption syndrome from any cause are diarrhea or frequent, loose, bulky, foul-smelling stools that have increased fat content and are often grayish (steatorrhea).

Activity C

PART 1: Key Terms

1. e	**2.** m	**3.** i	**4.** o	**5.** a
6. g	**7.** k	**8.** b	**9.** p	**10.** j
11. c	**12.** n	**13.** d	**14.** l	**15.** h
16. f				

PART 2: Laxative Classification and Action

1. b-5	**2.** d-3	**3.** e-6	**4.** a-1	**5.** c-2
6. f-4				

SECTION II: APPLYING YOUR KNOWLEDGE

Activity D

CASE STUDY: Appendicitis

1. Vague epigastric or periumbilical pain progresses to right lower quadrant pain and is usually accompanied by a low-grade fever and nausea, and sometimes by vomiting. Loss of appetite is common. In up to 50% of presenting cases, local tenderness is elicited at McBurney point when pressure is applied. Rebound tenderness may be present.
2. A pregnancy test should be performed to rule out pregnancy prior to any x-rays or medications administered.
3. The appendix has ruptured.

SECTION III: PRACTICING FOR NCLEX

Activity E

1. b	**2.** c	**3.** c	**4.** b	**5.** a
6. d	**7.** b	**8.** c	**9.** c	**10.** a
11. b	**12.** b	**13.** a	**14.** c	**15.** b

CHAPTER 42

SECTION I: ASSESSING YOUR UNDERSTANDING

Activity A

1. Obesity
2. 42.4
3. behavioral, environmental, physiologic, genetic

4. leptin
5. height, weight
6. 35, 40
7. lifestyle modifications

Activity B

1. According to the "thrifty gene" hypothesis, the human **genome** (i.e., the total complement of genes in humans) was sequenced during times when finding and storing food sources expended more energy than during contemporary times. Hunting for scarce food sources during prehistoric times consumed a lot of energy, and food sources were not abundant. Storing fat to provide energy sources during times of food scarcity was a physiologic adaptive response to these environmental challenges (Budd & Peterson, 2014).
2. Certain processed and high-caloric foods that contain fructose corn syrup, simple sugars, or trans fats are hypothesized to be **obesogenic.**
3. The following multicomponent behavioral intervention should be discussed with a patient that has a BMI in excess of 30 kg/m²: setting weight loss goals, improving diet habits, increasing physical activity, addressing barriers to change, self-monitoring, and strategizing ongoing lifestyle changes aimed at a healthy weight.
4. Physical activity recommendations for all adults (those with and without obesity) include at least 150 minutes of moderate-intensity aerobic exercise weekly or 75 minutes of vigorous-intensity aerobic exercise weekly. In addition, muscle-strengthening exercises that engage all major muscle groups should be done at least twice weekly (Fitch et al., 2013; Orringer et al., 2016).
5. Advising patients with sleep disturbances to plan to be in bed with lights out at least 7 hours prior to wake-up time, to create a dark, relaxing bedroom environment, to avoid activities that can cause arousal around bedtime (e.g., texting), and to avoid beverages with caffeine after lunchtime can all be helpful strategies aimed at ensuring a restful night's sleep that is consonant with weight reduction (Orringer et al., 2016).
6. Indications for antiobesity medications include a BMI >30 kg/m² or a BMI >27 kg/m² with concomitant morbidity that is related to being overweight (e.g., type 2 diabetes, hypertension) (Apovian et al., 2015; Bays, Seger, Primach, et al., 2016).

Activity C

1. b   2. d   3. a   4. e   5. c

SECTION II: APPLYING YOUR KNOWLEDGE

Activity D

CASE STUDY: Obesity

1. The following types of contraindication should be assessed for when discussing gastric bypass: reversible endocrine or other disorders that can cause obesity, current drug or alcohol abuse, uncontrolled, severe psychiatric illness, lack of comprehension of risks, benefits, expected outcomes, alternatives, and lifestyle changes required with bariatric surgery.
2. The following prescreening testing is performed prior to gastric bypass surgery: CBC, electrolytes, blood urea nitrogen (BUN), creatinine, sleep study, upper endoscopy, ECG, lipid profile, AST, ALT, glucose, hemoglobin A1C, iron, vitamin B_{12}, thiamine, folate, vitamin D, and calcium levels.
3. The complications of the Roux-en-Y bypass can include hemorrhage, venous thromboembolism, bile reflux, dumping syndrome, dysphagia, bowel or gastric outlet obstruction, and anastomotic leak.

SECTION III: PRACTICING FOR NCLEX

Activity E

1. b, c, e   2. c   3. d   4. a   5. b
6. a   7. d   8. b   9. c   10. d

CHAPTER 43

SECTION I: ASSESSING YOUR UNDERSTANDING

Activity A

1. 70
2. bleeding, bile peritonitis
3. blood
4. hepatitis C
5. chronic liver disease, hepatitis B, hepatitis C, cirrhosis
6. infection
7. portal vein
8. vitamin K
9. cholesterol
10. 90
11. Hepatitis C
12. Ruptured esophageal varices

Activity B

1. Refer to Chart 43-1, Age-Related Changes of the Hepatobiliary System, in the textbook.
2. Producing ketone bodies, synthesizing albumin, and participating in gluconeogenesis.
3. *Hemolytic jaundice* is the result of an increased destruction of red blood cells that overload the plasma with bilirubin so quickly that the liver cannot excrete the bilirubin as fast as it is formed. *Hepatocellular jaundice* is caused by the inability of damaged liver cells to clear normal amounts of bilirubin from the blood. *Obstructive jaundice* is usually caused by occlusion of the bile duct by a gallstone, an inflammatory process, a tumor, or pressure from an enlarged organ.
4. Fat emulsification in the intestines.
5. Unintentional exposure to HBsAg-positive blood, perinatal exposure, sexual contact with those who are positive for HBsAg.

6. Chloroform, gold compounds, and phosphorus.
7. Esophagus, lower rectum, and stomach.
8. Ascites, jaundice, and portal hypertension.

Activity C

1. c	**2.** e	**3.** b	**4.** a	**5.** d
6. g	**7.** f			

SECTION II: APPLYING YOUR KNOWLEDGE

Activity D

CASE STUDY: Liver Biopsy

1. Making sure that informed consent has been obtained and the permit is signed, compatible donor blood is obtained, vital signs are obtained and recorded, and coagulation studies are reviewed.
2. Recumbent, with her right upper abdomen exposed.
3. Instruct the patient to inhale and exhale deeply several times, finally to exhale, and to hold breath at the end of expiration.
4. The right side-lying position with a pillow placed under the right costal margin.

CASE STUDY: Paracentesis

1. 3 L.
2. Upright, with her feet resting on a support so that the puncture site will be readily visible.
3. Hypotension, oliguria, and pallor.

CASE STUDY: Alcoholic or Nutritional Cirrhosis

1. Palpation of a nodular liver that is decreased in size (less than 10 cm for a male).
2. 3500 calories.
3. 2000 to 2500 per 24 hours.

CASE STUDY: Liver Transplantation

1. Bleeding.
2. Nephrotoxicity, septicemia, and thrombocytopenia.
3. For patients with liver cancer anticipating surgery, support, education, and encouragement are provided to help them prepare psychologically for the surgery.

SECTION III: PRACTICING FOR NCLEX

Activity E

1. b	**2.** c, d	**3.** b	**4.** d	**5.** a
6. d	**7.** a	**8.** b	**9.** c	**10.** a
11. c	**12.** d	**13.** a	**14.** d	**15.** b

CHAPTER 44

SECTION I: ASSESSING YOUR UNDERSTANDING

Activity A

1. 30; 50
2. insulin, glucagon, somatostatin

3. amylase; trypsin; lipase
4. Calculous cholecystitis
5. bile duct injury
6. pancreatic necrosis
7. gallbladder
8. secretin
9. multiparous, obese, over 40

Activity B

1. If a gallstone obstructs the cystic duct, the gallbladder becomes distended, inflamed, and eventually infected (acute cholecystitis).
2. The bile, which is no longer carried to the duodenum, is absorbed by the blood and gives the skin and mucous membranes a yellow color.
3. Because of the short hospital stay with uncomplicated laparoscopic cholecystectomies, it is important to provide patient education about managing postoperative pain and reporting signs and symptoms of intra-abdominal complications, including loss of appetite, vomiting, pain, distention of the abdomen, and temperature elevation.
4. Patients with sepsis or severe cardiac, renal, pulmonary, or liver failure
5. Refer to Chart 50-3, Criteria for Predicting Severity of Pancreatitis, in the textbook.

Activity C

1. b	**2.** c	**3.** e	**4.** d	**5.** a

SECTION II: APPLYING YOUR KNOWLEDGE

Activity D

CASE STUDY: Cholecystectomy: Preoperative Situation

1. Antispasmodic agents and antibiotics, intravenous fluids, and nasogastric suctioning.
2. Lockhart should avoid foods high in fat, as well as eggs, cream, pork, fried foods, cheese, rich dressings, gas-forming vegetables, and alcohol.
3. Chenodeoxycholic acid may not be effective if taken with dietary cholesterol, estrogens, or oral contraceptives.

CASE STUDY: Cholecystectomy: Postoperative Situation

1. If the common bile duct is thought to be obstructed by a gallstone, an ERCP with sphincterotomy may be performed to explore the duct before laparoscopy.
2. Indicators of infection, leakage of bile into the peritoneal cavity, and obstruction of bile drainage
3. 4 to 6 weeks.

SECTION III: PRACTICING FOR NCLEX

Activity E

1. c	**2.** b, c, d	**3.** d	**4.** d	**5.** a
6. a	**7.** b	**8.** a, c, d	**9.** a, b, c	**10.** a
11. c	**12.** d	**13.** a	**14.** c	**15.** b
16. b				

CHAPTER 45

SECTION I: ASSESSING YOUR UNDERSTANDING

Activity A

1. negative feedback
2. hypothalamus
3. vasopressin, the excretion of water by the kidneys; oxytocin, milk ejection during lactation
4. acromegaly, gigantism
5. diabetes insipidus; excessive thirst (polydipsia), large volumes of dilute urine
6. thyroxine, triiodothyronine, and calcitonin
7. autoimmune thyroiditis (Hashimoto disease)
8. women; men
9. Graves disease
10. methimazole, propylthiouracil
11. Trousseau, Chvostek
12. corticosteroids, mineralocorticoids, androgens
13. kidney stones
14. Toxic nodular goiter

Activity B

1. Adrenocorticotropic hormone (ACTH), follicle-stimulating hormone (FSH), thyroid-stimulating hormone (TSH).
2. Answer should include four of the following: steroids, proteins or peptides, polypeptides and glycoproteins, amines and amino acids, and fatty acid derivatives.
3. The objectives in the management of hypothyroidism are to restore a normal metabolic state by replacing the missing hormone, and prevention of disease progression and complications.
4. Several routes are available for administering radiation to the thyroid or tissues of the neck, including oral administration of radioactive iodine and external administration of radiation therapy.

Activity C

1. h	2. g	3. i	4. d	5. a
6. c	7. f	8. e	9. j	10. b

SECTION II: APPLYING YOUR KNOWLEDGE

Activity D

CASE STUDY: Primary Hypothyroidism

1. Serum TSH, T$_3$ resin uptake test, immunoassay for antithyroid antibodies, radioactive iodine uptake, thyroid scan, radioscan, or scintiscan.
2. Extreme fatigue, hair loss, brittle nails, dry skin, and numbness and tingling of the fingers may occur. Hoarseness, menstrual disturbances, and weight gain are other potential clinical manifestations.
3. Encouraging frequent periods of rest throughout the day, offering her additional blankets to help prevent chilling, and using a cleansing lotion instead of soap for her skin.
4. Mrs. Conrad must be instructed that many over-the-counter and prescription medications interact with levothyroxine and caution must be maintained when taking anything. There is a decrease in thyroid hormone absorption when patients are also taking magnesium-containing antacids. See section heading "Prevention of Medication Interaction" in the textbook.

CASE STUDY: Hyperparathyroidism

1. Exophthalmos.
2. Increased sensitivity to catecholamines or to changes in neurotransmitter turnover.
3. The nurse instructs Ms. Boone to take the medication in the morning on an empty stomach 30 minutes before eating to avoid decrease in absorption associated with some foods such as walnuts, soybean flour, cottonseed meal, and dietary fiber. Ms. Boone is also informed that it may take several weeks until relief of symptoms occurs.

CASE STUDY: Subtotal Thyroidectomy

1. Semi-Fowler position, with his head supported by pillows.
2. Voice change.
3. IV calcium gluconate.

SECTION III: PRACTICING FOR NCLEX

Activity E

1. a	2. b	3. b, c, d	4. d	5. a, b, c
6. b	7. d	8. a	9. d	10. a, c, d
11. c	12. c	13. b	14. a	15. b
16. a, b, c				

CHAPTER 46

SECTION I: ASSESSING YOUR UNDERSTANDING

Activity A

1. 25.8
2. nontraumatic amputation, blindness, end-stage kidney disease
3. type 1 diabetes, type 2 diabetes, gestational diabetes
4. glycogenolysis, gluconeogenesis
5. osmotic diuresis
6. decreased
7. hyperglycemic hyperosmolar syndrome
8. 18
9. 105 mg/dL, 130 mg/dL
10. polyuria, polydipsia, polyphagia
11. elevated blood glucose level
12. seventh, 20
13. 24 to 28
14. Ketoacidosis
15. Hyperglycemia, ketosis, metabolic acidosis

Activity B

1. Because of increasing health care costs and an aging population.
2. Hyperglycemia develops during pregnancy because of the secretion of placental hormones, which causes insulin resistance.

3. Insulin resistance and impaired insulin secretion.
4. One risk involved in suddenly increasing fiber intake is that it may require adjusting the dosage of insulin or oral agents to prevent hypoglycemia. Other problems may include abdominal fullness, nausea, diarrhea, increased flatulence, and constipation if fluid intake is inadequate.
5. Insulin regulates the production and storage of glucose. In diabetes, either the pancreas stops producing insulin or the cells stop responding to insulin. Hyperglycemia results and can lead to acute metabolic complications such as diabetic ketoacidosis and hyperglycemic hyperosmolar nonketotic syndrome. Long-term complications can contribute to macrovascular or microvascular complications.
6. Answer should include the following: hypotension, profound dehydration, tachycardia, and variable neurologic signs (seizures, hemiparesis, and alteration of sensorium).
7. Sulfonylureas act by directly stimulating the beta cells of the pancreas to secrete insulin (cannot be used in patients with type 1 diabetes).

Activity C

1. c   **2.** a   **3.** b   **4.** e   **5.** d

SECTION II: APPLYING YOUR KNOWLEDGE

Activity D

CASE STUDY: Type 1 Diabetes

Refer to Table 46-3, Categories of Insulin, in the textbook.
1. Between 11:30 AM and 7:30 PM.
2. 16 to 20 hours.
3. Signs of hypoglycemia earlier than expected.

CASE STUDY: Hypoglycemia

1. Stress due to the breakup, lack of dietary intake.
2. Symptoms of rebound hypoglycemia.
3. Emotional changes, slurred speech and double vision, staggering gait, weakness, diaphoresis, and lack of coordination.
4. Eating regularly scheduled meals, eating snacks to cover the peak time of insulin, and increasing food intake when engaging in increased levels of physical exercise.

CASE STUDY: Diabetic Ketoacidosis

1. Monitoring urinary output by means of an indwelling catheter, evaluating serum electrolytes, testing for glucosuria and acetonuria, blood glucose testing, and vital signs.
2. 0.9% sodium chloride.
3. Hyperkalemia.
4. When hanging the insulin drip, the nurse must flush the insulin solution through the entire IV infusion set and discard the first 50 mL of fluid. Insulin molecules adhere to the inner surface of plastic IV infusion sets; therefore, the initial fluid may contain a decreased concentration of insulin.
5. Hypokalemia.

SECTION III: PRACTICING FOR NCLEX

Activity E

1. a, b, d	**2.** a	**3.** a	**4.** a	**5.** c
6. a	**7.** a	**8.** a, b, c	**9.** a	**10.** c
11. b	**12.** c	**13.** d	**14.** a, b, c	**15.** d
16. b				

CHAPTER 47

SECTION I: ASSESSING YOUR UNDERSTANDING

Activity A

1. nephron; cortex
2. 400 to 500
3. 300 mOsm/kg
4. aldosterone
5. increased
6. antidiuretic hormone (ADH)
7. 7.35 to 7.45; 4.5
8. urea; 20 to 30
9. creatinine clearance

Activity B

1. If the total number of functioning nephrons is less than 20% of normal, renal replacement therapy needs to be considered.
2. There are three narrowed areas of each ureter: the ureteropelvic junction, ureteral segment near the sacroiliac junction, and ureterovesical junction.
3. Amino acids and glucose are usually filtered at the level of the glomerulus and reabsorbed so that neither is excreted in the urine.
4. It is secreted by the posterior portion of the pituitary gland in response to changes in osmolality of the blood.
5. The regulation of sodium volume excreted depends on aldosterone, a hormone synthesized and released from the adrenal cortex.

Activity C

1. b	**2.** d	**3.** a	**4.** c	**5.** e

SECTION II: APPLYING YOUR KNOWLEDGE

Activity D

1. Before the biopsy is carried out, coagulation studies are conducted to identify any risk of postbiopsy bleeding.
2. The sedated patient is placed in a prone position with a sandbag under the abdomen.
3. IV fluids may be administered to help clear the kidneys and prevent clot formation.

SECTION III: PRACTICING FOR NCLEX

Activity E

1. a	**2.** b	**3.** c	**4.** a, b, c	**5.** a
6. a	**7.** b	**8.** a, b, c	**9.** a	**10.** b

CHAPTER 48

SECTION I: ASSESSING YOUR UNDERSTANDING

Activity A

1. Diabetes and hypertension
2. acute hypertensive and benign
3. creatinine, BUN
4. Hypertriglyceridemia
5. peritonitis
6. abdominal distention, paralytic ileus
7. weight
8. edema
9. 85
10. initiation, oliguria, diuresis, recovery
11. Nephrotic syndrome

Activity B

1. Cardiomegaly, a gallop rhythm, distended neck veins, and other signs and symptoms of heart failure may be present. Crackles can be heard in the bases of the lungs.
2. Clinical findings include a marked increase in protein (particularly albumin) in the urine (proteinuria), a decrease in albumin in the blood (hypoalbuminemia), diffuse edema, high serum cholesterol, and low-density lipoproteins (hyperlipidemia).
3. *Autosomal dominant PKD* is the most common inherited form. Symptoms usually develop between the ages of 30 and 40, but they can begin earlier, even in childhood. About 90% of all PKD cases are autosomal dominant PKD. *Autosomal recessive PKD* is a rare inherited form. Symptoms of autosomal recessive PKD begin in the earliest months of life or in utero.
4. The nurse assists the patient to prepare physically and psychologically for these procedures and monitors carefully for signs and symptoms of dehydration and exhaustion.
5. Factors that influence mortality include increased age, comorbid conditions, and preexisting kidney and vascular diseases and respiratory failure.

Activity C

1. a	2. b	3. c	4. e	5. d
6. j	7. h	8. f	9. g	10. i

SECTION II: APPLYING YOUR KNOWLEDGE

Activity D

CASE STUDY: Continuous Ambulatory Peritoneal Dialysis (CAPD)

1. The procedure allows the patient reasonable freedom and control of daily activities but requires a serious commitment to be successful.
2. Approximately four to five times per day with no night exchanges.
3. 10 to 15 minutes.

4. Mr. Edwards should adopt a diet that is high in protein.

CASE STUDY: Acute Kidney Injury

1. Reduced glomerular filtration, renal ischemia, and tubular damage.
2. 70 g/24 h.
3. A high-protein diet.
4. 6 to 12 months.

SECTION III: PRACTICING FOR NCLEX

Activity E

1. d	2. a	3. a, c, d	4. c	5. b
6. a	7. b	8. a	9. b	10. b
11. c	12. d	13. a	14. d	15. c

CHAPTER 49

SECTION I: ASSESSING YOUR UNDERSTANDING

Activity A

1. glycosaminoglycan (GAG); urinary immunoglobulin A (IgA); normal bacterial flora of the vagina and urethral area
2. *Escherichia coli, Pseudomonas, Enterococcus*
3. catheter-associated urinary tract infections (CAUTI)
4. bladder
5. stress incontinence
6. 1.5
7. infection
8. kidney failure
9. 3
10. pain

Activity B

1. See Chart 49-2, Risk Factors: Urinary Tract Infection, in the textbook.
2. Answer may include the following: high incidence of multiple chronic medical conditions, frequent use of antimicrobial agents, presence of infected pressure injuries, immunocompromised, cognitive impairment, immobility, and incomplete bladder emptying.
3. Answer may include the following: pregnancy, menopause, GI surgery, pelvic muscle weakness, incompetent urethra, immobility, high-impact exercise, diabetes, stroke, age-related changes, morbid obesity, cognitive disturbance, medications (diuretics, sedatives, etc.), and caregiver or toilet unavailable.
4. Answer may include the following: delirium/confusion, UTI, atrophic vaginitis, urethritis, prostatitis, medications, psychological factors, excessive urine production, limited or restricted activity, and stool impaction/constipation.
5. See Chart 49-10, Preventing Infection in the Patient with an Indwelling Urinary Catheter, in the textbook.

6. Answer includes the following: cigarette smoking, exposure to environmental carcinogens, recurrent or chronic bacterial infections of the urinary tract, bladder stones, high urine pH, high cholesterol intake, pelvic radiation, and other cancers related to the urinary tract.

Activity C

1. d   **2.** f   **3.** e   **4.** c   **5.** a
6. b

SECTION II: APPLYING YOUR KNOWLEDGE

Activity D

CASE STUDY: Acute Pyelonephritis

1. Urine for culture and sensitivity.
2. Physical examination reveals pain and tenderness in the area of the costovertebral angle.
3. An ultrasound or CT scan.

SECTION III: PRACTICING FOR NCLEX

Activity E

1. c   **2.** b   **3.** c   **4.** a   **5.** b, c, d
6. a   **7.** b   **8.** c   **9.** d   **10.** d
11. b, c, e **12.** a **13.** c **14.** d **15.** c

CHAPTER 50

SECTION I: ASSESSING YOUR UNDERSTANDING

Activity A

1. 11 to 13 years; 10 years
2. follicle-stimulating; luteinizing
3. 45 to 52; 51; 35
4. the luteinizing hormone
5. physical violence, sexual violence, stalking, and psychological aggression
6. human immune deficiency virus (HIV) and sexually transmitted infections (STIs)
7. endometrial biopsy
8. Metrorrhagia
9. estrogens, progesterones
10. diaphragm

Activity B

1. In women, chronic pelvic pain is often associated with physical violence, emotional neglect, and sexual abuse in childhood.
2. To prevent cervical cancer
3. A patient who has received anesthesia for a surgical cone biopsy is advised to rest for 24 hours after the procedure and to leave any vaginal packing in place until it is removed (usually the next day). The patient is instructed to report any excessive bleeding.
4. Hysteroscopy allows direct visualization of all parts of the uterine cavity by means of a lighted optical instrument.

5. Premenstrual syndrome (PMS) is a cluster of physical, emotional, and behavioral symptoms that are usually related to the luteal phase of the menstrual cycle.
6. The tube can be resected (salpingostomy) or removed (salpingectomy) along with an ovary (salpingo-oophorectomy); methotrexate may be used to "dissolve" the ectopic pregnancy if it is not ruptured. The conservative approach may include "milking the tube."
7. Possible causes are salpingitis, peritubal adhesions, structural abnormalities of the fallopian tube, previous ectopic pregnancy or tubal surgery, the presence of an IUD, and multiple previous abortions.

Activity C

1. f   **2.** d   **3.** h   **4.** a   **5.** e
6. g   **7.** c   **8.** b

SECTION II: APPLYING YOUR KNOWLEDGE

Activity D

1. The hot or warm flashes and night sweats reported by some women are thought to be caused by hormonal changes and denote vasomotor instability.
2. Hormone therapy (HT) or menopausal hormonal therapy (previously referred to as hormone replacement therapy [HRT]) has been found to increase some health disorders and to be less effective in preventing others than previously believed. Although HT decreases hot flashes and reduces the risk of osteoporotic fractures as well as colorectal cancer, studies have shown that it increases the risk of breast cancer, heart attack, stroke, and blood clots. Thus, the benefits of HT are inadequate given the increased risk of these other disorders.
3. Problematic hot flashes have been treated with low-dose venlafaxine and other medications. Similarly, vitamin B_6 and vitamin E may be effective. Some women have expressed interest in other alternative treatments (e.g., natural estrogens, progestins, black cohosh, ginseng, dongquai, soy products, several other herbal preparations); however, few data exist about their safety or effectiveness.

SECTION III: PRACTICING FOR NCLEX

Activity E

1. a   **2.** c   **3.** c   **4.** a   **5.** a
6. a   **7.** b   **8.** c   **9.** a, b, d   **10.** a
11. b   **12.** a   **13.** d   **14.** b

CHAPTER 51

SECTION I: ASSESSING YOUR UNDERSTANDING

Activity A

1. *Lactobacillus acidophilus*
2. estrogen

3. fishlike
4. premature labor, premature rupture of membranes, endometritis
5. skin, cervix, vagina, anus, penis, oral cavity
6. 100
7. condylomata
8. dysplasia
9. metronidazole, tinidazole
10. douche
11. lifestyle changes, weight loss, pharmacology

Activity B

1. Refer to Chart 51-1, Risk Factors: Vulvovaginal Infections, in the textbook.
2. Estrogen breaks down glycogen into lactic acid, which is responsible for producing a low vaginal pH. A pH level of 3.5 to 4.5 suppresses bacterial growth.
3. Treatments include antifungal agents such as miconazole, nystatin, clotrimazole, and terconazole cream.
4. PID is a condition of the pelvic cavity that may involve the uterus, fallopian tubes, ovaries, pelvic peritoneum, or pelvic vascular system.
5. Vulvovaginal candidiasis occurs more commonly in pregnancy or with a systemic condition such as diabetes or human immune deficiency virus (HIV) infection, or when patients are taking medications such as corticosteroids or oral contraceptives.

Activity C

1. f	2. d	3. p	4. e	5. h
6. c	7. n	8. o	9. i	10. a
11. j	12. m	13. k	14. b	15. l
16. g				

SECTION II: APPLYING YOUR KNOWLEDGE

Activity D

CASE STUDY: Bacterial Vaginosis

1. Risk factors include douching after menses, smoking, multiple sex partners, and other sexually transmitted infections (STIs) (also referred to as sexually transmitted diseases [STDs]).
2. A vaginal pH of over 4.7.
3. Patients are strongly advised to abstain from alcohol during treatment and for 24 hours after taking metronidazole.

CASE STUDY: Pelvic Inflammatory Disease

1. Pelvic or generalized peritonitis, abscesses, strictures, and fallopian tube obstruction may develop. There is also the potential for bacteremia with septic shock; chronic pelvic and abdominal pain; and recurring PID.
2. Broad-spectrum antibiotic therapy is prescribed, usually a combination of ceftriaxone, azithromycin, and doxycycline.
3. Neisseria gonorrhoeae bacterium and Chlamydia trachomadis.

SECTION III: PRACTICING FOR NCLEX

Activity E

1. d	2. d	3. a, b, c	4. a	5. b
6. d	7. d	8. b	9. c	10. d
11. a, b, c	12. c	13. a	14. a	15. a

CHAPTER 52

SECTION I: ASSESSING YOUR UNDERSTANDING

Activity A

1. second, sixth
2. Cooper ligament
3. 10
4. Gynecomastia
5. breast-feeding

Activity B

1. Refer to Chart 52-2, Patient Education: Breast Self-Examination, in the textbook.
2. The nurse plays a critical role in BSE education, a modality used for the early detection of breast cancer. BSE can be taught in a variety of settings—either on a one-to-one basis or in a group. It can also be initiated by a health care provider during a patient's routine physical examination. Current practice is shifting from teaching BSE to promoting breast self-awareness, a woman's attentiveness to the normal appearance and feel of her breasts.
3. Variations in breast tissue occur during the menstrual cycle, pregnancy, and the onset of menopause.
4. Nipple discharge in a woman who is not lactating may be related to many causes, such as carcinoma, papilloma, pituitary adenoma, cystic breasts, and various medications. Oral contraceptives, pregnancy, hormone therapy (HT), chlorpromazine-type medications, and frequent breast stimulation may be contributing factors. In some athletic women, nipple discharge may occur during running or aerobic exercises.
5. Research suggests that racial disparities in cancer mortality are driven in large part by differences in socioeconomic status.

Activity C

1. e	2. g	3. a	4. c	5. b
6. d	7. f			

SECTION II: APPLYING YOUR KNOWLEDGE

Activity D

CASE STUDY: Total Mastectomy (Simple Mastectomy)

1. Upper outer quadrant.
2. Common sensations include tenderness, soreness, numbness, tightness, pulling, and twinges. These sensations may occur along the chest wall, in the axilla, and along the inside aspect of the upper

arm. After mastectomy, some patients experience phantom sensations and report a feeling that the breast or nipple is still present.

3. The nurse first assesses the patient's readiness and provides gentle encouragement. It is important to maintain the patient's privacy while assisting her as she views the incision; this allows her to express feelings safely to the nurse. Asking the patient what she perceives, acknowledging her feelings, and allowing her to express her emotions are important nursing actions. Reassuring the patient that her feelings are a normal response to breast cancer surgery may be comforting.

SECTION III: PRACTICING FOR NCLEX

Activity E

1. b	**2.** a	**3.** c	**4.** a	**5.** b
6. b	**7.** a	**8.** c	**9.** a	**10.** a, b, c
11. c	**12.** a	**13.** c	**14.** b	**15.** d

CHAPTER 53

SECTION I: ASSESSING YOUR UNDERSTANDING

Activity A

1. prostate-specific antigen (PSA), digital rectal examination (DRE)
2. *Escherichia coli*
3. androgen deprivation therapy (ADT), Lupron, Zoladex, Eulexin, Casodex, Nilandron
4. hemorrhage, infection, DVT, catheter obstruction, sexual dysfunction
5. human chorionic gonadotropin, alpha-fetoprotein
6. spermatogenesis, testosterone
7. Libido, potency
8. kidney, bladder, prostate, penis
9. prostate-specific antigen (PSA)
10. Retrograde ejaculation
11. Urinary incontinence
12. Phosphodiesterase-5 (PDE-5) inhibitors

Activity B

1. Answer may include the following: fever, perineal prostatic pain, dysuria, and urinary tract symptoms (frequency, urgency, hesitancy, and nocturia).
2. Answer may include the following: frequency of urination, nocturia, urgency and a sensation that the bladder has not emptied completely, hesitancy in starting urination, abdominal straining, a decrease in the volume and force of the urinary stream, recurring urinary tract infections, interruption of the urinary stream, and dribbling.
3. Factors to consider in choosing a penile prosthesis are the patient's activities of daily living, social activities, and the expectations of the patient and his partner. Ongoing counseling for the patient and his partner is usually necessary to help them adapt to the prosthesis.

Activity C

1. c	**2.** f	**3.** e	**4.** a	**5.** d
6. h	**7.** g	**8.** b		

SECTION II: APPLYING YOUR KNOWLEDGE

Activity D

CASE STUDY: Prostatectomy

1. Depending on the type of surgery, the patient may experience sexual dysfunction related to erectile dysfunction, decreased libido, and fatigue. These issues may become a concern to the patient soon after surgery or in the weeks to months of rehabilitation. With nerve-sparing radical prostatectomy, the likelihood of recovering the ability to have erections is better for men who are younger and men in whom both neurovascular bundles are spared. A decrease in libido is usually related to the impact of the surgery on the body. Reassurance that the usual level of libido will return after recuperation from surgery is often helpful for the patient and his partner. The patient should be aware that he may experience fatigue during rehabilitation from surgery. This fatigue may also decrease his libido and alter his enjoyment of usual activities.
2. Patients experiencing bladder spasms may report an urgency to void, a feeling of pressure or fullness in the bladder, and bleeding from the urethra around the catheter.
3. Medications that relax the smooth muscles can help ease the spasms, which can be intermittent and severe; these medications include flavoxate and oxybutynin. Warm compresses to the pubis or sitz baths may also relieve the spasms.

SECTION III: PRACTICING FOR NCLEX

Activity E

1. a	**2.** b	**3.** a	**4.** a	**5.** a, b, c
6. b	**7.** c	**8.** d	**9.** a	**10.** c
11. b	**12.** c	**13.** c	**14.** a	**15.** b

CHAPTER 54

SECTION I: ASSESSING YOUR UNDERSTANDING

Activity A

1. Human sexuality
2. Sexual orientation
3. XX, estrogen, XY, testosterone
4. federal-level data
5. social, historical, cultural
6. sex steroids/hormones

Activity B

1. In people who are transgender women (male-to-female), the previous effects of androgens on the skeleton (average greater height; size and shape of hands, feet, and jaw; and pelvic structure) cannot be reversed by hormones.

2. Spironolactone, cyproterone acetate, GnRH agonists (e.g., goserelin, buserelin, triptorelin), and 5-alpha reductase inhibitors (e.g., finasteride, dutasteride).
3. Progestogen is typically not recommended due to the higher incidence of breast cancer and cardiovascular disease.
4. Changes in scalp hair, skin oiliness, facial and body hair, voice, body fat composition, muscle mass, menses, clitoris, and vagina.
5. Laser hair removal is the leading therapy option for long-term results and works on the principle of selective photothermolysis, whereby photons destroy the hair follicle while sparing the surrounding tissue (Thomas & Houreld, 2019). The main risk of this procedure is overheating resulting in redness, blisters, and burns. Treatments should be avoided when photosensitizing medications are being used, such as acne medications (e.g., isotretinoin, minocycline, doxycycline), antibiotics (e.g., tetracyclines, sulfonamides, quinolones), and spironolactone. Nurses should review a patient's medication list and identify those that are photosensitive. Electrolysis involves the use of an electric current that destroys the root of individual hair follicles. This treatment is more time consuming and more painful than laser hair removal. The main risks of electrolysis are redness and pigment changes. To help manage the pain during laser hair removal and electrolysis, topical anesthetics (lidocaine-containing products) and acetaminophen are used.
6. To prevent complications and infection and to ensure patency of the neovaginal cavity.

Activity C

1. d   **2.** a   **3.** e   **4.** b   **5.** f
6. c

SECTION II: APPLYING YOUR KNOWLEDGE

Activity D

CASE STUDY: Care of the Transgender Female Undergoing Orchiectomy and Vaginoplasty

1. To create a perineogenital complex as feminine in appearance and function as possible and free of poorly healed areas, scars, and neuromas.
2. To prevent complications and infection and to ensure patency of the neovaginal cavity.
3. The patient will have the vaginal dilator in place for 5 days continuously; then, the dilator is periodically removed, and daily cleansing of the neovaginal cavity begins.
4. Education on how to dilate and cleanse their vaginal cavity for 3 to 6 months.

SECTION III: PRACTICING FOR NCLEX

Activity E

1. b, c, d, e   **2.** c   **3.** b, c, d   **4.** a   **5.** a
6. d   **7.** c, d   **8.** b   **9.** a   **10.** c

CHAPTER 55

SECTION I: ASSESSING YOUR UNDERSTANDING

Activity A

1. epidermis, dermis, subcutaneous tissue
2. keratinocytes, Merkel cells, Langerhans cells
3. 2 to 3 weeks
4. adipose, temperature
5. alopecia
6. Sebaceous, sweat
7. D
8. sclera, mucous membrane
9. hypoxia
10. Radiation, conduction, convection

Activity B

1. Melanin is controlled by a hormone secreted from the hypothalamus of the brain called *melanocyte-stimulating hormone*.
2. The hair of the skin provides thermal insulation in mammals. This function is enhanced during cold or fright by piloerection, caused by contraction of the tiny erector muscles attached to the hair follicle.
3. The receptor endings of nerves in the skin allow the body to constantly monitor the conditions of the immediate environment. They sense temperature, pain, light touch, and pressure.
4. Answer may include dryness, wrinkling, uneven pigmentation, and various proliferative lesions. Cellular changes associated with aging include a thinning at the junction of the dermis and epidermis.

Activity C

1. h   **2.** i   **3.** j   **4.** g   **5.** d
6. f   **7.** c   **8.** a   **9.** e   **10.** b

SECTION II: APPLYING YOUR KNOWLEDGE

Activity D

1. The color of the lesions; redness, heat, pain, or swelling; size and location of the involved area; pattern of eruption; and distribution of the lesion.
2. Diabetic dermopathy.
3. Because of changes in peripheral nerves, patients with diabetes do not always sense minor injuries to the lower legs and feet. Infections can begin and, if left untreated, may lead to ulcerations. Ulcerations are often not noticed and become quite large before being treated.

SECTION III: PRACTICING FOR NCLEX

Activity E

1. b   **2.** a   **3.** a   **4.** a   **5.** b
6. c   **7.** c   **8.** d   **9.** d   **10.** b
11. a   **12.** d   **13.** b   **14.** b   **15.** d

CHAPTER 56

SECTION I: ASSESSING YOUR UNDERSTANDING

Activity A

1. acne
2. passive, interactive, active
3. débridement
4. anti-inflammatory, antipruritic, vasoconstrictive
5. sweat glands
6. *Sarcoptes scabiei*
7. *Staphylococcus aureus*
8. autoimmune
9. Gentle removal of the scales
10. topical, phototherapy, systemic
11. Infection

Activity B

1. Answer should include the following: prevent additional damage, prevent secondary infection, revise the inflammatory process, and relieve symptoms.
2. Moisture-retentive dressings have a high moisture vapor transmission rate. Some dressings even have reservoirs to hold excessive exudate.
3. Cytokines are proteins with mitogenic activity that release increased amounts of growth factors into a wound. This process stimulates cell growth and granulation of skin.
4. Foam dressings are nonadherent, thus the nurse must apply a secondary dressing to keep them in place.
5. Keratoconjunctivitis, sepsis, and multiple organ dysfunction syndrome (MODS) are potential complications of TEN and SJS.
6. Risk factors for malignant melanoma include: Caucasian skin color (particularly fairer-skinned or freckled, blue-eyed, blond or red-haired people of Celtic or Scandinavian origin); history of sunburns, particularly in childhood; previous history of melanoma (multiple primary melanomas are not uncommon); family history of melanoma (10% of patients diagnosed with melanoma have a positive family history of melanoma); personal or family history of multiple atypical nevi (formerly called dysplastic nevi); and family history of astrocytoma or pancreatic cancer.

Activity C

1. e	**2.** f	**3.** g	**4.** d	**5.** i
6. j	**7.** l	**8.** k	**9.** b	**10.** h
11. m	**12.** n	**13.** o	**14.** c	**15.** a

SECTION II: APPLYING YOUR KNOWLEDGE

Activity D

CASE STUDY: Acne Vulgaris

1. Diet is not believed to play a major role in therapy. However, the elimination of a specific food or food product associated with a flare-up of acne, such as chocolate, cola, fried foods, or milk products, should be promoted.

2. Tetracycline.
3. Major nursing activities include patient education, particularly in proper skin care techniques, and managing potential problems related to the skin disorder or therapy. Providing positive reassurance, listening attentively, and being sensitive to the feelings of the patient with acne are essential for the patient's psychological well-being and understanding of the disease and treatment plan.

CASE STUDY: Malignant Melanoma

1. A superficial spreading melanoma.
2. Excisional biopsy.
3. Metastasis is probable. The primary provider will include education about biopsy and treatment options.

SECTION III: PRACTICING FOR NCLEX

Activity E

1. d	**2.** c	**3.** b	**4.** a, b, c	**5.** a
6. a	**7.** a	**8.** c	**9.** c	**10.** a
11. d	**12.** b	**13.** d	**14.** c	**15.** b, c, d

CHAPTER 57

SECTION I: ASSESSING YOUR UNDERSTANDING

Activity A

1. young children, older adults
2. one third
3. Hypovolemia
4. the depth of the injury, the extent of injured body surface area
5. acute respiratory failure, acute respiratory distress syndrome (ARDS)
6. sepsis
7. 0.5, 1.0 mL/kg/hr
8. *Pseudomonas,* methicillin-resistant *Staphylococcus, Acinetobacter*
9. silver sulfadiazine, silver nitrate, mafenide acetate
10. increased temperature, tachycardia, widened pulse pressure, flushed, dry skin in nonburned areas

Activity B

1. Advances in burn care over the past 80 years have contributed to significant improvements in morbidity and mortality of patients with burns. These advances include the introduction of systemic antibiotics and topical antimicrobials, advances in fluid resuscitation, aggressive nutrition, early excision and wound closure, the introduction of engineered tissue therapies, advances in critical-care therapies, and the advent of specialized burn centers.
2. The central area of the wound is termed the *zone of coagulation* due to the characteristic coagulation necrosis of cells that occurs. The surrounding zone, the *zone of stasis,* describes an area of

injured cells that may remain viable but, with persistent decreased blood flow, will undergo necrosis within 24 to 48 hours. The *zone of hyperemia,* the outermost zone, sustains minimal injury and may fully recover over time.

3. The first is a thermal effect, which results in cutaneous burn injuries. The second effect is damage to the cellular DNA, which may be localized or affect the whole body.

4. Carbon monoxide, a byproduct of the combustion of organic materials, combines with hemoglobin to form carboxyhemoglobin. Carboxyhemoglobin competes with oxygen for available hemoglobin-binding sites.

5. Primary survey, prevention of shock, prevention of respiratory distress, detection and treatment of concomitant injuries, wound assessment, and initial care.

6. The depth of the injury depends on the temperature of the burning agent and the duration of contact with the agent.

7. Inhalation injury below the vocal cords results from inhaling the products of incomplete combustion or noxious gases, and is often the source of death at the scene of a fire.

8. The secondary survey focuses on obtaining a history, the completion of the total body system assessment, initial fluid resuscitation, and provision of psychosocial support of the conscious patient.

9. Preventive treatment modalities are used to prevent scar contractures and excess hypertrophic tissue. Compression is introduced early in burn wound treatment. Elastic bandage wraps are used initially to help promote adequate circulation, but they can also be used as the first form of compression for scar management, followed by elasticized tubular bandage until the patient can be measured for a customized garment.

10. Fluid overload may occur when fluid is mobilized from the interstitial compartment back into the intravascular compartment. If the cardiac system cannot compensate for the excess volume, congestive heart failure may result.

Activity C

1. b	2. f	3. c	4. e	5. d
6. a	7. g			

SECTION II: APPLYING YOUR KNOWLEDGE

Activity D

1. Indicators of possible inhalation injury include the following: injury occurring in an enclosed space; burns of the face or neck; singed nasal hair; hoarseness, high-pitched voice change, and stridor; soot in sputum; dyspnea or tachypnea and other signs of reduced oxygen levels (hypoxemia); and erythema and blistering of the oral or pharyngeal mucosa.

2. Intubation and mechanical intubation, possible escharotomy to allow adequate chest expansion.

3. 1944 mL: 2 mL lactated Ringer × patient's weight in kilograms (72) × %TBSA (13.5), second-, third-, and fourth-degree burns.

SECTION III: PRACTICING FOR NCLEX

Activity E

1. b	2. c	3. d	4. c	5. a
6. a	7. 2400 mL	8. a, b, d	9. d	10. b
11. a, b, d	12. c	13. c	14. a	15. c
16. b	17. c			

CHAPTER 58

SECTION I: ASSESSING YOUR UNDERSTANDING

Activity A

1. 10 to 21 mm Hg
2. Ishihara polychromatic plates
3. pallor (lack of blood supply), cupping of the optic nerve disc
4. laser trabeculoplasty, laser iridotomy
5. Laser scanning polarimetry
6. irrigation with normal saline
7. *Streptococcus pneumoniae, Haemophilus influenzae, Staphylococcus aureus*
8. "pink eye," or dilation of the conjunctival blood vessels
9. diabetic retinopathy
10. cytomegalovirus (CMV)
11. Lipoid, aqueous, mucoid
12. ptosis

Activity B

1. Visual acuity is tested for both near (14 inches away) and distance (20 feet away) vision and performed on each eye separately with a standardized Snellen chart for distance and a Rosenbaum pocket screener for near vision.

2. Patients are cautioned to avoid squeezing the eyelids, holding the breath, or performing a Valsalva maneuver, as these may result in abnormally increased IOP.

3. The Amsler grid is a test often used for patients with macular problems, such as macular degeneration.

Activity C

PART I

1. b	2. c	3. f	4. j	5. a
6. e	7. g	8. d	9. h	10. i

PART II

1. g	2. n	3. e	4. l	5. o
6. a	7. b	8. j	9. c	10. k
11. d	12. m	13. f	14. i	15. h

SECTION II: APPLYING YOUR KNOWLEDGE

Activity D

CASE STUDY: Cataract Surgery

1. Smoking, diabetes, alcohol abuse, and inadequate intake of antioxidant vitamins over time.
2. Painless blurring of vision, sensitivity to glare, and functional impairment due to reduced visual acuity.
3. She cannot lie on the affected side for two nights.

SECTION III: PRACTICING FOR NCLEX

Activity E

1. a, b, c	**2.** c	**3.** d	**4.** d	**5.** d
6. c	**7.** a, b, c	**8.** c	**9.** a, b, c	**10.** a
11. c	**12.** c	**13.** c	**14.** a	**15.** b

CHAPTER 59

SECTION I: ASSESSING YOUR UNDERSTANDING

Activity A

1. cochlea
2. organ of Corti
3. eighth
4. 30
5. 70, 90
6. functional
7. 85, 90
8. 50
9. seventh
10. eighth

Activity B

1. Hearing is conducted over two pathways: air and bone. Sounds transmitted by air conduction travel over the air-filled external and middle ear through vibration of the tympanic membrane and ossicles. Sounds transmitted by bone conduction travel directly through bone to the inner ear, bypassing the tympanic membrane and ossicles.
2. Rhine, Weber, and Whisper tests.
3. Inspection of the external, middle, and inner ear.
4. Frequency, pitch, and intensity.
5. A tympanogram, or impedance audiometry, measures middle ear muscle reflex to sound stimulation and compliance of the tympanic membrane by changing the air pressure in a sealed ear canal.

Activity C

1. h	**2.** a	**3.** i	**4.** g	**5.** c
6. j	**7.** f	**8.** b	**9.** d	**10.** e

SECTION II: APPLYING YOUR KNOWLEDGE

Activity D

CASE STUDY: Mastoid Surgery

1. The patient's mastoid pressure dressing can be removed 24 to 48 hours after surgery.
2. Although infrequently injured, the facial nerve, which runs through the middle ear and mastoid, is at some risk for injury during mastoid surgery. As the patient awakens from anesthesia, any evidence of facial paresis should be reported to the primary provider.
3. Constant, throbbing pain accompanied by fever may indicate infection and should be reported to the primary provider.

CASE STUDY: Ménière's Disease

1. Answer may include vertigo, tinnitus, fluctuating and progressive sensorineural hearing loss, a feeling of pressure or fullness in the ear, and episodic and incapacitating vertigo accompanied by nausea and vomiting.
2. Limit foods high in salt or sugar. Be aware of foods with hidden salts and sugars. Limit alcohol and caffeine. Avoid foods with monosodium glutamate (MSG).
3. Aspirin or aspirin products.

SECTION III: PRACTICING FOR NCLEX

Activity E

1. a	**2.** c	**3.** b	**4.** a	**5.** c
6. c	**7.** a	**8.** b	**9.** a, c, d	**10.** b
11. d	**12.** a	**13.** b	**14.** d	**15.** a

CHAPTER 60

SECTION I: ASSESSING YOUR UNDERSTANDING

Activity A

1. Serotonin
2. dopamine
3. frontal
4. temporal
5. frontal
6. hypothalamus
7. pituitary
8. thalamus
9. 150
10. C8, L3
11. acetylcholine
12. cerebellum

Activity B

1. This barrier is formed by the endothelial cells of the brain's capillaries, which form continuous tight junctions, creating a barrier to macromolecules and many compounds.
2. The *autonomic nervous system* regulates the activities of internal organs such as the heart, lungs, blood vessels, digestive organs, and glands. Maintenance and restoration of internal homeostasis is largely the responsibility of the autonomic nervous system.
3. Flaccid paralysis and atrophy of the affected muscles.

4. Destruction or dysfunction of the basal ganglia leads not to paralysis but to muscle rigidity, disturbances of posture, and difficulty initiating or changing movement.

Activity C

Neurotransmitters and Nervous System Response

1. e **2.** f **3.** d **4.** c **5.** a
6. b

Cranial Nerves

Nerve No.	Column I	Column II
I	Olfactory	Smell
II	Optic	Vision
III	Oculomotor	Eye movement
IV	Trochlear	Eye movement
V	Trigeminal	Facial sensation
VI	Abducens	Eye movement
VII	Facial	Taste and expression
VIII	Vestibulocochlear	Hearing and equilibrium
IX	Glossopharyngeal	Taste
X	Vagus	Swallowing, gastric motility, and secretion
XI	Spinal accessory	Trapezius and sternomastoid muscles
XII	Hypoglossal	Tongue movement

SECTION II: APPLYING YOUR KNOWLEDGE

Activity D

CASE STUDY: Mental Status

1. Institute safety and fall prevention measures.
2. Procedures and preparations needed for diagnostic tests are explained, taking into account the possibility of impaired hearing and slowed responses in the older adult. Providing instruction at an unrushed pace and using reinforcement enhance learning and retention. Material should be short, concise, and concrete. Vocabulary is matched to the patient's ability, and terms are clearly defined. The older adult patient requires adequate time to receive and respond to stimuli, learn, and react. These measures allow comprehension, memory, and formation of association and concepts.
3. Delirium (transient mental confusion, usually with delusions and hallucinations) is seen in older adult patients who have underlying central nervous system damage or are experiencing an acute condition such as infection, adverse medication reaction, or dehydration. Drug toxicity and depression may produce impairment of attention and memory, and should be evaluated as a possible cause of mental

status change. Delirium must be differentiated from dementia, which is a chronic and irreversible deterioration of cognitive status.

SECTION III: PRACTICING FOR NCLEX

Activity E

1. a	**2.** c	**3.** c	**4.** b, c, d	**5.** b
6. a	**7.** b	**8.** d	**9.** a	**10.** d
11. b	**12.** b	**13.** b	**14.** c	**15.** c

CHAPTER 61

SECTION I: ASSESSING YOUR UNDERSTANDING

Activity A

1. locked-in syndrome
2. pneumonia, aspiration, respiratory failure
3. a change in the level of consciousness (LOC)
4. brain stem herniation, diabetes insipidus, syndrome of inappropriate antidiuretic hormone (SIADH)
5. brain herniation resulting in death
6. cerebral edema, pain, seizures, increased ICP, neurologic status
7. cerebrovascular disease
8. status epilepticus

Activity B

1. An altered LOC is present when the patient is not oriented, does not follow commands, or needs persistent stimuli to achieve a state of alertness. LOC is gauged on a continuum, with a normal state of alertness and full cognition on one end and coma on the other end.
2. Answer should include five of the following: respiratory distress, pneumonia, aspiration, pressure injury, deep vein thrombosis, and contractures.
3. A neurologic examination should include evaluation of mental status, cranial nerve function, cerebellar function, reflexes, and motor and sensory function, as well as the score of the Glasgow Coma Scale.
4. Before and after suctioning, the patient is adequately ventilated to prevent hypoxia.
5. Alertness is measured by the patient's ability to open the eyes spontaneously or in response to a vocal or noxious stimulus (pressure or pain).

Activity C

1. a and f **2.** c and e **3.** b **4.** a **5.** c

SECTION II: APPLYING YOUR KNOWLEDGE

Activity D

CASE STUDY: Optimizing Cerebral Perfusion Pressure

1. Proper positioning helps reduce ICP. The patient's head is kept in a neutral (midline) position, maintained with the use of a cervical collar if necessary, to promote venous drainage. Elevation of the head

is maintained at 30 to 45 degrees unless contraindicated. Extreme rotation of the neck and flexion of the neck are avoided, because compression or distortion of the jugular veins increases ICP. Extreme hip flexion is also avoided, because this position causes an increase in intra-abdominal and intrathoracic pressures, which can produce an increase in ICP.

2. Stool softeners may be prescribed. When Alex is awake and alert, a high-fiber diet may be indicated. Abdominal distention, which increases intra-abdominal and intrathoracic pressure and ICP, should be noted. Enemas and cathartics are avoided if possible. When moving or being turned in bed, ask Alex to exhale (which opens the glottis) to avoid the Valsalva maneuver.

3. Space activities to avoid stress and strain. Maintain a calm atmosphere and decrease environmental stimuli.

SECTION III: PRACTICING FOR NCLEX

Activity E

1. d	**2.** a	**3.** c	**4.** b	**5.** c
6. a, b, c	**7.** d	**8.** c	**9.** d	**10.** c
11. a, c, d	**12.** c	**13.** a	**14.** d	**15.** c

CHAPTER 62

SECTION I: ASSESSING YOUR UNDERSTANDING

Activity A

1. stroke, brain attack
2. 4.5
3. fifth
4. carotid endarterectomy
5. Arteriosclerosis
6. hemiplegia
7. brain tissue, the ventricles, the subarachnoid space
8. rebleeding or hematoma expansion, cerebral vasospasm, acute hydrocephalus, seizures
9. hypertension
10. Ischemic, hemorrhagic

Activity B

1. Atrial fibrillation.
2. Small, penetrating artery thrombotic stroke affect one or more vessels, and is the most common type of ischemic stroke.
3. The DASH diet is high in fruits and vegetables, moderate in low-fat dairy products, and low in animal protein (has a substantial amount of plant protein from legumes and nuts).
4. By dissolving the blood clot that is blocking blood flow to the brain.

Activity C

1. d	**2.** h	**3.** e	**4.** a	**5.** b
6. g	**7.** c	**8.** f		

SECTION II: APPLYING YOUR KNOWLEDGE

Activity D

1. Before receiving t-PA, the patient is assessed using the National Institutes of Health Stroke Scale (NIHSS), a standardized assessment tool that helps evaluate stroke severity.
2. The nurse will administer 6.48 mg. (The dosage for t-PA is 0.9 mg/kg, with a maximum dose of 90 mg. Ten percent of the calculated dose is administered as an IV bolus over 1 minute.)
3. Bleeding is the most common side effect of t-PA administration, thus the patient is closely monitored for any bleeding (IV insertion sites, urinary catheter site, endotracheal tube, nasogastric tube, urine, stool, emesis, and other secretions).

SECTION III: PRACTICING FOR NCLEX

Activity E

1. a	**2.** a	**3.** c	**4.** a	**5.** c
6. d	**7.** a, b, d	**8.** b	**9.** a	**10.** c
11. d	**12.** b	**13.** c	**14.** a, b, c	**15.** a

CHAPTER 63

SECTION I: ASSESSING YOUR UNDERSTANDING

Activity A

1. brain, blood, cerebrospinal fluid
2. Monro–Kellie doctrine
3. linear, comminuted, depressed, frontal, temporal, basilar
4. CT scan
5. hematoma (either epidural, subdural, or intracerebral)
6. coma, hypertension, bradycardia, bradypnea
7. coma, absence of brain stem reflexes, apnea
8. concussion
9. eye opening, verbal responses, motor responses to verbal commands or painful stimuli
10. systemic infections, neurosurgical infections, heterotrophic ossification
11. 5th cervical, 6th cervical, 7th cervical, 12th thoracic, 1st lumbar

Activity B

1. In Brown-Séquard syndrome, ipsilateral paralysis or paresis is noted, together with ipsilateral loss of touch, pressure, and vibration, and contralateral loss of sensation of pain and temperature.
2. The most common causes of TBI are falls (35.2%), motor vehicle crashes (17.3%), being struck by objects (16.5%), and assaults (10%).
3. *Primary injury* is the initial damage to the brain that results from a traumatic event. This may include contusions, lacerations, and torn blood vessels due to impact, acceleration/deceleration, or foreign object penetration. *Secondary injury* evolves

over the ensuing hours and days after an initial injury and results from inadequate delivery of nutrients and oxygen to the cells. These processes include intracranial hemorrhage, cerebral edema, increased intracranial pressure, hypoxic brain damage, and infection.

4. A grade 1 concussion has symptoms of transient confusion, no loss of consciousness, and duration of mental status abnormalities on examination that resolve in less than 15 minutes.

5. Monitoring includes observing the patient for a decrease in LOC, worsening headache, dizziness, seizures, abnormal pupil response, vomiting, irritability, slurred speech, and numbness or weakness in the arms or legs.

Activity C

1. c	2. f	3. h	4. e	5. i
6. b	7. g	8. j	9. d	10. a

SECTION II: APPLYING YOUR KNOWLEDGE

Activity D

CASE STUDY: Spinal Cord Injury

1. Independent in transfers and wheelchair.

2. A major aspect of nursing care is educating the patient and family about complications and strategies to minimize risks. UTIs, contractures, infected pressure injury, and sepsis may necessitate hospitalization. Other late complications that may occur include lower extremity edema, joint contractures, respiratory dysfunction, and pain. To avoid these and other complications, the patient and a family member are educated about skin care, catheter care, range-of-motion exercises, breathing exercises, and other care techniques.

3. The diet for the patient with tetraplegia or paraplegia should be high in protein, vitamins, and calories to ensure minimal wasting of muscle and the maintenance of healthy skin, and high in fluids to maintain well-functioning kidneys. Excessive weight gain and obesity should be avoided, because they further limit mobility.

SECTION III: PRACTICING FOR NCLEX

Activity E

1. c	2. a	3. d	4. c	5. b
6. a	7. c	8. d	9. a, b, c, d	10. a, b, d
11. b	12. b	13. a	14. c	15. d

CHAPTER 64

SECTION I: ASSESSING YOUR UNDERSTANDING

Activity A

1. meningitis, brain abscesses, various types of encephalitis, Creutzfeldt–Jakob disease (CJD), variant CJD

2. areflexia, ascending weakness
3. herpes simplex virus (HSV), acyclovir
4. immunologic assessment, electroencephalogram (EEG), magnetic resonance imaging (MRI)
5. myelin sheath
6. immunomodulating, immunosuppressive
7. acetylcholine receptors
8. double vision, ptosis
9. *Streptococcus pneumoniae*, *Neisseria meningitidis*
10. Syndrome of inappropriate antidiuretic hormone (SIADH), hyponatremia

Activity B

1. Risks for an unfavorable outcome include older age, a heart rate of greater than 120 bpm, decreased score on the Glasgow Coma Scale, cranial nerve palsies, and a positive Gram stain 1 hour after presentation to the hospital.

2. *Demyelination* refers to the destruction of myelin, the fatty and protein material that surrounds nerve fibers in the brain and spinal cord. This destruction results in impaired transmission of nerve impulses.

3. Avoiding hot temperatures, effective treatment of depression and anemia, and occupational and physical therapies may help control fatigue. Additional strategies include a balance of rest and activities, good nutrition to avoid being overweight and obese, and a healthy lifestyle, including avoidance of alcohol and cigarette smoking.

Activity C

1. b	2. b	3. e	4. d	5. f
6. f	7. g	8. h	9. h	10. d

SECTION II: APPLYING YOUR KNOWLEDGE

Activity D

CASE STUDY: Multiple Sclerosis

1. Exacerbations and remissions are characteristic of MS. During exacerbations, new symptoms appear and existing ones worsen; during remissions, symptoms decrease or disappear. Relapses may be associated with emotional and physical stress, which Mrs. Singh is experiencing related to her clinical and classroom schedule.

2. Side effects include mood swings, weight gain, and electrolyte imbalances.

3. Nursing assessment should include neurologic deficits, secondary complications, and the impact of the disease on the patient and family. The patient's mobility and balance are observed to determine whether there is risk of falling. Assessment of function is carried out both when the patient is well rested and when fatigued. The patient is assessed for weakness, spasticity, visual impairment, incontinence, and disorders of swallowing and speech. Additional areas of assessment include how MS has affected the patient's lifestyle, how the patient is coping, adherence to the prescribed medication regimen, and what the patient would like to improve.

SECTION III: PRACTICING FOR NCLEX

Activity E

1. a, b, c   **2.** a   **3.** b   **4.** a   **5.** c
6. d   **7.** c   **8.** b, c, d   **9.** a   **10.** c
11. a   **12.** b   **13.** b   **14.** c   **15.** a

CHAPTER 65

SECTION I: ASSESSING YOUR UNDERSTANDING

Activity A

1. lung, breast, lower gastrointestinal tract, pancreas, kidney, skin
2. headache, vomiting (with or without nausea), papilledema
3. motor, sensory, cranial nerve dysfunction
4. intramedullary
5. Answer may include five of the following seven: Parkinson's disease, Huntington disease, Alzheimer's disease, amyotrophic lateral sclerosis, muscular dystrophies, degenerative disc disease, and postpolio syndrome.
6. tremor, rigidity, bradykinesia, postural instability
7. fatigue, progressive muscle weakness, cramps, fasciculations (twitching), incoordination
8. progressive muscle wasting and weakness, abnormal elevation in blood muscle enzymes
9. C5 to C6, C6 to C7
10. hematoma at the surgical site, causing cord compression; neurologic deficit and recurrent or persistent pain after surgery

Activity B

1. A variety of physiologic changes can occur, such as increased ICP and cerebral edema, seizure activity and focal neurologic signs, hydrocephalus, and altered pituitary function.
2. Brain tumors are classified according to origin: those arising from the covering of the brain, those developing in or on the cranial nerves, those originating within brain tissue, and metastatic lesions originating elsewhere in the body.
3. Primary brain tumors originate from cells within the brain. Secondary, or metastatic, brain tumors develop from structures outside the brain and are twice as common as primary brain tumors.
4. Computer-assisted stereotactic (three-dimensional) biopsy is used to diagnose deep-seated brain tumors and to provide a basis for treatment and prognosis. Stereotactic approaches involve the use of a three-dimensional frame that allows very precise localization of the tumor; a stereotactic frame and multiple imaging studies (x-rays, CT scans, or MRIs) are used to localize the tumor and verify its position. Brain-mapping technology helps determine how close diseased areas of the brain are to structures essential for normal brain function.

5. Although symptoms are variable, a slow, unilateral resting tremor is present in the majority of patients at the time of diagnosis.

Activity C

1. d   **2.** c   **3.** g   **4.** a   **5.** h
6. f   **7.** b   **8.** e

SECTION II: APPLYING YOUR KNOWLEDGE

Activity D

CASE STUDY: Parkinson's Disease

1. A progressive program of daily exercise will increase muscle strength, improve coordination and dexterity, reduce muscular rigidity, and prevent contractures that occur when muscles are not used.
2. Walking, riding a stationary bicycle, swimming, and gardening are all exercises that help maintain joint mobility. Stretching (stretch–hold–relax) and range-of-motion exercises promote joint flexibility. Postural exercises are important to counter the tendency of the head and neck to be drawn forward and down. A physical therapist may be helpful in developing an individualized exercise program and can provide instruction to the patient and caregiver on exercising safely. Faithful adherence to an exercise and walking program helps delay the progress of the disease. Warm baths and massage, in addition to passive and active exercises, help relax muscles and relieve painful muscle spasms that accompany rigidity.
3. Carbidopa is often added to levodopa to avoid metabolism of levodopa before it can reach the brain.
4. The goals for the patient may include improving functional mobility, maintaining independence in activities of daily living, achieving adequate bowel elimination, attaining and maintaining acceptable nutritional status, achieving effective communication, and developing positive coping mechanisms.

CASE STUDY: Huntington Disease

1. The most prominent clinical features of the disease that this patient is experiencing are chorea (rapid, jerky involuntary movements) and impaired voluntary movement. Other prominent features include intellectual decline and, often, personality changes.
2. The Huntington's Disease Society of America helps patients and families by providing information, referrals, family and public education, and support for research.
3. SSRIs and tricyclics have been recommended for control of psychiatric symptoms. The threat of suicide is present particularly early in the course of the disease. Psychotic symptoms usually respond to antipsychotic medications. Psychotherapy aimed at allaying anxiety and reducing stress may be beneficial.

SECTION III: PRACTICING FOR NCLEX

Activity E

1. a, b, c	**2.** c	**3.** d	**4.** b	**5.** b
6. a	**7.** d	**8.** b	**9.** d	**10.** c
11. c	**12.** a	**13.** a	**14.** c	**15.** b

CHAPTER 66

SECTION I: ASSESSING YOUR UNDERSTANDING

Activity A

1. 50
2. measles, mumps, rubella, pertussis, tetanus, hepatitis B, varicella
3. fever, transient lymphadenopathy, hypersensitivity reaction
4. World Health Organization (WHO), Centers for Disease Control and Prevention (CDC)
5. coagulase-negative *staphylococci,* diphtheroids; *Staphylococcus aureus, Pseudomonas aeruginosa*
6. *Clostridium difficile,* methicillin-resistant *Staphylococcus aureus* (MRSA), vancomycin-resistant *Enterococcus* (VRE)
7. pneumococcus, meningococcus
8. skin, urethra, cervix, vagina, rectum, oropharynx

Activity B

1. These essentials are a causative organism, a reservoir of available organisms, a portal or mode of exit from the reservoir, a mode of transmission from reservoir to host, a susceptible host, and a mode of entry to the host.
2. *Infectious disease* is the state in which the infected host displays a decline in wellness due to the infection. An *infection* is a condition in which the host interacts physiologically and immunologically with a microorganism.
3. Spread of microorganisms by the hands of health care workers.
4. Avoidance of percutaneous injury.
5. When hospitalized, a patient with tuberculosis should be in an airborne infection isolation room (AIIR), engineered to provide negative air pressure, rapid turnover of air, and air either highly filtered or exhausted directly to the outside. Health care providers should wear an N95 respirator (i.e., protective mask) at all times while in the patient's room. The nurse should be able to validate negative pressure when it is in place by reading a pressure manometer placed outside the room or by witnessing that a tissue held at the gap between the door and the floor will be pulled toward the room.

Activity C

1. a	**2.** d	**3.** b	**4.** e	**5.** f
6. c	**7.** g	**8.** h		

SECTION II: APPLYING YOUR KNOWLEDGE

Activity D

1. Chlamydia.
2. In women, pelvic inflammatory disease (PID), ectopic pregnancy, endometritis, and infertility are possible complications of either *N. gonorrhoeae* or *Chlamydia trachomatis* infection.
3. Diagnostic methods used in *N. gonorrhoeae* infection include Gram stain (appropriate only for male urethral samples), culture, and nucleic acid amplification tests (NAATs).
4. Along with reinforcing the importance of abstinence, when appropriate, education should address limiting the number of sexual partners and using condoms for barrier protection. Young women and pregnant women should also be instructed about the importance of routine screening for chlamydia.

SECTION III: PRACTICING FOR NCLEX

Activity E

1. b	**2.** c	**3.** a	**4.** c	**5.** a, c, d
6. b	**7.** d	**8.** a	**9.** b	**10.** a
11. c	**12.** c	**13.** d	**14.** a	**15.** c

CHAPTER 67

SECTION I: ASSESSING YOUR UNDERSTANDING

Activity A

1. primary
2. Emergency Medical Treatment and Active Labor Act (EMTALA)
3. speak, breathe, cough, 3 to 5
4. self-protection
5. muscle cramps, profound diaphoresis, profound thirst
6. 5, 85
7. 1, 9
8. 4, 12
9. 500, 1000, normal saline solution

Activity B

1. Endotracheal intubation is indicated to establish an airway for a patient who cannot be adequately ventilated with an oropharyngeal airway, bypass an upper airway obstruction, prevent aspiration, permit connection of the patient to a resuscitation bag or mechanical ventilator, or facilitate the removal of tracheobronchial secretions.
2. Lactated Ringer solution is initially useful because it approximates plasma electrolyte composition and osmolality, allows time for blood typing and screening, restores circulation, and serves as an adjunct to blood component therapy.
3. For older adult patients, especially those in extended-care facilities, sedatives and hypnotic medications,

diseases affecting motor coordination (e.g., Parkinson's disease), and mental dysfunction (e.g., dementia, mental retardation) are risk factors for asphyxiation by food.

4. A quick neurologic assessment may be performed using the AVPU mnemonic:
   - *A*—*a*lert; is the patient alert and responsive?
   - *V*—*v*erbal; does the patient respond to verbal stimuli?
   - *P*—*p*ain; does the patient respond only to painful stimuli?
   - *U*—*u*nresponsive; is the patient unresponsive to all stimuli, including pain?

5. A basic and widely used triage system that has been in use for many years utilized three categories: emergent, urgent, and nonurgent. In this system, emergent patients have the highest priority, urgent patients are those with serious health problems but not immediately life-threatening ones, and nonurgent patients are those with episodic illnesses.

Activity C

1. g **2.** h **3.** b **4.** f **5.** d
6. a **7.** c **8.** e

SECTION II: APPLYING YOUR KNOWLEDGE

Activity D

CASE STUDY: Heat Stroke

1. Clinical manifestations of heat stroke may include profound central nervous system (CNS) dysfunction (manifested by confusion, delirium, bizarre behavior, coma, seizures); elevated body temperature (40.6°C [105°F] or higher); hot, dry skin; and usually anhidrosis (absence of sweating), tachypnea, hypotension, and tachycardia.

2. The main goal is to reduce the high body temperature as quickly as possible, because mortality in heat stroke or morbid progression to heat stroke with less serious forms of heat-induced illnesses is directly related to the duration of hyperthermia. For the patient with heat stroke, simultaneous treatment focuses on stabilizing oxygenation using the CABs (*c*irculation, *a*irway, and *b*reathing) (formerly called the ABCs) of basic life support. This includes establishing intravenous (IV) access for fluid administration.

3. Urine output is measured frequently because acute tubular necrosis may occur as a complication of heat stroke from rhabdomyolysis (myoglobin in the urine).

SECTION III: PRACTICING FOR NCLEX

Activity E

1. b **2.** d **3.** b **4.** b **5.** b
6. a, b, c **7.** c **8.** a, b, d **9.** c **10.** b, c, d
11. a **12.** a **13.** c **14.** c **15.** c

CHAPTER 68

SECTION I: ASSESSING YOUR UNDERSTANDING

Activity A

1. environmental forces
2. Department of Health and Human Services (HHS), Department of Defense, Department of Homeland Security
3. Food and Drug Administration (FDA)
4. Communication
5. anthrax, smallpox
6. ciprofloxacin, doxycycline
7. 13

Activity B

1. The ICS is a management tool for organizing personnel, facilities, equipment, and communication for any emergency. Its activation during emergencies is mandated by the federal government. Successful incident management requires equipment compatibility, effective communication, adequate distribution of resources, and clear differentiation of members' roles. The ICS ensures that any hazardous substances used during an MCI are identified promptly and that appropriate personal protection equipment is distributed. In addition to all of these responsibilities, the ICS is also responsible for determining when an MCI has ended.

2. Preservation, acceleration, expansion, and allocation.

3. Disaster tags, which are numbered and include triage priority, name, address, age, location and description of injuries, and treatments or medications given, are used to communicate patient information. The tag should be securely placed on the patient and remain with the patient at all times. The tag number and the patient's name, if known, are recorded in a disaster log.

4. Some cultural considerations include language differences, a variety of religious preferences (hygiene, diet, and medical treatment), rituals of prayer, traditions for burying the dead, and the timing of funeral services.

5. The nurse can assist through active listening and providing emotional support, giving information, and referring patients to therapists or social workers. Experience has shown that few victims of disaster seek these services, and early intervention minimizes psychological consequences. Nurses can also discourage victims from subjecting themselves to repeated exposure to the event through media replays and news articles, as well as encourage them to return to normal activities and social roles when appropriate (ENA, 2020).

6. *Level A* protection is worn when the highest level of respiratory, skin, eye, and mucous membrane protection is required. This includes a self-contained breathing apparatus (SCBA) and a fully encapsulating, vapor-tight, chemical-resistant suit with chemical-resistant gloves and boots.

Level B protection requires the highest level of respiratory protection but a lesser level of skin and eye protection than with level A situations. This level of protection includes the SCBA and a chemical-resistant suit, but the suit is not vapor tight.

Level C protection requires the air-purified respirator, which uses filters or sorbent materials to remove harmful substances from the air. A chemical-resistant coverall with splash hood, chemical-resistant gloves, and boots are included in level C protection.

Level D protection is the typical work uniform and is used for nuisance contamination only; it does not provide adequate protection in cases in which respiratory or skin threats are present. Other PPE such as gloves or mask may be required based on the situation.

Activity C

Triage Categories During a Mass Casualty Incident (MCI)

1. c	**2.** d	**3.** a	**4.** a	**5.** d
6. c	**7.** c	**8.** b	**9.** a	**10.** a
11. d	**12.** d	**13.** b	**14.** b	

SECTION II: APPLYING YOUR KNOWLEDGE

Activity D

1. Disaster tags, which are numbered and include triage priority, name, address, age, location and description of injuries, and treatments or medications administered, are used to communicate patient information.
2. In a disaster situation when health care providers are faced with a large number of casualties, the fundamental principle guiding resource allocation is to do the greatest good for the greatest number of people.
3. Traffic control within the facility is one of the most important components of managing the disaster and resources.

SECTION III: PRACTICING FOR NCLEX

Activity E

1. c	**2.** b	**3.** c	**4.** b	**5.** b
6. d	**7.** a	**8.** a	**9.** b	**10.** c
11. c	**12.** d	**13.** a	**14.** c	**15.** a